Anti-Photoagaing and Photo-Protective Compounds from Marine Organisms

Anti-Photoagaing and Photo-Protective Compounds from Marine Organisms

Special Issue Editors

Kyung-Hoon Shin
Se-Kwon Kim

MDPI • Basel • Beijing • Wuhan • Barcelona • Belgrade

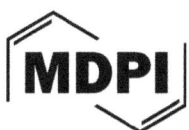

Special Issue Editors

Kyung-Hoon Shin
Hanyang University
Korea

Se-Kwon Kim
Korea Maritime and Ocean University
Korea

Editorial Office
MDPI
St. Alban-Anlage 66
4052 Basel, Switzerland

This is a reprint of articles from the Special Issue published online in the open access journal *Marine Drugs* (ISSN 1660-3397) from 2018 to 2019 (available at: https://www.mdpi.com/journal/marinedrugs/special_issues/Anti-Photoagaing_Photo-protective_compounds_Marine_Organisms).

For citation purposes, cite each article independently as indicated on the article page online and as indicated below:

LastName, A.A.; LastName, B.B.; LastName, C.C. Article Title. *Journal Name* **Year**, *Article Number*, Page Range.

ISBN 978-3-03928-044-5 (Pbk)
ISBN 978-3-03928-045-2 (PDF)

© 2020 by the authors. Articles in this book are Open Access and distributed under the Creative Commons Attribution (CC BY) license, which allows users to download, copy and build upon published articles, as long as the author and publisher are properly credited, which ensures maximum dissemination and a wider impact of our publications.

The book as a whole is distributed by MDPI under the terms and conditions of the Creative Commons license CC BY-NC-ND.

Contents

About the Special Issue Editors vii

Preface to "Anti-Photoaging and Photo-Protective Compounds from Marine Organisms" . . ix

Tobias Weinrich, Yanan Xu, Chiziezi Wosu, Patricia J. Harvey and Glen Jeffery
Mitochondrial Function, Mobility and Lifespan Are Improved in *Drosophila melanogaster* by Extracts of 9-*cis*-β-Carotene from *Dunaliella salina*
Reprinted from: *Mar. Drugs* **2019**, *17*, 279, doi:10.3390/md17050279 1

Yea Seong Ryu, Pincha Devage Sameera Madushan Fernando, Kyoung Ah Kang, Mei Jing Piao, Ao Xuan Zhen, Hee Kyoung Kang, Young Sang Koh and Jin Won Hyun
Marine Compound 3-Bromo-4,5-dihydroxybenzaldehyde Protects Skin Cells against Oxidative Damage via the Nrf2/HO-1 Pathway
Reprinted from: *Mar. Drugs* **2019**, *17*, 234, doi:10.3390/md17040234 10

Francisca de la Coba, José Aguilera, Nathalie Korbee, María Victoria de Gálvez, Enrique Herrera-Ceballos, Félix Álvarez-Gómez and Félix L. Figueroa
UVA and UVB Photoprotective Capabilities of Topical Formulations Containing Mycosporine-like Amino Acids (MAAs) through Different Biological Effective Protection Factors (BEPFs)
Reprinted from: *Mar. Drugs* **2019**, *17*, 55, doi:10.3390/md17010055 22

Marina Pozzolini, Enrico Millo, Caterina Oliveri, Serena Mirata, Annalisa Salis, Gianluca Damonte, Maria Arkel and Sonia Scarfì
Elicited ROS Scavenging Activity, Photoprotective, and Wound-Healing Properties of Collagen-Derived Peptides from the Marine Sponge *Chondrosia reniformis*
Reprinted from: *Mar. Drugs* **2018**, *16*, 465, doi:10.3390/md16120465 41

Long-Yan Li, Yu-Qin Zhao, Yu He, Chang-Feng Chi and Bin Wang
Physicochemical and Antioxidant Properties of Acid- and Pepsin-Soluble Collagens from the Scales of Miiuy Croaker (*Miichthys Miiuy*)
Reprinted from: *Mar. Drugs* **2018**, *16*, 394, doi:10.3390/md16100394 67

Young-In Kim, Won-Seok Oh, Phil Hyun Song, Sungho Yun, Young-Sam Kwon, Young Joon Lee, Sae-Kwang Ku, Chang-Hyun Song and Tae-Ho Oh
Anti-Photoaging Effects of Low Molecular-Weight Fucoidan on Ultraviolet B-Irradiated Mice
Reprinted from: *Mar. Drugs* **2018**, *16*, 286, doi:10.3390/md16080286 86

Lei Wang, WonWoo Lee, Jae Young Oh, Yong Ri Cui, BoMi Ryu and You-Jin Jeon
Protective Effect of Sulfated Polysaccharides from Celluclast-Assisted Extract of *Hizikia fusiforme* Against Ultraviolet B-Induced Skin Damage by Regulating NF-κB, AP-1, and MAPKs Signaling Pathways In Vitro in Human Dermal Fibroblasts
Reprinted from: *Mar. Drugs* **2018**, *16*, 239, doi:10.3390/md16070239 99

Thanh Sang Vo, Se-Kwon Kim, BoMi Ryu, Dai Hung Ngo, Na-Young Yoon, Long Giang Bach, Nguyen Thi Nhat Hang and Dai Nghiep Ngo
The Suppressive Activity of Fucofuroeckol-A Derived from Brown Algal *Ecklonia stolonifera* Okamura on UVB-Induced Mast Cell Degranulation
Reprinted from: *Mar. Drugs* **2018**, *16*, 1, doi:10.3390/md16010001 111

Hakuto Kageyama and Rungaroon Waditee-Sirisattha
Antioxidative, Anti-Inflammatory, and Anti-Aging Properties of Mycosporine-Like Amino Acids: Molecular and Cellular Mechanisms in the Protection of Skin-Aging
Reprinted from: *Mar. Drugs* **2019**, *17*, 222, doi:10.3390/md17040222 . . . . **120**

Ji Hye Kim, Jae-Eun Lee, Kyoung Heon Kim and Nam Joo Kang
Beneficial Effects of Marine Algae-Derived Carbohydrates for Skin Health
Reprinted from: *Mar. Drugs* **2018**, *16*, 459, doi:10.3390/md16110459 . . . . **138**

Ratih Pangestuti, Evi Amelia Siahaan and Se-Kwon Kim
Photoprotective Substances Derived from Marine Algae
Reprinted from: *Mar. Drugs* **2018**, *16*, 399, doi:10.3390/md16110399 . . . . **158**

About the Special Issue Editors

Kyung-Hoon Shin, Ph.D., is currently Professor at the Department of Marine Sciences and Convergent Technology, and Director of the Institute of Ocean and Atmospheric Sciences, Hanyang University. He received his B.Sc. and M.Sc. degrees from Hanyang University, South Korea, and got his M.Sc. from Nagoya University and Ph.D. degrees from Hokkaido University, Japan. He worked as a research scientist in Frontier Observational Research System of Global Change/International Arctic Research Center, University of Alaska Fairbanks (dispatched from Japan Marine Science and Technology Center, JAMSTEC), and obtained the Outstanding Research Accomplishment Award of Frontier Observational Research System for Global Change/JAMSTEC in 2002. He served as the Editor-in-Chief of the Korean Journal of Ecology and Environment in 2011–2018, and is Associated Editor of Geochemical Journal since 2016. Based on his research performance (total 175 research papers), he received numerous academic awards during the last 10 years. He won the best paper award of Korean Society of Oceanography in 2011, the Outstanding Research Academic Award of Korean Society of Limnology, and the Best Paper Award of Korean Federation of Science and Technology Societies in 2012, the Best Academic Award of Hanyang University, the Yeochon Academic Award for Ecology in 2015, and the Best Cited Paper Award of Hanyang University in 2018. His broad scientific interests include stable isotope ecology, marine biogeochemistry, organic carbon cycle, environmental safety and food forensics, organic geochemistry, pollution trace, environmental chemistry and contaminant bioaccumulation, production and fate of bio-toxins.

Se-Kwon Kim, Ph.D., is presently Distinguished Professor at Korea Maritime and Ocean University and Research Advisor of Kolmar Korea Company. He has also previously held positions as Distinguished Professor at the Department of Marine Bio Convergence Science and Technology and Director of Marine Bioprocess Research Center (MBPRC) at Pukyong National University, Busan, South Korea. He received his M.Sc. and Ph.D. degrees from Pukyong National University and conducted his postdoctoral studies at the Laboratory of Biochemical Engineering, University of Illinois, Urbana-Champaign, Illinois, USA. He was later a Visiting Scientist at the Memorial University of Newfoundland and University of British Colombia in Canada. Dr. Kim served as President of the 'Korean Society of Chitin and Chitosan' in 1986–1990, and the 'Korean Society of Marine Biotechnology' in 2006–2007. To the credit of his research, he won the best paper award from the American Oil Chemists' Society in 2002. Dr. Kim was also the chairman for '7th Asia-Pacific Chitin and Chitosan Symposium', which was held in South Korea in 2006. He was the Chief Editor in the 'Korean Society of Fisheries and Aquatic Science' during 2008–2009. In addition, he is the board member of International Society of Marine Biotechnology Associations (IMBA) and International Society of Nutraceuticals and Functional Food (ISNFF). His major research interests are investigation and development of bioactive substances from marine resources. His immense experience of marine bio-processing and mass-production technologies for marine bio-industry is the key asset of holding majorly funded Marine Bio projects in Korea. Furthermore, he expended his research fields up to the development of bioactive materials from marine organisms for their applications in oriental medicine, cosmeceuticals, and nutraceuticals. To date, he has authored around 750 research papers, 70 books, and 120 patents.

Preface to "Anti-Photoagaing and Photo-Protective Compounds from Marine Organisms"

Ultraviolet radiation can damage, darken, and wrinkle the skin of organisms on Earth. In recent years, significant progress had been achieved in the utilization of marine-derived compounds in cosmeceutical development due to their unique and potential uses as cures for various skin-based diseases. Secondary metabolites, vitamins, carbohydrates, proteins, peptides and enzymes, lipids, and phenolic compounds from marine organisms have demonstrated effective protection against UVB-induced damage in skin. These compounds can potentially be developed as cosmeceuticals for use as anti-photoaging, anti-wrinkle, UV-blocking, and skin-whitening agents. The current Special Issue of *Marine Drugs* highlights the advances in recent research regarding marine organism-derived anti-photoaging and photoprotective compounds. In this volume, a total of eight regular articles and two reviews are included, covering novel anti-photoaging and photoprotective effects of various bioactive compounds. For examples, the included articles introduce the suppressive activity of fucofuroeckol-A derived from brown algal *Ecklonia stolonifera* on UVB-induced mast cell degranulation; the UVB-protective effect of sulfated polysaccharides from celluclast-assisted extract of Hizikia fusiforme; the anti-photoaging effects of low molecular-weight fucoidan; the beneficial effects of marine algae-derived carbohydrates for skin health; the elicited ROS scavenging activity and photoprotective and wound-healing properties of collagen-derived peptides from the marine sponge *Chondrosia reniformis*; the protective effects of 3-bromo-4,5-dihydroybenzaldehyde against oxidative damage; and the improved mitochondrial function, mobility, and lifespan conferred by extracts of 9-*cis*-β-carotene from *Dunaliella salina*. In addition, two reviews cover the photoprotective substances derived from marine algae and the beneficial effects of marine algae-derived carbohydrates for skin health. This Special Issue provides valuable information in cosmeceutical product development and increases the value of marine products at the industrial level

Kyung-Hoon Shin, Se-Kwon Kim
Special Issue Editors

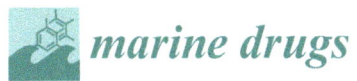

Article

Mitochondrial Function, Mobility and Lifespan Are Improved in *Drosophila melanogaster* by Extracts of 9-*cis*-β-Carotene from *Dunaliella salina*

Tobias Weinrich [1], Yanan Xu [2], Chiziezi Wosu [2], Patricia J. Harvey [2] and Glen Jeffery [1,*]

1. Institute of Ophthalmology, University College London, 11-43 Bath Street, London EC1V 9EL, UK; t.weinrich@ucl.ac.uk
2. School of Science, University of Greenwich, Central Avenue, Chatham ME4 4TB, UK; Y.Xu@greenwich.ac.uk (Y.X.); Chiziezi.Wosu@greenwich.ac.uk (C.W.); P.J.Harvey@greenwich.ac.uk (P.J.H.)
* Correspondence: g.jeffery@ucl.ac.uk

Received: 5 April 2019; Accepted: 8 May 2019; Published: 10 May 2019

Abstract: Carotenoids are implicated in alleviating ageing and age-related diseases in humans. While data from different carotenoids are mixed in their outcomes, those for 9-*cis*-β-carotene indicate general positive effects, although basic data on its biological impact are limited. Here, we show that supplementation with 9-*cis*-β-carotene in ageing *Drosophila melanogaster* improved mitochondrial function in terms of ATP production and whole-body respiration and extended mean lifespan. It also resulted in improved mobility. These data provide a potential biological rational for the beneficial effects of dietary supplementation with 9-*cis*-β-carotene. These effects may be based on the maintenance of a sound mitochondrial function.

Keywords: ageing; 9-*cis*-β-carotene; mitochondrial function; mobility; lifespan; *Drosophila melanogaster*; microalgae; *Dunaliella salina*

---

1. Introduction

Ageing is regulated by intrinsic and extrinsic factors [1]. Harman [2] proposed that a key driver of the ageing process is declining mitochondrial function that results in reduced production of ATP, the energy source that underpins cellular function. This in turn is associated with increased production of reactive oxygen species (ROS) and formation of a hyperoxidant state that contributes to systemic inflammation and increases the pace of ageing [1,2].

Diet is a key extrinsic factor that impacts on both the quality of life and its length. Carotenoids are natural organic pigments found in all photosynthetic organisms, including algae, and are able to interact with free radical and oxygen singlets. They are not synthesized in animals who depend on dietary intake to maintain an adequate supply of carotenoids. Maintaining carotenoid levels has many biological advantages, as they are strong anti-oxidants because of their conjugated double-bond structure and have anti-tumour and anti-inflammatory properties [3]. Despite evidence of their positive impact in the prevention of age-related diseases, results of human trials remain controversial. In part, this is due to their numerous types and diverse nature. Further, their use in human trials suffers from confounding issues associated with human heterogeneity. Consequently, it is important to assess their impact in tightly controlled experiments that reduce these variables.

Carotenoids are characterised by a polyene backbone consisting of a series of conjugated C=C bonds: alterations in the backbone modifying the number of conjugated double bonds or the addition of chemical functional groups alter their reactivity [4]. Carotenes such as α- and β-carotene contain exclusively carbon and hydrogen atoms, whilst xanthophylls such as lutein and zeaxanthin also contain oxygen. Multiple geometric (*cis*/*trans* or Z/E) isomers are also possible, although the more stable all-*trans* configuration is more common, and methods for the synthetic production of all-*trans* but not *cis* isomers are well established [5,6].

Dunaliella salina (*D. salina*) is one of the richest sources of natural carotenoids and accumulates a high content of β-carotene (up to 10% of the dry biomass), of which 9-*cis*-β-carotene makes up ~50% of total β-carotene. Recent studies with algal preparations enriched in 9-*cis*-β-carotene have proved to be promising, showing beneficial effects on retinal dystrophies such as retinitis pigmentosa [7] as well as atherosclerosis, diabetes, and psoriasis [8–10]; also, Sher et al. [11] demonstrated positive effects using synthetic 9-*cis*-β-carotene. However, we do not know what the impact of 9-*cis*-β-carotene has on fundamental mitochondrial metrics, which are known to be involved in the regulation of ageing.

Hence, here we investigated the effect of *D. salina* extracts rich in 9-*cis*-β-carotene on lifespan, mobility and mitochondrial function of *Drosophila melanogaster*. We also asked which components of the extract were responsible for any improvements in these metrics.

2. Results

HPLC profiles of the different carotenoid extracts are shown in Figure 1a. The identity of 9-*cis*-β-carotene was verified by UV-Vis spectral features (maxima in nm at 424, 446 and 472 nm) coupled to the retention time relative to all-*trans* β-carotene determined by HPLC (Figure 1b,c) and by mass spectrometric analysis (m/z = 536.439). All-*trans*-β-carotene and 9-*cis*-β-carotene are the most abundant carotenes in algal extracts, with only small amounts of other carotenoids, including lutein, zeaxanthin, α-carotene, and phytoene. Their concentrations are shown in Table 1. The two algal extracts obtained after supercritical CO_2 extraction had similar profiles but differ slightly in the relative amounts of the two β-carotene isomers. The supercritical CO_2 extracts had a 9-*cis*-/all-*trans*-β-carotene ratio of ~0.8 (sample 1) and ~1.4 (sample 2) and reflected seasonal batch-to-batch variation in carotenoid productivity of the alga grown outdoors. By contrast the high 9-*cis*-β-carotene extract had a very high 9-*cis*-/all-*trans*-β-carotene ratio of ~2.4 and a much lower relative concentration of α-carotene. As extracts were painted onto the surfaces of corn-yeast agar meal, the concentration of carotenoids in corn-yeast agar meal was also analysed. No carotenes were detected, and the concentrations of lutein (0.007 µg mL^{-1}) and zeaxanthin (0.003 µg mL^{-1}) were negligible compared with the amounts present in the extracts.

The impact of *D. salina* carotenoid extract on lifespan was investigated and compared with those of synthetic all-*trans*-β-carotene and un-extracted *D. salina* powder along with controls. This is shown in Figure 2a,b. In males (Figure 2a), there was an overall increase in the median lifespan when they were fed the extracts. However, these differences were only significant for 10 µM total β-carotene solutions, which induced a 32.6% increase in median life span. No concentration determined an increase in absolute lifespan, as animals in both experimental and control groups were dead by around day 80. Hence, the positive impact was on increasing the probability of survival in middle-aged and late-middle-aged flies. However, treatment with un-extracted *D. salina* powder had a significant detrimental effect on lifespan, decreasing the median lifespan by approximately 25% compared with controls. In female flies (Figure 2b), there was also a significant increase in median lifespan with the 10 µM carotenoid solution, although of a slightly lower magnitude than in male flies. However, unlike in male flies, the un-extracted *D. salina* powder had no impact on females.

Treatments that improve lifespan are often associated with functional improvements. When seven-week-old, the same groups as above that were examined for lifespan were tested for mobility by assessing negative geotaxis following one week of supplementation. Figure 2c,d shows the locomotor function at 8 weeks of age for the different treatment groups and for both sexes. As with lifespan, the impact of the extract was greater in males than in females, but in both sexes, the solution applied at 10 µM with respect to total β-carotene was the most effective dose at improving the climbing ability, although, in males, this was matched by the 100 µM solution. Again, as with lifespan, the un-extracted *D. salina* had a significant negative impact on males but not on females when compared with the controls. A similar observation of negative effects using whole algal biomass was reported by Ross and Dominy [12], who showed that whilst biomass supplements prepared from washed and dried *Spirulina platensis* had a deleterious effect on the growth of chicks fed 10 and 20% algae as part of their diet, *Spirulina* biomass up to 12% could substitute for other protein sources in broiler diets and would mediate good growth and feed efficiency.

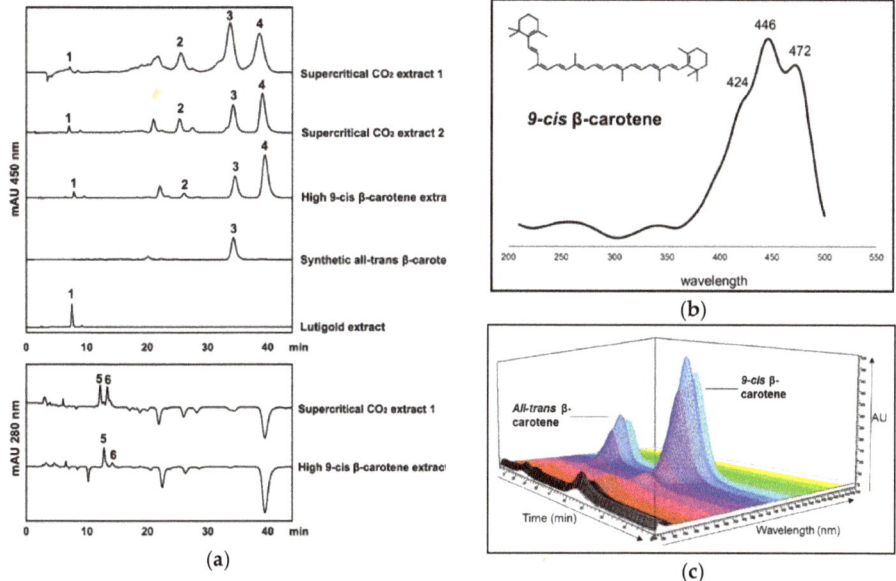

Figure 1. (a) HPLC chromatograms of ethanol extracts of carotenoids at 450 nm and 280 nm showing the carotenoid profiles. The major peaks shown are: 1, lutein; 2, α-carotene; 3, all-*trans*-β-carotene; 4, 9-*cis*-β-carotene; 5, 15-*cis*-phytoene; 6, all-*trans*-phytoene; mAU, milli-Absorbance Units. (b) UV-Visible spectrum of 9-*cis*-β-carotene; (c) 3D image showing spectral features and relative retention times for all-*trans*-β-carotene and 9-*cis*-β-carotene after HPLC chromatography.

Table 1. Concentrations of individual carotenoids in the working ethanol extracts. Volumes of 100 μL of working ethanol extracts were sprayed onto the surface of fly feed every 2 days. DS, *Dunaliella salina*.

Test Sample	Concentration of Carotenoid			
	All-*trans*-β-carotene (μM)	9-*cis*-β-carotene (μM)	α-carotene (μM)	Lutein (μM)
Synthetic all-*trans*-β-carotene	5.59	-	-	-
Lutigold	-	-	-	0.07
Supercritical CO$_2$ DS extract 1 (~10 μM with respect to carotene)	5.40	4.28	1.26	0.07
Supercritical CO$_2$ DS extract 2	6.71	8.94	2.01	0.35
High 9-*cis*-β-carotene extract	5.59	13.22	0.88	0.44

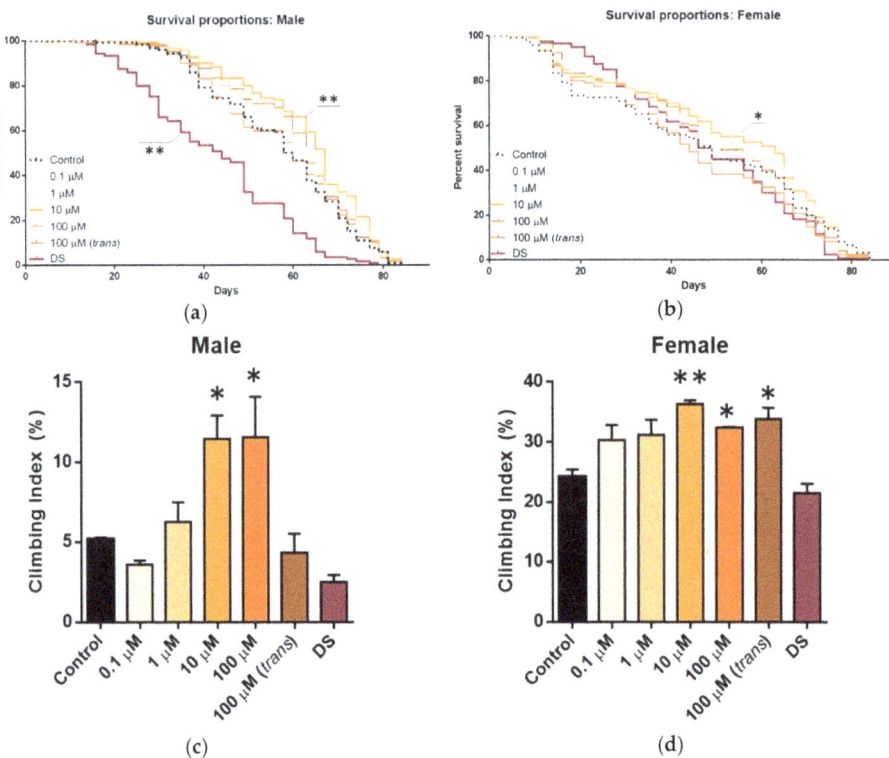

Figure 2. Lifespan (**a** and **b**) and locomotor activity (**c** and **d**) in flies treated with *D. salina* extract, *D. salina* powder and synthetic all-*trans*-β-carotene. DS Extract 1 was applied at different concentrations with respect to β-carotene content (varying from 0.1 to 100 μM) and synthetic all-*trans*-β-carotene (100 μM *trans*), and effect on lifespan of male flies (**a**) and females (**b**) was recorded ($n = 120$ flies in each group), Long-rank Mantel Cox test. In (**c**) and (**d**), locomotor activity assessed by negative geotaxis in seven-week-old flies treated since birth ($n = 40$ flies in each group), one-way ANOVA, multiple comparisons Bonferroni; * $p < 0.05$, ** $p < 0.01$).

These combined results identified algal extracts with 10 μM total carotene as the most effective concentration for improved lifespan and mobility. Hence, we treated male flies, in which the effects were more marked, to assess the impact of natural carotenoid supplementation upon mitochondria (Figure 3). This time, we used a *D. salina* extract (DS Extract 2) which contained a greater concentration of 9-*cis*-β-carotene relative to all-*trans*-β-carotene and set the concentration of all-*trans*-β-carotene to match that used in the previous experiment. Whole-body metabolic rate was measured via CO_2 production, and total body ATP levels were also measured. Whole metabolic rate is used as a surrogate marker for mitochondrial respiration. In treated flies, the metabolic rate increased by 27% (Figure 3a), and ATP levels increased by 26.5% compared with the control group (Figure 3b). Consequently, these data are consistent with natural β-carotene extracts from *D. salina* enriched in 9-*cis*-β-carotene improving mitochondrial function.

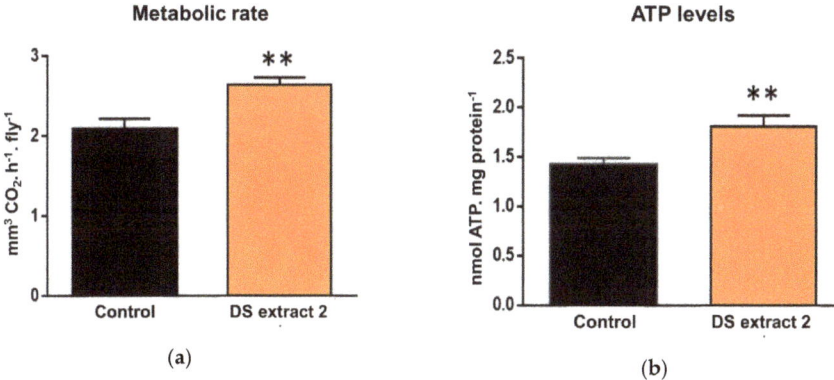

Figure 3. Effects of 14-day DS extract 2 supplementation in aged flies: metabolic rate (**a**) and ATP levels (**b**). The treatment with DS carotenoids extract enriched in 9-*cis*-β-carotene significantly improved mitochondrial function compared with untreated flies; metabolic rate was measured as a marker of (**a**) mitochondrial respiration and (**b**) ATP levels. Six replicates containing five flies each. Results are mean + SEM; ** $p < 0.01$.

D. salina extracts contain different carotenoids, including all-*trans*-β-carotene, 9-*cis*-β-carotene and lutein. To confirm the identity of the component responsible for the observed biological improvements, we fed flies with the different carotenoids and assessed locomotor function (Figure 4). Because of the inability to get a stable purified 9-*cis*-β-carotene sample, an extract with very high 9-*cis*-/all-*trans*-β-carotene ratio was used. The results confirmed that 9-*cis*-β-carotene was responsible for the biological improvements.

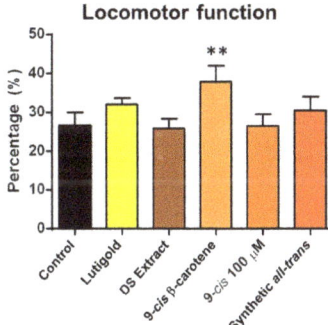

Figure 4. Fourteen-day supplementation in aged flies with different carotenoids from *D. salina*, DS Extract (6.71 µM all-*trans*-β-carotene and 8.94 µM 9-*cis*-β-carotene), 9-*cis*-β-carotene (5.59 µM all-*trans*-β-carotene and 13.22 µM 9-*cis*-β-carotene); Lutigold (0.07 µM lutein) and synthetic all-*trans*-β-carotene (5.59 µM all-*trans*-β-carotene). Effects on locomotor function assessed by negative geotaxis after administration of different carotenoids supplements. Only flies in the group treated with high concentration of 9-*cis*-β-carotene significantly improved their climbing index by 36.8%. All other groups had climbing indexes similar to that of the control group; $n = 60$ flies per group. Results are mean +SEM. ** $p < 0.01$.

3. Discussion

This study demonstrates that 9-*cis*-β-carotene derived from extracts of a natural alga improves mitochondrial function, mean lifespan and mobility in *D. melanogaster*. Nagpal and Abraham [13] recently showed that a synthetic sample of all-*trans*-β-carotene exerted antigenotoxic and antioxidant effects in *Drosophila*; however 9-*cis*-β-carotene has a higher antioxidant activity than all-*trans*-β-carotene and may also be more efficient than all-*trans*-β-carotene in vivo [14,15].

The potential protective effects of different carotenoids have been the subject of debate, with data both in favour of their use and against it. However, they have not analysed the combined metrics used in this study. The amplitude of the effects on lifespan was different in females and males, indicative of physiological differences between sexes. This sex difference was highlighted when flies were treated with only the un-extracted *D. salina* powder. This resulted in a significant reduction in lifespan and locomotor activity in males but had less impact on females.

The carotenoid literature is complex, with a large number of variables between studies. Studies vary in the application of different carotenoids at different concentrations on different species and over different periods. Treatments have been tested in models in which the physiology of the organism has been challenged in some way via external agents and in natural models where there has been no external challenge. Further, while lifespan has often been examined, other readouts have varied. This makes a coherent synthesis of the literature difficult to perform. Experiments on lifespan in mice failed to find significant differences [16], while experiments in invertebrates appeared more promising, including those in *Caenorhabditis elegans* [17] and *Tenebrio molitor* [18]. Positive results have been found in *Drosophila* in some studies [19,20] but not others [21]. However, these studies have not examined 9-*cis*-β-carotene.

It is thought that carotenoids play a role in the protection of the human central retina because they produce pigments that protect against short-wavelength light. β-carotene is strongly associated with this process. However, the overall evaluation of carotenoids in humans has been clouded by the association of synthetic all-*trans*-β-carotene with lung cancer [22]. This has significantly marred the development of carotenes for human health. However, our study has revealed consistent biological improvement in flies using the geometric isomer 9-*cis*-β-carotene derived from the marine microalga *D. salina*, and this may have wider cross-species translation. There is a growing literature across species showing that 9-*cis*-β-carotene supplementation has a positive impact. In mice, it prevents atherosclerotic progression when the animals are given a high-fat diet [23], and this is consistent with the demonstration that, in humans, it increases high-density lipoprotein (HDL)-cholesterol [24]. In humans suffering from retinitis pigmentosa, a degenerative disease of the retina, where disrupted mitochondrial dysfunction is implicated [25,26], 9-*cis*-β-carotene improves retinal function [7]. Likewise, in fundus albipunctatus, which is a retinal dystrophy, 9-*cis*-β-carotene again improved retinal function [27], whilst Sher et al. [11] showed that 9-*cis*-β-carotene inhibited photoreceptor degeneration in cultures of eye cup receptors. That these are retinal studies may be significant, because the retina has the greatest concentration of mitochondria in the body and shows a marked decline of mitochondria with age [28], leaving significant room for therapeutic action to any agent that has the ability to improve mitochondrial function.

In spite of the highly complex nature of the carotene literature, there is now clear evidence that potentially positive impacts may derive from the use of 9-*cis*-β-carotene, from fly through mouse and to man. These are likely due to its influence over mitochondrial function. Given the pivotal role of mitochondria in ageing and many diseases, either as a primary or a secondary mechanism, this may be of significance.

4. Materials and Methods

4.1. Carotenoid Extracts

These were derived from biomass of *D. salina* cultured in open raceway ponds by Monzon Biotech, Spain, harvested, then freeze-dried and extracted using supercritical CO_2 by $NATECO_2$ (Germany). The extracts were diluted in ethanol before use. DS extract 1 and DS extract 2 were extracted from two batches of biomass that were harvested in different seasons, and consequently they present minor differences in the relative composition of all-*trans*- and 9-*cis*-β-carotene, as shown in Table 1. Further carotenoid extracts containing very high 9-*cis*-β-carotene content were prepared in laboratory incubators according to a patented cultivation process with red light treatment (GB2017019440-Production of *Dunaliella*) of *D. salina* strain CCAP 19/41. The biomass was harvested in batches in 50 mL centrifugation tubes by centrifugation at $3000 \times g$ for 10 min. The cells were ruptured via ultrasonication and vortexed in ethanol to provide an extract that was then clarified by centrifugation at $3000 \times g$ for 10 min, and the supernatant was aliquoted into 14 amber glass bottles for fly feeding. Lyophilised *D. salina* biomass which was not extracted was also used as a control. Lutein was from Holland and Barrett (Lutigold UK), and all-*trans*-β-carotene from Sigma-Aldrich (UK).

The carotenoid composition of the extracts was analysed using high-performance liquid chromatography with diode array detection (HPLC–DAD). Each extract in ethanol was filtered through a 0.45 µm syringe filter into amber HPLC vials and then analysed using a YMC30 250 × 4.9 mm I.D S-5 µm HPLC column. The column temperature was set at 25 °C, and the flow rate of the mobile phase at 1 mL min^{-1}, with isocratic elution with 80% methanol/20% methyl *tert*-butyl ether (MTBE) with a pressure of 88 bar. 9-*cis*-β-carotene was identified from the analysis of UV-Vis spectral features and from *m/z* data obtained using a Waters Acquity UPCC (Waters, Elstree, UK) instrument fitted with a Diode Array Detector and connected to a Synapt G2 HDMS (Waters, Elstree, UK). The Synapt G2 was fitted with an electrospray source and operated in positive ion mode over a mass range of 50–800 *m/z* units. Wavelength-dependent absorption was measured using the DAD, operating in the wavelength range 200–700 nm. Inlet conditions A: scCO$_2$; B: methanol + 0.1% formic acid (*v/v*); make-up solvent/methanol + 0.1% formic acid (*v/v*); column: acquity UPLC HSS C18 SB, 3.0 × 100 mm, 1.8 µm particle size. Processing was carried out using MassLynx v4.1.

Absorbance at 450 nm was used to quantify all-*trans*-β-carotene, 9-*cis*-β-carotene, α-carotene and lutein, and absorbance at 280 nm was used to quantify phytoene. Carotenoids standards of synthetic β-carotene, α-carotene, lutein and phytoene were obtained from Sigma-Aldrich (UK), and the concentrations of 9-*cis*- and all-*trans*-β-carotene, α-carotene, lutein and phytoene in the extracts were estimated using the standard curves.

In initial experiments, four different concentrations of *D. salina* extract (DS Extract 1, ratio of 9-*cis*-/all-*trans*-β-carotene, 0.8) were dissolved in 100% ethanol to give a range of concentrations with respect to total β-carotene (9-*cis*- + all-*trans*-β-carotene), i.e., 100 µM, 10 µM, 1 µM and 0.1 µM. A further set of experiments was conducted with a *D. salina* extract (DS Extract 2, ratio 9-*cis*-/all-*trans*-β-carotene, 1.4), and with a highly concentrated 9-*cis* extract prepared from laboratory cultivation, (ratio 9-*cis*-/all-*trans*-β-carotene, 2.4), each used at the same relative concentration of all-*trans*-β-carotene in ethanol as for DS Extract 1. Synthetic all-*trans*-β-carotene was used at the same relative concentration of all-*trans*-β-carotene in ethanol as for DS Extract 1, and Lutigold was tested at the same concentration of lutein determined in DS Extract 1 (see Table 1). Finally, normal corn meal/agar/sucrose/yeast was substituted by a lyophilised *D. salina* compound in 1% agar, on a kcal like-for-like substitution. Volumes of 100 µL of each concentration were sprayed on top of normal food, for each group. The control group consisted of 100% ethanol only. The samples were feed every 2 days until the end of each experiment.

4.2. Drosophila Melanogaster

Wild-type male and female *D. melanogaster* Dahomey were used. These were separately housed in standard fly vials containing a normal cornmeal/sugar/yeast/agar medium maintained at 25 °C, 12 h L/D. To determine the effects of the *D. salina* extract on longevity, 150 flies were collected for each experimental group (experimental groups N = 7, 30 flies per vial, with 5 vials per group) separated into males and females. The number of dead flies was counted three times per week, and the remaining flies were transferred to fresh vials. Survival patterns were calculated using the Kaplan–Meier method and are presented as survival curves. The mean, median, minimum and maximum lifespans were determined.

Locomotor activity was assessed at eight weeks of age separately in males and females in the same groups as above ($N = 7$). The measurements were performed using the negative geotaxis assay following one week of diet supplementation. Briefly, the flies were placed in empty polystyrene vials marked at 8 cm of height and gently tapped to the bottom. The number of flies that climbed above the mark in 20 s after being tapped to the bottom were counted. The test was performed 10 times for each group of 10 flies.

Whole-animal metabolic rate was assessed by measuring CO_2 production in lab-made respirometers following a protocol previously described [29]. In each group, there were five replicates containing five flies. Metabolic rate was measured over 120 min.

4.3. Data Analysis

Data collected were analysed with GraphPad Prism v.6, and statistical analysis was undertaken using two-way Mann–Whitney *U* test unless otherwise stated. A $p < 0.05$ value was considered significant, and data presented are mean + SEM.

Author Contributions: Conceptualization, all; Fly experiments, T.W., Preparation and analysis of carotenoids, P.J.H., Y.X., C.W.; Writing-Original Draft Preparation, G.J., P.J.H.; Writing-Review & Editing, all; Supervision, G.J., P.J.H.; Funding Acquisition, P.J.H.

Funding: This research was funded by the grant EU KBBE.2013.3.2-02 programme (D-Factory: 368 613870) and by the Biotechnology and Biological Science Research Council grant BB/N000250/1.

Acknowledgments: Monzon Biotech, Spain, contributed freeze-dried samples of *D. salina* biomass from open pond raceways, which were extracted with supercritical CO_2 by Hopfenveredlung St. Johann GmbH (NATECO2).

Conflicts of Interest: The authors declare no conflict of interest.

References

1. López-Otín, C.; Blasco, M.A.; Partridge, L.; Serrano, M.; Kroemer, G. The hallmarks of aging. *Cell* **2013**, *153*, 1194–1217. [CrossRef] [PubMed]
2. Harman, D. The free radical theory of aging: Effect of age on serum copper levels. *J. Gerontol.* **1965**, *20*, 151–153. [CrossRef]
3. Honarvar, N.M.; Saedisomeolia, A.; Abdolahi, M.; Shayeganrad, A.; Sangsari, G.T.; Rad, B.H.; Muench, G. Molecular Anti-inflammatory Mechanisms of Retinoids and Carotenoids in Alzheimer's Disease: A Review of Current Evidence. *J. Mol. Neurosci.* **2016**, *61*, 289–304. [CrossRef] [PubMed]
4. Milani, A.; Basirnejad, M.; Shahbazi, S.; Bolhassani, A. Carotenoids: Biochemistry, pharmacology and treatment. *Br. J. Pharmacol.* **2017**, *174*, 1290–1324. [CrossRef] [PubMed]
5. Gong, M.; Bassi, A. Carotenoids from microalgae: A review of recent developments. *Biotechnol. Adv.* **2016**, *34*, 1396–1412. [CrossRef] [PubMed]
6. Rodriguez-Amaya, D.B. Structures and Analysis of Carotenoid Molecules. In *Subcellular Biochemistry*; Springer International Publishing: Basel, Switzerland, 2016; pp. 71–108.
7. Rotenstreich, Y.; Belkin, M.; Sadetzki, S.; Chetrit, A.; Ferman-Attar, G.; Sher, I.; Harari, A.; Shaish, A.; Harats, D. Treatment with 9-*cis* β-carotene-rich powder in patients with retinitis pigmentosa: A randomized crossover trial. *JAMA Ophthalmol.* **2013**, *131*, 985–992. [CrossRef]
8. Levy, Y.; Zaltsberg, H.; Ben-Amotz, A.; Kanter, Y.; Aviram, M. Dietary supplementation of a natural isomer mixture of beta-carotene inhibits oxidation of LDL derived from patients with diabetes mellitus. *Ann. Nutr. Metab.* **2000**, *44*, 54–60. [CrossRef]
9. Greenberger, S.; Harats, D.; Salameh, F.; Lubish, T.; Harari, A.; Trau, H.; Shaish, A. 9-*cis*-rich β-carotene powder of the alga Dunaliella reduces the severity of chronic plaque psoriasis: A randomized, double-blind, placebo-controlled clinical trial. *J. Am. Coll. Nutr.* **2012**, *31*, 320–326. [CrossRef]
10. Bechor, S.; Zolberg Relevy, N.; Harari, A.; Almog, T.; Kamari, Y.; Ben-Amotz, A.; Harats, D.; Shaish, A. 9-*cis* β-Carotene Increased Cholesterol Efflux to HDL in Macrophages. *Nutrients* **2016**, *8*, 435. [CrossRef]
11. Sher, I.; Tzameret, A.; Peri-Chen, S.; Edelshtain, V.; Ioffe, M.; Sayer, A.; Buzhansky, L.; Gazit, E.; Rotenstreich, Y. Synthetic 9-*cis*-beta-carotene inhibits photoreceptor degeneration in cultures of eye cups from rpe65rd12 mouse model of retinoid cycle defect. *Sci. Rep.* **2018**, *8*, 6130. [CrossRef] [PubMed]

12. Ross, E.; Dominy, W. The nutritional value of dehydrated, blue-green algae (*Spirulina plantensis*) for Poultry. *Poult. Sci.* **1990**, *69*, 794. [CrossRef]
13. Nagpal, I.; Abraham, S.K. Protective effects of tea polyphenols and β-carotene against γ-radiation induced mutation and oxidative stress in *Drosophila melanogaster*. *Genes Environ.* **2017**, *39*, 24. [CrossRef]
14. Levin, G.; Mokady, S. Antioxidant activity of 9-*cis* compared to all-*trans* β-carotene *in vitro*. *Free Radic. Biol. Med.* **1994**, *17*, 77. [CrossRef]
15. Jaime, L.; Mendiola, J.; Ibáñez, E.; Martin-Alvarez, P.; Cifuentes, A.; Reglero, G.; Señoráns, F. Beta-carotene isomer composition of sub- and supercritical carbon dioxide extracts. Antioxidant activity measurement. *J. Agric. Food Chem.* **2007**, *55*, 10585. [CrossRef]
16. Massie, H.R.; Ferreira, J.R.; DeWolfe, L.K. Effect of dietary beta-carotene on the survival of young and old mice. *Gerontology* **1986**, *32*, 189–195. [CrossRef]
17. Yazaki, K.; Yoshikoshi, C.; Oshiro, S.; Yanase, S. Supplemental cellular protection by a carotenoid extends lifespan via Ins/IGF-1 signaling in Caenorhabditis elegans. *Oxid. Med. Cell Longev.* **2011**, *2011*, 596240–596249. [CrossRef]
18. Dhinaut, J.; Balourdet, A.; Teixeira, M.; Chogne, M.; Moret, Y. A dietary carotenoid reduces immunopathology and enhances longevity through an immune depressive effect in an insect model. *Sci. Rep.* **2017**, *7*, 12429. [CrossRef]
19. Moskalev, A.; Shaposhnikov, M.; Zemskaya, N.; Belyi, A.; Dobrovolskaya, E.; Patova, A.; Guvatova, Z.; Lukyanova, E.; Snezhkina, A.; Kudryavtseva, A. Transcriptome analysis reveals mechanisms of geroprotective effects of fucoxanthin in Drosophila. *BMC Genom.* **2018**, *19*, 77. [CrossRef]
20. Lashmanova, E.; Proshkina, E.; Zhikrivetskaya, S.; Shevchenko, O.; Marusich, E.; Leonov, S.; Melerzanov, A.; Zhavoronkov, A.; Moskalev, A. Fucoxanthin increases lifespan of Drosophila melanogaster and Caenorhabditis elegans. *Pharmacol. Res.* **2015**, *100*, 228–241. [CrossRef]
21. Massie, H.R.; Williams, T.R. Singlet oxygen and aging in Drosophila. *Gerontology* **1980**, *26*, 16–21. [CrossRef]
22. Satia, J.A.; Littman, A.; Slatore, C.G.; Galanko, J.A.; White, E. Long-term use of beta-carotene, retinol, lycopene, and lutein supplements and lung cancer risk: Results from the VITamins And Lifestyle (VITAL) study. *Am. J. Epidemiol.* **2009**, *169*, 815–828. [CrossRef]
23. Harari, A.; Abecassis, R.; Relevi, N.; Levi, Z.; Ben-Amotz, A.; Kamari, Y.; Harats, D.; Shaish, A. Prevention of atherosclerosis progression by 9-*cis*-β-carotene rich alga *Dunaliella* in apoE-deficient mice. *Biomed. Res. Int.* **2013**, *2013*. [CrossRef]
24. Shaish, A.; Harari, A.; Hananshvili, L.; Cohen, H.; Bitzur, R.; Luvish, T.; Ulman, E.; Golan, M.; Ben-Amotz, A.; Gavish, D.; et al. 9-*cis* beta-carotene-rich powder of the alga *Dunaliella bardawil* increases plasma HDL-cholesterol in fibrate-treated patients. *Atherosclerosis* **2006**, *189*, 215–221. [CrossRef]
25. Ferrari, S.; Di Iorio, E.; Barbaro, V.; Current, D.P. 2011 Retinitis pigmentosa: Genes and disease mechanisms. *Curr. Genom.* **2011**, *12*, 238–249.
26. Mansergh, F.C.; Millington-Ward, S.; Kennan, A.; Kiang, A.S.; Humphries, M.; Farrar, G.J.; Humphries, P.; Kenna, P.F. Retinitis pigmentosa and progressive sensorineural hearing loss caused by a C12258A mutation in the mitochondrial MTTS2 gene. *Am. J. Hum. Genet.* **1999**, *64*, 971–985. [CrossRef]
27. Rotenstreich, Y.; Harats, D.; Shaish, A.; Pras, E.; Belkin, M. Treatment of a retinal dystrophy, fundus albipunctatus, with oral 9-*cis*-{beta}-carotene. *Br. J. Ophthalmol.* **2010**, *94*, 616–621. [CrossRef]
28. Gkotsi, D.; Begum, R.; Salt, T.; Lascaratos, G.; Hogg, C.; Chau, K.-Y.; Schapira, A.H.V.; Jeffery, G. Recharging mitochondrial batteries in old eyes. Near infra-red increases ATP. *Exp. Eye Res.* **2014**, *122*, 50–53. [CrossRef]
29. Yatsenko, A.S.; Marrone, A.K.; Kucherenko, M.M.; Shcherbata, H.R. Measurement of metabolic rate in Drosophila using respirometry. *J. Vis. Exp.* **2014**, e51681. [CrossRef]

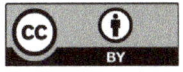

© 2019 by the authors. Licensee MDPI, Basel, Switzerland. This article is an open access article distributed under the terms and conditions of the Creative Commons Attribution (CC BY) license (http://creativecommons.org/licenses/by/4.0/).

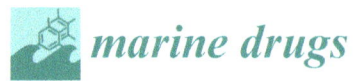

Article

Marine Compound 3-Bromo-4,5-dihydroxybenzaldehyde Protects Skin Cells against Oxidative Damage via the Nrf2/HO-1 Pathway

Yea Seong Ryu, Pincha Devage Sameera Madushan Fernando, Kyoung Ah Kang, Mei Jing Piao, Ao Xuan Zhen, Hee Kyoung Kang, Young Sang Koh and Jin Won Hyun *

School of Medicine and Jeju Research Center for Natural Medicine, Jeju National University, Jeju 63243, Korea; rmj5924@naver.com (Y.S.R.); sameeramadhu91@gmail.com (P.D.S.M.F.); legna07@naver.com (K.A.K.); meijing0219@hotmail.com (M.J.P.); zhenaoxuan705@gmail.com (A.X.Z.); pharmkhk@jejunu.ac.kr (H.K.K.); yskoh7@jejunu.ac.kr (Y.S.K.)
* Correspondence: jinwonh@jejunu.ac.kr; Tel.: +82-64-754-3838

Received: 14 March 2019; Accepted: 17 April 2019; Published: 19 April 2019

Abstract: In this study, we aimed to illustrate the potential bio-effects of 3-bromo-4,5-dihydroxybenzaldehyde (3-BDB) on the antioxidant/cytoprotective enzyme heme oxygenase-1 (HO-1) in keratinocytes. The antioxidant effects of 3-BDB were examined via reverse transcription PCR, Western blotting, HO-1 activity assay, and immunocytochemistry. Chromatin immunoprecipitation analysis was performed to test for nuclear factor erythroid 2-related factor 2 (Nrf2) binding to the antioxidant response element of the HO-1 promoter. Furthermore, the 3-(4,5-dimethylthiazol-2-yl)-2,5-diphenyltetrazolium bromide assay showed that the cytoprotective effects of 3-BDB were mediated by the activation of extracellular signal-regulated kinase (ERK) and protein kinase B (PKB, Akt) signaling. Moreover, 3-BDB induced the phosphorylation of ERK and Akt, while inhibitors of ERK and Akt abrogated the 3-BDB-enhanced levels of HO-1 and Nrf2. Finally, 3-BDB protected cells from H_2O_2- and UVB-induced oxidative damage. This 3-BDB-mediated cytoprotection was suppressed by inhibitors of HO-1, ERK, and Akt. The present results indicate that 3-BDB activated Nrf2 signaling cascades in keratinocytes, which was mediated by ERK and Akt, upregulated HO-1, and induced cytoprotective effects against oxidative stress.

Keywords: keratinocytes; 3-bromo-4,5-dihydroxybenzaldehyde; heme oxygenase-1; nuclear factor erythroid 2-related factor 2; cytoprotection

1. Introduction

The balance between reactive oxygen species (ROS) production and eradication of their toxicity is crucial to maintaining the skin redox balance. The skin is one of the most important targets of oxidative stress due to ROS from exposure to environmental stimuli and endogenous reactions [1,2]. ROS are a group of free radicals which affect macromolecules (DNA, lipids, and proteins), resulting in the generation of other reactive species [3,4]. ROS are generated during normal metabolism and rapidly induce antioxidant enzymes to maintain cellular homeostasis. The skin possesses an antioxidant defense system; however, it can be disrupted by excessive ROS, leading to oxidative damage, atopic dermatitis, premature skin aging, and skin cancer [5]. As a cytoprotective signaling mechanism, the Kelch-like ECH-associated protein 1 (Keap1)-nuclear factor erythroid 2-related factor 2 (Nrf2) pathway can help prevent and treat oxidative damage and related diseases [6].

Under normal conditions, Nrf2 has a short half-life and is continuously subjected to ubiquitination and degradation via the sequestration of the negative regulator Keap1 [7]. However, under conditions of oxidative stress, Nrf2 ubiquitination and degradation are blocked, thus allowing for Nrf2 phosphorylation and nuclear translocation [8]. In the nucleus, Nrf2 binds to the antioxidant response element (ARE) in the promoter region of target genes, including heme oxygenase-1 (HO-1), thereby inducing their expression [9].

HO-1 is an antioxidant enzyme that is induced as a response to cellular oxidative stress, and it regulates the rate-limiting step of heme catabolism, resulting in the production of carbon monoxide, ferrous iron, and biliverdin. Biliverdin is further degraded to bilirubin by the action of biliverdin reductase [10]. Intracellular ROS are neutralized by the end products of heme catabolism, indicating the antioxidant properties of these products [11]. HO-1 gene expression has been shown to be regulated at the transcriptional level and enhanced by Nrf2 nuclear translocation [12–14], resulting from the activation of various signal transduction pathways, including extracellular signal-regulated kinase (ERK) and protein kinase B (PKB, Akt). HO-1 pla ys an important role in cytoprotection against oxidative damage [15–17]. In addition, HO-1 provides cytoprotection against ROS in the skin [18,19].

The natural antioxidant compound 3-bromo-4,5-dihydroxybenzaldehyde (3-BDB) has been isolated from marine red algae such as *Rhodomela confervoides*, *Polysiphonia morrowii*, and *Polysiphonia urceolata* [20–22]. The 3-BDB compound exerts radical scavenging and antiviral effects against different types of viruses such as infectious pancreatic necrosis virus and fish pathogenic infectious hematopoietic necrosis virus [21,22], while also exerting photoprotective effects on human keratinocytes that are exposed to ultraviolet B-mediated oxidative stress [23]. However, the mechanisms underlying the cytoprotective effects of 3-BDB against oxidative stress are unclear.

In this study, we investigated the mechanisms underlying 3-BDB-mediated cytoprotection against oxidative stress in human keratinocytes, with a primary focus on the stimulatory effects of 3-BDB on HO-1 activity. Furthermore, we analyzed the roles of the ERK- and Akt-Nrf2 signaling cascades in this cytoprotection and HO-1 induction.

2. Results

2.1. HO-1 Activity and Expression Are Induced by 3-BDB in a Concentration- and Time-Dependent Manner

HaCaT cells were pretreated with 3-BDB at selected concentrations of 10 μM, 20 μM, 30 μM, 40 μM and 50 μM to determine its effects on HO-1 expression. HO-1 mRNA and protein expression levels were enhanced upon treatment with 10 μM 3-BDB and they were further increased with treatment up to 30 μM 3-BDB compared with the levels in the untreated control cells (Figure 1a). However, 40 μM and 50 μM 3-BDB downregulated HO-1 mRNA and protein expression relative to the expression with 30 μM 3-BDB. It has been reported that 3-BDB is not cytotoxic at lower concentrations (10 μM, 20 μM, and 30 μM). However, 3-BDB was shown to be cytotoxic at higher concentrations (40 μM and 50 μM) [24]. Consistent with the mRNA and protein levels, HO-1 activity was upregulated upon 3-BDB treatment (Figure 1b), exhibiting a peak at 30 μM. According to these results, we decided to use 30 μM 3-BDB as the optimum concentration for subsequent experiments.

To examine the time-dependent effects of 3-BDB, HaCaT cells were pretreated with 30 μM 3-BDB and HO-1 expression was observed for 24 h. HO-1 mRNA and protein was upregulated within three hours following 3-BDB treatment (Figure 1c). This temporal upregulation was closely associated with an increase in HO-1 activity over time (Figure 1d). These results suggest that 3-BDB has a biological antioxidant effect in HaCaT cells.

2.2. Protein Expression, Nuclear Translocation, and ARE Binding of Nrf2 Are Enhanced by 3-BDB

Several cytoprotective enzymes are regulated by the transcription factor Nrf2. HO-1 is also regulated by Nrf2. Accordingly, we examined whether 3-BDB stimulates phosphorylation and nuclear translocation of Nrf2. Treatment with 3-BDB upregulated Nrf2 expression and increased Nrf2 phosphorylation, indicating that 3-BDB temporally increased the nuclear accumulation of Nrf2 (Figure 2a). Nrf2 nuclear translocation induced by 3-BDB was further supported by immunocytochemical analysis (Figure 2b). Furthermore, when untreated cells were compared with 3-BDB treated cells, a significant enhancement in Nrf2 binding to the ARE in the HO-1 promoter region was observed in the treated cells, which was assessed with a chromatin immunoprecipitation (ChIP) assay (Figure 2c). Keap1 was downregulated after treatment with 3-BDB in a time-dependent manner (Figure 2d).

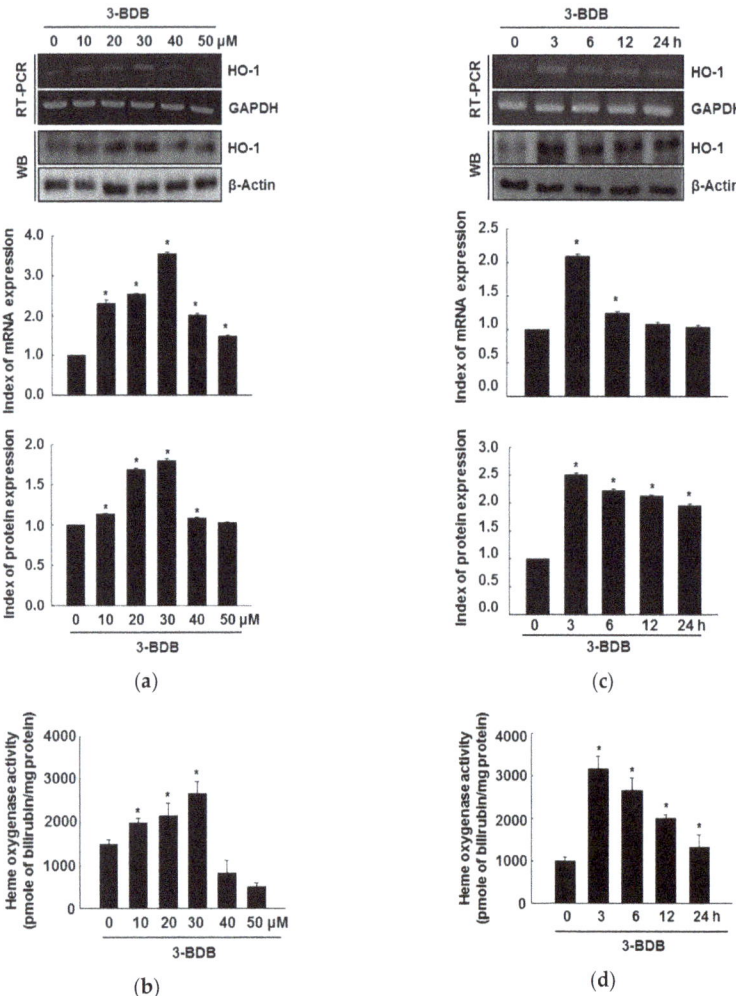

Figure 1. Effects of 3-bromo-4,5-dihydroxybenzaldehyde (3-BDB) on the levels and bioactivity of heme oxygenase-1 (HO-1) in a concentration- and time-dependent manner. HaCaT cells were pretreated with 3-BDB and incubated for 24 h with the indicated concentrations. (**a,c**) RT-PCR and Western blotting (WB) were used to analyze the HO-1 mRNA and protein expression. Glyceraldehyde-3-phosphate dehydrogenase (GAPDH) was used as the loading control. (**b,d**) The amount of bilirubin formed was used as an indicator, to assess HO-1 activity. * Significant difference compared to the control ($p < 0.05$).

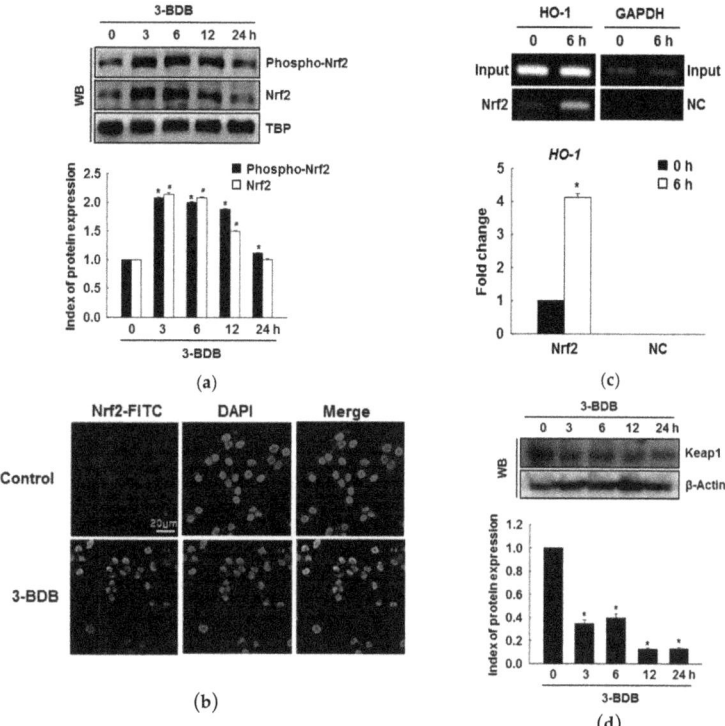

Figure 2. Effect of 3-BDB (30 μM) on the protein expression, nuclear translocation, and Nrf2 binding to antioxidant response element. (**a**) The expressions of phospho-Nrf2 and Nrf2 were detected by Western blotting of nuclear extracts. (**b**) Cells with Nrf2 are shown in green; the nuclei are shown in blue. Merged images show the nuclear translocation of Nrf2. Green represented Nrf2-fluorescein isothiocyanate (FITC) stained cells and blue represented 4′,6-diamidino-2-phenylindole (DAPI) stained nucleus. (**c**) Binding of Nrf2 to the ARE sequence in the HO-1 promoter was analyzed via chromatin immunoprecipitation (ChIP) followed by PCR. NC: negative control. (**d**) Keap1 expression was analyzed via Western blotting. * Significant difference compared to the control ($p < 0.05$).

2.3. The Compound 3-BDB Induces HO-1 by Mediating Nrf2

To investigate whether target gene transcription is upregulated by Nrf2, we evaluated Nrf2 and HO-1 expression after short hairpin RNA (shRNA)-mediated Nrf2 knockdown. Nrf2 silencing abrogated 3-BDB-induced HO-1 expression (Figure 3a). Moreover, treatment of mouse embryonic fibroblasts (MEFs) derived from Nrf2-deficient mice with 3-BDB attenuated the increase in Nrf2 and HO-1 levels (Figure 3b).

2.4. The Compound 3-BDB Activates Expression of HO-1 and Nrf2 via Phosphorylation of ERK and Akt

Treatment with 3-BDB (30 μM) significantly enhanced the phosphorylation of ERK and Akt in a time-dependent manner within 30 min of treatment (Figure 4a). To further examine whether ERK and Akt activation are caused by the cytoprotective effects of 3-BDB, cells were pretreated with U0126 and LY294002 (ERK inhibitor and Akt inhibitor, respectively) one hour before treatment with 3-BDB. U0126 and LY294002 notably attenuated HO-1 expression and Nrf2 phosphorylation upon 3-BDB treatment (Figure 4b,c). These results suggest that the protective effect of 3-BDB is mediated by ERK and Akt signaling, an important upstream signaling pathway that regulates Nrf2/HO-1.

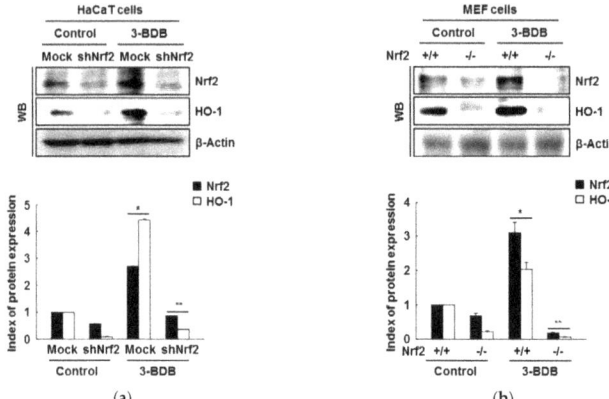

Figure 3. Role of Nrf2 in the 3-BDB (30 µM)-mediated enhancement of Nrf2 and HO-1 expression. (**a**) HaCaT cells were transfected with shRNA-control and shRNA-Nrf2 plasmids and treated with 3-BDB. Western blotting was used to analyze the proteins in the whole cell lysates. (**b**) Nrf2-WT or Nrf2-deficient mouse embryonic fibroblast (MEF) cells were treated 3-BDB, and Western blotting was used to measure the levels of HO-1 and Nrf2. * Significant difference compared with control ($p < 0.05$); ** significant difference compared with 3-BDB-treated cells ($p < 0.05$).

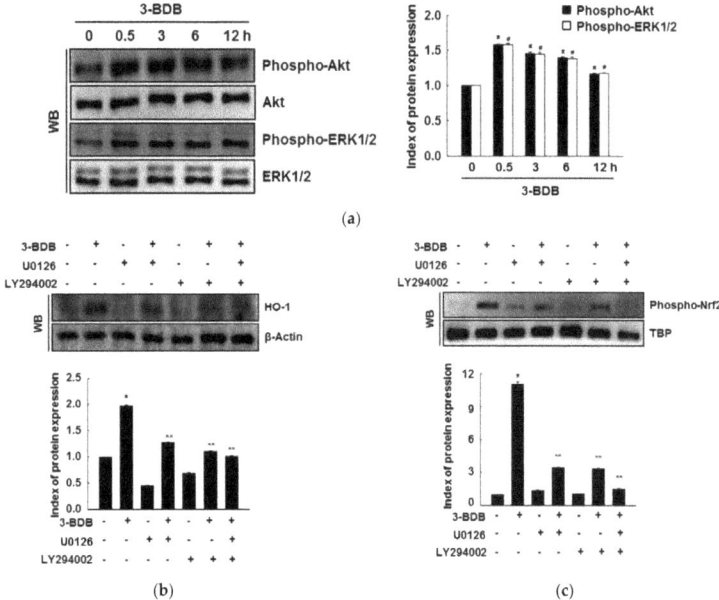

Figure 4. The extracellular signal-regulated kinase (ERK) and the protein kinase B (Akt) signaling pathways are affected by 3-BDB (30 µM) treatment. (**a**) After treatment with 3-BDB, total protein lysates were collected and analyzed for the levels of phospho-Akt, Akt, phospho-ERK1/2, and ERK1/2 with Western blotting using specific antibodies. (**b**) HO-1 and (**c**) phospho-Nrf2 levels were analyzed via Western blotting. U0126 and LY294002 are an ERK inhibitor and a PI3K inhibitor, respectively. * Significant difference compared with control ($p < 0.05$); ** significant difference compared with 3-BDB-treated cells ($p < 0.05$).

2.5. Cytoprotective Effects of 3-BDB Are Mediated by Activation of ERK and Akt Signaling

To determine whether the cytoprotective effect of 3-BDB is related to the upregulation of HO-1 activity, HaCaT cells were pretreated with zinc protoporphyrin (ZnPP), a HO-1 inhibitor. ZnPP markedly inhibited the protective effect of 3-BDB against H_2O_2- or UVB-induced cytotoxicity, suggesting that HO-1 induction is responsible for the enhancement of cell viability in 3-BDB-pretreated cells under oxidative stress (Figure 5a,b). Thus, the cytoprotection by 3-BDB probably involves HO-1.

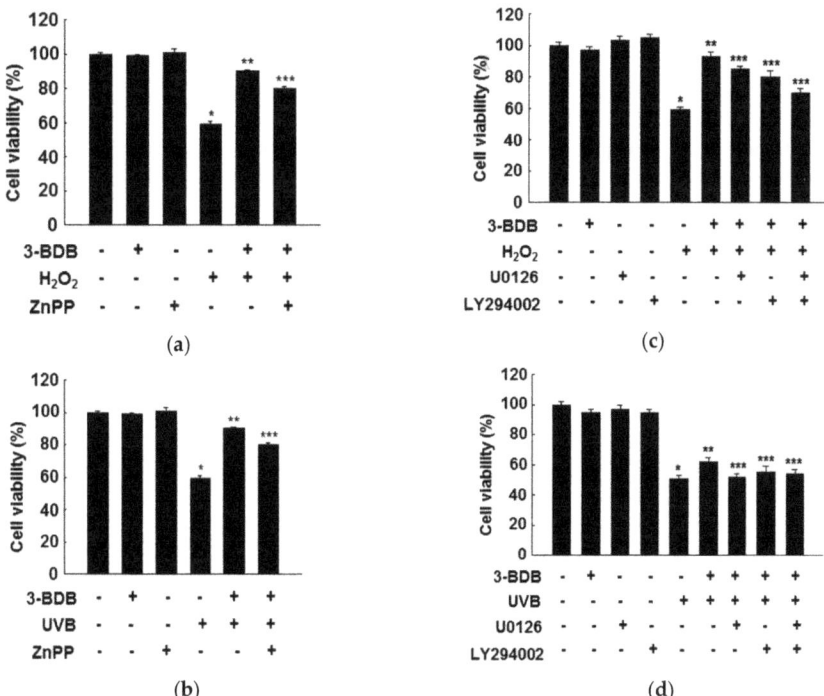

Figure 5. Cytoprotective effect of 3-BDB (30 μM) against cellular oxidative stress. HaCaT cells were pretreated with zinc protoporphyrin (ZnPP), along with 3-BDB, and exposed to (**a**) H_2O_2 or (**b**) UVB radiation. Cells were pretreated with U0126 or LY294002 and/or 3-BDB and exposed to (**c**) H_2O_2 or (**d**) UVB radiation. Cell viability was analyzed after 24 h by the 3-(4,5-dimethylthiazol-2-yl)-2,5-diphenyltetrazolium bromide (MTT) assay. * Significant difference compared with control ($p < 0.05$); ** significant difference compared with H_2O_2- or UVB-treated cells ($p < 0.05$); *** significant difference compared with 3-BDB + H_2O_2- or 3-BDB + UVB -treated cells ($p < 0.05$).

Furthermore, we examined whether ERK and PI3K/Akt signaling regulates HO-1 and Nrf2 expression in response to oxidative stress. The protection of 3-BDB against H_2O_2 and UVB exposure was suppressed by U0126 and LY294002. (Figure 5c,d). We hypothesize that the protective effect of 3-BDB is regulated by ERK and Akt signaling pathways, which induce HO-1 and Nrf2 expression.

3. Discussion

The epidermis and its associated cells are equipped with essential protective mechanisms, especially antioxidant systems that protect from oxidative stress. A previous study reported that 3-BDB has the ability to ameliorate redox reaction-mediated damage, especially within cells and tissues. In addition, 3-BDB was suggested to be a powerful antioxidant in human keratinocytes [25] and it exhibited antiviral activity against hematopoietic necrosis virus [21]. It has also been reported that 3-BDB can reduce intracellular ROS generation through harmful stimuli (hydrogen peroxide and UVB radiation), superoxide anion generation (xanthine/xanthine oxidase system), and hydroxyl radical generation (Fenton reaction). It has been specifically mentioned that 3-BDB can protect human keratinocytes from UVB-induced oxidative stress [23]. Keratinocytes are most frequently exposed to endogenous and exogenous pro-oxidant agents with deleterious effects on the skin.

HO-1, an inducible cytoprotective enzyme involved in cellular defense, plays a crucial role in adaptation to oxidative stress in different cell types. Several studies have reported that upregulated HO-1 was involved in the cellular defense system as a response to oxidative stress [26]. The present study shows that 3-BDB significantly upregulates levels of HO-1 mRNA and protein and HO-1 activity via the ARE sequence in the promoter region of HO-1. Furthermore, the inhibition of HO-1 eradicated the protective effect of 3-BDB against oxidative stress-mediated cellular damage. These data indicate that HO-1 upregulation in keratinocytes is responsible for the 3-BDB-mediated protective effect against oxidative stress.

Several compounds extracted from natural products have an ability to induce Nrf2-mediated HO-1 levels through the activation of Akt and ERK. For example, furotrilliumoside isolated from *Trillium tschonoskii* Maxim, sophoraflavonone G from *Sophora alopecuroides*, and morin isolated from Chinese herbs suppress oxidative stress by regulating the mitogen-activated protein kinase (MAPK), Akt, and Nrf2/HO-1 signaling pathways [27–29]. We previously reported that 7,8-dihydroxyflavone and eckol induce the Nrf2-mediated antioxidant enzyme HO-1 by activating ERK and Akt signaling pathways [26,30]. The present results indicate that 3-BDB has particularly potent protective effects.

Nrf2 modulates expression of phase II enzymes and is considered an upstream transcription factor [31]. Under normal conditions, Nrf2 is sequestered in the cytoplasm through its binding to Keap1. Oxidative and electrophilic stress provokes physiological responses, which leads to dissociation of Nrf2 from its docking protein and translocation to the nucleus [7,8]. The nuclear translocation of Nrf2 upregulates antioxidant genes, thus playing a crucial role in the induction of HO-1; it may provide an important therapeutic strategy against oxidative stress-mediated cell damage [32]. In the present study, 3-BDB treatment significantly upregulated Nrf2 expression and nuclear translocation, and it downregulated Keap1. However, because of the short half-life of Nrf2, it was downregulated in response to 3-BDB at 12 h. These results show that 3-BDB may retard Keap1-dependent Nrf2 degradation. Furthermore, the present results indicate that upregulation of HO-1 expression is regulated by Nrf2 activation in keratinocytes. Similarly, docosahexaenoic acid increases Keap1 degradation and prevents Keap1-mediated inactivation of Nrf2 [33].

Several studies have reported that ERK and Akt signaling pathways are involved in HO-1 expression and in Nrf2-dependent transcription in several cell types in response to oxidative stress. For instance, natural antioxidant compounds increase ERK and Akt phosphorylation, further inducing Nrf2 and HO-1 [28,30,34]. In the present study, ERK and Akt signaling induced HO-1 expression and Nrf2 phosphorylation. As shown in Figure 6, our results suggest that ERK and Akt regulate 3-BDB-induced Nrf2/HO-1 expression via ARE. Moreover, selective inhibitors of ERK and Akt pathways attenuated 3-BDB-induced HO-1 and phospho-Nrf2 levels by blocking ERK and Akt phosphorylation. These results suggest that Nrf2 downregulates ERK and Akt pathways. However, ERK and Akt are potentially important factors in the cellular signal transduction associated with the initiation of Nrf2 and transcriptional recruitment of HO-1 in keratinocytes. Further, a previous study has reported that 3-BDB potentially enhances antioxidants such as reduced glutathione [35].

The present results show that both ERK and Akt inhibitors significantly attenuate 3-BDB-induced phospho-Nrf2 and HO-1 by blocking ERK and Akt phosphorylation. This suggests that activation of several protein kinases, including ERK and Akt, results in Nrf2 phosphorylation and promotes the dissociation of Nrf2 from Keap1, thus activating the Nrf2 response to 3-BDB and Nrf2 accumulation in the nucleus. Furthermore, it has been reported that 3-BDB notably attenuated UVB-mediated intracellular ROS generation and cellular apoptosis [23].

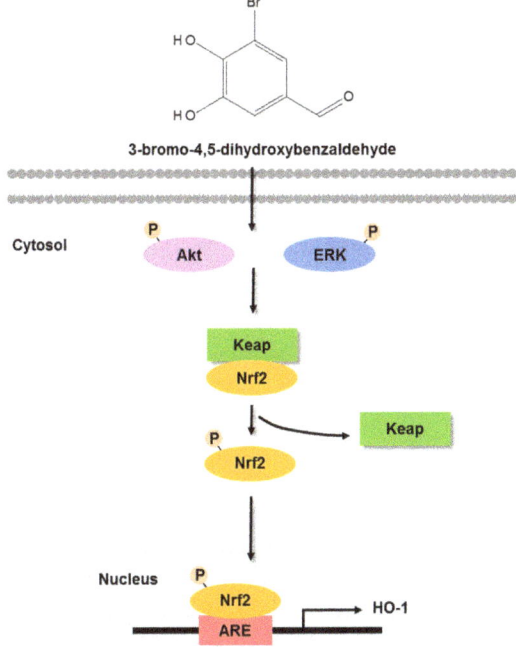

Figure 6. The compound 3-BDB protects human keratinocytes from oxidative stress by upregulating ERK and Akt, which allows Nrf2 to induce the transcription of the antioxidant enzyme HO-1.

Our results confirm that 3-BDB protects keratinocytes from damage due to oxidative stress. It exerts considerable antioxidant effects through the upregulation of ERK and Akt, allowing Nrf2 to induce the transcription of the antioxidant enzyme HO-1 (Figure 6). These findings provide novel insights into therapeutic approaches based on antioxidant compounds. The compound 3-BDB is suggested as a therapeutic candidate for skin aging, UVB-mediated skin damage, and inflammatory diseases of the skin.

4. Materials and Methods

4.1. Materials

The compounds 3-(4,5-dimethylthiazol-2-yl)-2,5-diphenyltetrazolium bromide (MTT) and ZnPP were purchased from Sigma Chemical Co. (St. Louis, MO, USA). Calbiochem (San Diego, CA, USA) provided U0126 and LY294002. Santa Cruz Biotechnology (Santa Cruz, CA, USA) supplied primary HO-1, β-actin, Nrf2, ERK, and phospho-ERK antibodies. Cell Signaling Technology (Beverly, MA, USA) supplied primary phospho-Akt (Ser 473) and Akt antibodies. Epitomics Inc. (Burlingame, CA, USA) provide the secondary rabbit-specific antibody. Other reagents were purchased as analytical grade.

4.2. Cell Culture

The human keratinocyte cell line HaCaT was purchased from Cell Lines Service (Heidelberg, Germany). Mouse MEFs from Nrf2 wild-type (Nrf2$^{+/+}$) and Nrf2-null (Nrf2$^{-/-}$) mice were provided by Professor Young Sam Keum (University of Dongguk, Seoul, Republic of Korea). Cells were cultured in Dulbecco's Modified Eagle's Medium (DMEM), with 10% FBS, streptomycin (100 μg/mL), and penicillin (100 units/mL) at 37 °C with 5% CO_2 in a humidified atmosphere.

4.3. Reverse Transcription-Polymerase Chain Reaction (RT-PCR)

Cells (1 × 10^5 cells/mL) were cultured in 100-mm dishes. After 16 h, the cells were treated with 3-BDB (10 µM, 20 µM, 30 µM, 40 µM, or 50 µM). At predetermined time points, total RNA was isolated with TRIzol® reagent (GibcoBRL, Grand Island, NY, USA). The PCR program for HO-1 and the housekeeping gene glyceraldehyde 3-phosphate dehydrogenase (GAPDH) was as follows: 35 cycles of 94 °C for 45 s, 53 °C for 45 s, and 72 °C for 60 s. The primer pairs (Bionics, Seoul, Republic of Korea) were as follows (forward and reverse, respectively): HO-1, 5′-GAGAATGCTGAGTTCATG-3′ and 5′-ATGTTGAGCAGGAAGGC-3′; GAPDH, 5′-GTGGGCCGCCCTAGGCACCAGG-3′ and 5′-GGAGGAAGAGGATGCGGCAGTG-3′. The amplified products were resolved on 1% agarose gels, stained with ethidium bromide, and photographed under UV light [19].

4.4. HO-1 Activity

A previously described method was followed to assess HO-1 activity [24]. Briefly, we homogenized the cells in sucrose solution (0.25 M) with potassium phosphate buffer (pH 7.4, 50 mM) on ice. Then, we centrifuged the samples: 200× g for homogenates, 9000× g and 15,000× g sequentially for supernatants. The resulting pellet was suspended in potassium phosphate buffer (pH 7.4, 50 mM) and the total amount of protein in the suspension was quantified. The reaction mixture (200 µL) consisting of cell lysate (500 µg/mL), hemin (0.2 mM), rat liver cytosol (0.5 mg/mL), $MgCl_2$ (0.2 mM), glucose-6-phosphate (2 mM), glucose-6-phosphate dehydrogenase (1 U/mL), NADPH (1 mM), and potassium phosphate buffer (pH 7.4, 50 mM) was incubated for 1 h at 37 °C. Chloroform (0.5 mL) was used to terminate the reaction. The absorbance of the chloroform layer at 464 nm and 530 nm was measured by a spectrophotometer to investigate the formation of bilirubin from the hemin substrate.

4.5. Western Blotting

Cells were seeded in 60-mm culture dishes. After 16 h, the cells were cocultured with 3-BDB (30 µM). The cells were then harvested at the indicated time points. After washing with phosphate-buffered saline (PBS) twice, the cells were lysed by incubating in lysis buffer for 30 min. After centrifuging, the lysate was used to detect protein levels. The proteins were separated via SDS-PAGE in a 10% resolving gel. The separated proteins were transferred to nitrocellulose membranes (Bio-Rad, Hercules, CA, USA). Then, the membranes were incubated with primary and then secondary antibodies (Pierce, Rockland, IL, USA). Images of Western blots were obtained on a LAS-3000 (Fujifilm, Tokyo, Japan) using an enhanced chemiluminescence Western blotting detection kit (Amersham, Little Chalfont, Buckinghamshire, UK) [36].

4.6. Nuclear Extract Preparation

At predetermined time points, the cells were harvested. The harvested cells were lysed on ice using 1 mL lysis buffer (Tris-HCl (pH 7.9,10 mM), NaCl (10 mM), $MgCl_2$ (3 mM), and N P-40 (1%)) for 4 min. The lysate was centrifuged, and the pellets were suspended in extraction buffer (20 mM N-2-hydroxyethylpiperazine-N′-2-ethanesulfonic acid (HEPES), pH 7.9), 20% glycerol, 1.5 mM $MgCl_2$, 300 mM NaCl, 0.2 mM ethylenediaminetetraacetic acid (EDTA), 1 mM dithiothreitol (DTT), and 1 mM phenylmethylsulfonyl fluoride (PMSF)). The samples were maintained on ice and then centrifuged. The resulting supernatants were used to measure protein concentrations and were then stored at −70 °C [33]

4.7. Immunocytochemistry

Initially, cells that had been seeded on coverslips were fixed with paraformaldehyde (4%). PBS containing 0.1% Triton X-100 was used to permeabilize the cells for 2.5 min. Then, the cells were incubated in PBS blocking medium for 1 h followed by anti-Nrf2 primary antibody for 2 h and fluorescein isothiocyanate (FITC)-conjugated secondary antibody (Jackson ImmunoResearch

Laboratories, West Grove, PA, USA) for 1 h. The cells were stained with DAPI (Vector, Burlingame, CA, USA) and mounted on microscope slides. A Zeiss confocal microscope (Carl Zeiss, Oberkochen, Germany) and Zeiss LSM 510 software (Version 2.8, Carl Zeiss) were used to acquire the images [33].

4.8. Chromatin Immunoprecipitation (ChIP) Analysis

The Simple ChIP™ Enzymatic Chromatin IP kit (Cell Signaling Technology, Danvers, MA, USA) was used to conduct the ChIP assay. Cellular proteins were crosslinked with 1% formaldehyde and then digested with nuclease for 12 min at 37 °C. The digested chromatin was incubated with primary anti-Nrf2 antibody and normal rabbit IgG overnight at 4 °C with continuous shaking. ChIP-grade protein G magnetic beads were used to collect the immunoprecipitated complexes. The immunoprecipitate was eluted with ChIP elution buffer after washing the beads. The eluent was incubated at 65 °C for 30 min to reverse the crosslinking. Subsequently, proteinase K was added, and the reaction was incubated at 65 °C for 2 h. Spin columns were used to purify the immunoprecipitated DNA fragments. The DNA collected from the immunoprecipitated complexes was subjected to 35 cycles of PCR. The primers for the HO-1 gene promoter were as follows (forward and reverse, respectively): 5′-CCAGAAAGTGGGCATCAGCT-3′ and 5′-GTCACATTTATGCTCGGCGG-3′. The PCR products were resolved on 1% agarose gels, stained with ethidium bromide, and photographed under UV light to visualize the DNA bands [33].

4.9. MTT Assay

The MTT assay was performed to assess the cytotoxicity of 3-BDB by checking cell viability. The MTT assay detects viable cells by the reduction of tetrazolium salt by mitochondrial dehydrogenases [33]. Cells (3×10^5 cells/well) were cultured in a 96-well plate and treated for 2 h with 30 µM 3-BDB, ZnPP (the inhibitor of HO-1,10 µM), U0126 (the inhibitor of ERK, 10 nM), and LY294002 (the inhibitor of Akt, 5 µM), with 1 mM H_2O_2 or 30 mJ/cm^2 UVB for another 1 h. After 24 h, we added 2 mg/mL MTT stock solution per well in a total reaction volume of 250 µL. After 2.5 h, the formazan crystals in the cells were dissolved in dimethyl sulfoxide. The absorbance was measured at 540 nm using a scanning multi-well spectrophotometer [37].

4.10. Statistical Analysis

Data were represented as means ± standard error. Multiple-group comparisons were performed using analysis of variance, followed by Tukey's post-hoc tests. A value of $p < 0.05$ was considered statistically significant.

Author Contributions: Y.S.R. and J.W.H. designed the experiments and wrote the paper. K.A.K., M.J.P., P.D.S.M.F., and A.X.Z. performed the experiments. H.K.K. and Y.S.K. contributed reagents, materials, and analytical tools.

Funding: This study was supported by a grant from the Basic Research Laboratory Program (NRF-2017R1A4A1014512) of the National Research Foundation of Korea (NRF) funded by the Korean government (MSIP).

Conflicts of Interest: The authors have declared no conflict of interest.

References

1. Wanger, F.A.; Carels, C.E.; Lundvig, D.M. Targeting the redox balance in inflammatory skin conditions. *Int. J. Mol. Sci.* **2013**, *14*, 9126–9167.
2. Rinnerthaler, M.; Bischof, J.; Steubel, M.K.; Trost, A.; Richter, K. Oxidative stress in aging human skin. *Biomolecules* **2015**, *5*, 545–589. [CrossRef] [PubMed]
3. Terra, V.A.; Souza-Neto, F.P.; Pereira, R.C.; Silva, T.N.; Costa, A.C.; Luiz, R.C.; Cecchini, R.; Cecchini, A.L. Time-dependent reactive species formation and oxidative stress damage in the skin after UVB irradiation. *J. Photochem. Photobiol. B Biol.* **2012**, *109*, 34–41. [CrossRef]
4. Moloney, J.N.; Cotter, T.G. ROS signalling in the biology of cancer. *Semin. Cell Dev. Biol.* **2018**, *80*, 50–64. [CrossRef] [PubMed]

5. Godic, A.; Polisak, B.; Adamic, M.; Dahmane, R. The role of antioxidants in skin cancer prevention and treatment. *Oxid. Med. Cell. Longev.* **2014**, *2014*, 860479. [CrossRef] [PubMed]
6. Kang, M.I.; Dobayashi, A.; Wakabayashi, N.; Kim, S.G.; Yamamoto, M. Scaffolding of Keap1 to the actin cytoskeleton controls the function of Nrf2 as key regulator of cytoprotective phase 2 genes. *Proc. Natl. Acad. Sci. USA* **2004**, *101*, 2046–2051. [CrossRef] [PubMed]
7. Dinkova-Kostova, A.T.; Abramov, A.Y. The emerging role of Nrf2 in mitochondrial function. *Free Radic. Biol. Med.* **2015**, *88*, 179–188. [CrossRef]
8. Leinonen, H.M.; Kansanen, E.; Polonen, P.; Heinaniemi, M.; Levonen, A.L. Role of the Keap1-Nrf2 pathway in cancer. *Adv. Cancer Res.* **2014**, *122*, 281–320. [PubMed]
9. Bryan, H.K.; Olayanju, A.; Goldring, C.E.; Park, B.K. The Nrf2 cell defence pathway: Keap1-dependent and -independent mechanisms of regulation. *Biochem. Pharmacol.* **2013**, *85*, 705–717. [CrossRef] [PubMed]
10. Lee, S.E.; Yang, H.; Jeong, S.I.; Jin, Y.H.; Park, C.S.; Park, Y.S. Induction of heme oxygenase-1 inhibits cell death in crotonaldehyde-stimulated HepG2 cells via the PKC- δ-p38-Nrf2 pathway. *PLoS ONE* **2012**, *7*, e41676. [CrossRef] [PubMed]
11. Aayadi, H.; Mittal, S.P.K.; Deshpande, A.; Gore, M.; Ghaskadbi, S.S. Cytoprotective effect exerted by geraniin in HepG2 cells is through microRNA mediated regulation of BACH-1 and HO-1. *BMB Rep.* **2017**, *50*, 560–565. [CrossRef] [PubMed]
12. Shi, X.; Zhou, B. The role of Nrf2 and MAPK pathways in PFOS-induced oxidative stress in zebrafish embryos. *Toxicol. Sci.* **2010**, *115*, 391–400. [CrossRef] [PubMed]
13. Kim, J.K.; Jang, H.D. Nrf2-mediated HO-1 induction coupled with the ERK signaling pathway contributes to indirect antioxidant capacity of caffeic acid phenethyl ester in HepG2 cells. *Int. J. Mol. Sci.* **2014**, *15*, 12149–12165. [CrossRef] [PubMed]
14. Kundu, J.; Chae, I.G.; Chun, K.S. Fraxetin induces heme oxygenase-1 expression by activation of Akt/Nrf2 or AMP-activated protein kinase α/Nrf2 pathway in HaCaT cells. *J. Cancer Prev.* **2016**, *21*, 135–143. [CrossRef] [PubMed]
15. Lee, M.H.; Cha, H.J.; Choi, E.O.; Han, M.H.; Kim, S.O.; Kim, G.Y.; Hong, S.H.; Park, C.; Moon, S.K.; Jeong, S.J.; et al. Antioxidant and cytoprotective effects of morin against hydrogen peroxide-induced oxidative stress are associated with the induction of Nrf-2-mediated HO-1 expression in V79-4 chinese hamster lung fibroblasts. *Int. J. Mol. Med.* **2017**, *39*, 672–680. [CrossRef] [PubMed]
16. Han, D.; Chen, W.; Gu, X.; Shan, R.; Zou, J.; Liu, G.; Shahid, M.; Gao, J.; Han, B. Cytoprotective effect of chlorogenic acid against hydrogen peroxide-induced oxidative stress in MC3T3-E1 cells through PI3K/Akt-mediated Nrf2/HO-1 signaling pathway. *Oncotarget* **2017**, *8*, 14680–14692. [CrossRef]
17. Li, T.; Chen, B.; Du, M.; Song, J.; Cheng, X.; Wang, X.; Mao, X. Casein glycomacropeptide hydrolysates exert cytoprotective effect against cellular oxidative stress by up-regulating HO-1 expression in HepG2 cells. *Nutrients* **2017**, *9*, 31. [CrossRef]
18. Kim, K.C.; Lee, I.K.; Kang, K.A.; Piao, M.J.; Ryu, M.J.; Kim, J.K.; Lee, N.H.; Hyun, J.W. Triphlorethol-A from *Ecklonia cava* up-regulates the oxidant sensitive 8-oxoguanine DNA glycosylase 1. *Mar. Drugs* **2014**, *12*, 5357–5371. [CrossRef]
19. Ryu, M.J.; Kang, K.A.; Piao, M.J.; Kim, K.C.; Zheng, J.; Yao, C.W.; Cha, J.W.; Hyun, C.L.; Chung, H.S.; Park, J.C.; et al. Effect of 7,8-dihydroxyflavone on the up-regulation of Nrf2-mediated heme oxygenase-1 expression in hamster lung fibroblasts. *In Vitro Cell. Dev. Biol. Anim.* **2014**, *50*, 549–554. [CrossRef]
20. Fan, X.; Xu, N.J.; Shi, J.G. Bromophenols from the red alga *Rhodomela confevoides*. *J. Nat. Prod.* **2003**, *66*, 455–458. [CrossRef]
21. Kim, S.Y.; Kim, S.R.; Oh, M.J.; Jung, S.J.; Kang, S.Y. In vitro antiviral activity of red alga, *Polysiphonia morrowii* extract and its bromophenols against fish pathogenic infectious hematopoietic necrosis virus and infectious pancreatic necrosis virus. *J. Microbiol.* **2011**, *49*, 102–106. [CrossRef]
22. Li, K.; Li, X.M.; Ji, N.Y.; Wang, B.G. Bromopenols from the marine red alga *Polysiphonia urceolata* with DPPH radical scavenging activity. *J. Nat. Prod.* **2008**, *71*, 28–30. [CrossRef] [PubMed]
23. Hyun, Y.J.; Piao, M.J.; Zhang, R.; Choi, Y.H.; Chae, S.; Hyun, J.W. Photo-protection by 3-bromo-4,5-dihydroxyfenzaldehyde against ultraviolet B-induced oxidative stress in human keratinocytes. *Ecotoxicol. Environ. Saf.* **2014**, *83*, 71–78. [CrossRef] [PubMed]

24. Piao, M.J.; Kang, K.A.; Ryu, Y.S.; Shilinkova, K.; Park, J.E.; Hyun, Y.; Zhen, A.; Kang, H.; Koh, Y.; Ahn, M.; et al. The red algae compound 3-bromo-4,5-dihydroxybenzaldehyde protects human keratinocytes on oxidative stress-related molecules and pathways activated by UVB irradiation. *Mar. Drugs* **2017**, *15*, 268. [CrossRef] [PubMed]
25. Ji, N.; Lou, H.; Gong, X.; Fu, T.; Ni, S. Treatment with 3-bromo-4,5-dihydroxybenzaldehyde improves cardiac function by inhibiting macrophage infiltration in mice. *Korean Circ. J.* **2018**, *48*, 933–943. [CrossRef] [PubMed]
26. Ryu, M.J.; Kang, K.A.; Piao, M.J.; Kim, K.C.; Zheng, J.; Yao, C.W.; Cha, J.W.; Chung, H.S.; Kim, S.; Jung, C.E.; et al. 7,8-Dihydroxyflavone protects human keratinocytes against oxidative stress-induced cell damage via the ERK and PI3K/Akt-mediated Nrf2/HO-1 signaling pathways. *Int. J. Mol. Med.* **2014**, *33*, 964–970. [CrossRef] [PubMed]
27. Guo, C.; Yang, L.; Wan, C.X.; Xia, Y.Z.; Zhang, C.; Chen, M.H.; Wang, Z.D.; Li, Z.R.; Li, X.M.; Geng, Y.D.; et al. Anti-neuroinflammatory effect of sophoraflavanone G from *Sophora alopecuroides* in LPS-activated BV2 microglia by MAPK, JAK/STAT and Nrf2/HO-1 signaling pathways. *Phytomedicine* **2016**, *23*, 1629–1637. [CrossRef]
28. Yan, T.; Yu, X.; Sun, X.; Meng, D.; Jia, J.M. A new steroidal saponin, furotrilliumoside from *Trillium tschonoskii* inhibits lipopolysaccharide-induced inflammation in Raw264.7 cells by targeting PI3K/Akt, MARK and Nrf2/HO-1 pathways. *Fitoterapia* **2016**, *115*, 37–45. [CrossRef]
29. Jung, J.S.; Choi, M.J.; Lee, Y.Y.; Moon, B.I.; Park, J.S.; Kim, H.S. Suppression of lipopolysaccharide-induced neuroinflammation by morin via MAPK, PI3K/Akt, and PKA/HO-1 signaling pathway modulation. *J. Agric. Food Chem.* **2017**, *65*, 373–382. [CrossRef] [PubMed]
30. Kim, K.C.; Kang, K.A.; Zhang, R.; Piao, M.J.; Kim, G.Y.; Kang, M.Y.; Lee, S.J.; Lee, N.H.; Surh, Y.J.; Hyun, J.W. Up-regulation of Nrf2-mediated heme oxygenase-1 expression by eckol, a phlorotannin compound, through activation of Erk and PI3K/Akt. *Int. J. Biochem. Cell Biol.* **2010**, *42*, 297–305. [CrossRef]
31. Xu, X.; Li, H.; Hou, X.; Li, D.; He, S.; Wan, C.; Yin, P.; Liu, M.; Liu, F.; Xu, J. Punicalagin induces Nrf2/HO-1 expression via upregulation of PI3K/AKT pathway and inhibits LPS-induced oxidative stress in RAW264.7 macrophages. *Mediat. Inflamm.* **2015**, *2015*, 380218.
32. Chen, B.; Lu, Y.; Chen, Y.; Cheng, J. The role of Nrf2 in oxidative stress-induced endothelial injuries. *J. Endocrinol.* **2015**, *225*, R83–R99. [CrossRef] [PubMed]
33. Bang, H.Y.; Park, S.A.; Saeidi, S.; Na, H.K.; Surh, Y.J. Docosahexaenoic acid induces expression of heme oxygenase-1 and NAD(P)H: Quinone oxidoreductase through activation of Nrf2 in human mammary epithelial cells. *Molecules* **2017**, *22*, 969. [CrossRef] [PubMed]
34. Lin, C.C.; Yang, C.C.; Chen, Y.W.; Hsiao, L.D.; Yang, C.M. Arachidonic acid induces ARE/Nrf2-dependent heme oxygenase-1 transcription in rat brain astrocytes. *Mol. Neurobiol.* **2018**, *55*, 3328–3343. [CrossRef] [PubMed]
35. Kim, K.C.; Hyun, Y.J.; Hewage, S.R.K.M.; Piao, M.J.; Kang, K.A.; Kang, H.K.; Koh, Y.S.; Ahn, M.J.; Hyun, J.W. 3-Bromo-4,5-dihydroxybenzaldehyde enhances the level of reduced glutathione via the Nrf2-mediated pathway in human keratinocytes. *Mar. Drugs* **2017**, *15*, 291. [CrossRef]
36. Lee, H.; Cheong, K.A.; Kim, J.Y.; Kim, N.H.; Noh, M.; Lee, A.Y. IL-1 receptor antagonist reduced chemical-induced keratinocyte apoptosis through antagonism to IL-1α/IL-1β. *Biomol. Ther.* **2018**, *26*, 417–423. [CrossRef] [PubMed]
37. Song, I.B.; Gu1, H.; Han, H.J.; Lee, N.Y.; Cha, J.Y.; Son, Y.K.; Kwon, K. Effects of 7-MEGATM 500 on oxidative stress, inflammation, and skin regeneration in H_2O_2-treated skin cells. *Toxicol. Res.* **2018**, *34*, 103–110. [CrossRef]

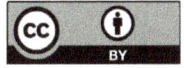

© 2019 by the authors. Licensee MDPI, Basel, Switzerland. This article is an open access article distributed under the terms and conditions of the Creative Commons Attribution (CC BY) license (http://creativecommons.org/licenses/by/4.0/).

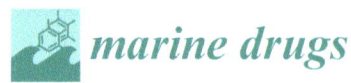

Article

UVA and UVB Photoprotective Capabilities of Topical Formulations Containing Mycosporine-like Amino Acids (MAAs) through Different Biological Effective Protection Factors (BEPFs)

Francisca de la Coba [1,2,*], José Aguilera [3,4], Nathalie Korbee [1], María Victoria de Gálvez [3,4], Enrique Herrera-Ceballos [3,4], Félix Álvarez-Gómez [1] and Félix L. Figueroa [1,2]

1. Department of Ecology and Geology, Faculty of Science, University of Malaga, Campus Universitario de Teatinos s/n, E-29071 Malaga, Spain; nkorbee@uma.es (N.K.); felix_alvarez000@hotmail.com (F.A.-G.); felix_lopez@uma.es (F.L.F.)
2. Photobiology Laboratory, Central Service for Research Support (SCAI), University of Malaga, Campus Universitario de Teatinos s/n, E-29071 Malaga, Spain
3. Photobiological Dermatology Laboratory, Medical Research Centre, University of Malaga, Campus Universitario de Teatinos s/n, E-29071 Malaga, Spain; jaguilera@uma.es (J.A.); mga@uma.es (M.V.d.G.); eherrera@uma.es (E.H.-C.)
4. Department of Dermatology and Medicine, Faculty of Medicine, University of Malaga, Campus Universitario de Teatinos s/n, E-29071 Malaga, Spain
* Correspondence: pdlacoba@uma.es; Tel.: +34-952-133-337

Received: 13 November 2018; Accepted: 3 January 2019; Published: 14 January 2019

Abstract: The safety and stability of synthetic UV-filters and the procedures for evaluating the photoprotective capability of commercial sunscreens are under continuous review. The influence of pH and temperature stressors on the stability of certain Mycosporine-like amino acids (MAAs) isolated at high purity levels was examined. MAAs were highly stable at room temperature during 24 h at pH 4.5–8.5. At 50 °C, MAAs showed instability at pH 10.5 while at 85 °C, progressive disappearances were observed for MAAs through the studied pH range. In alkaline conditions, their degradation was much faster. Mycosporine-serinol and porphyra-334 (+shinorine) were the most stable MAAs under the conditions tested. They were included in four cosmetically stable topical sunscreens, of which the Sun Protection Factor (SPF) and other Biological Effective Protection Factors (BEPFs) were calculated. The formulation containing these MAAs showed similar SPF and UVB-BEPFs values as those of the reference sunscreen, composed of synthetic UV absorbing filters in similar percentages, while UVA-BEPFs values were slightly lower. Current in vitro data strongly suggest that MAAs, as natural and safe UV-absorbing and antioxidant compounds, have high potential for protection against the diverse harmful effects of solar UV radiation. In addition, novel complementary in vitro tests for evaluation of commercial sunscreens efficacy are proposed.

Keywords: Biological Effective Protection Factors (BEPFs); mycosporine-like amino acids; photoprotection; pH-thermo stability; UV- mediated action spectra

1. Introduction

Terrestrial solar ultraviolet radiation (UVR) (295–400 nm) comprises UVA (320–400 nm) and UVB (295–320 nm). Although UVB accounts for no more than 5% of terrestrial UVR, their clinical effects on normal human skin are typically much greater than those of UVA. These effects, which are mostly adverse, may be acute or chronic. The most notable acute alterations caused by UVB radiation include erythema (sunburn), pigmentation (tanning), oedema, skinfold thickening, sunburn cells (SBC) formation, phototoxic reactions, photosensitivity and photoimmunosuppression [1]. Chronic effects include photocarcinogenesis and photoaging, also mediated by UVA [2]. All effects are underpinned by molecular or cellular effects such as DNA damage, generation of reactive oxygen species (ROS) (i.e., singlet oxygen, superoxide, peroxyl and hydroxyl radicals, peroxynitrite), melanogenesis, apoptosis, depletion of Langerhans cells, and expression of many genes and related proteins. On the other hand, the main widely-established benefit of UVR on the skin is the photosynthesis of vitamin D that is initiated by the UVB-induced conversion of epidermal 7-dehydrocholesterol into vitamin D3. Other positive effects are photo-adaptation (natural protection for the skin), immunosuppression of acquired immunity, induction of innate immunity, and recently identified, a reduction in blood pressure by UVA [3,4].

Recently, several effects of blue light (400–450 nm) on human skin have been reported, such as changes in pigmentation and erythema, thermal damage and free radical production [5,6]. In addition, near infrared radiation (A: 700–1400 nm) is associated with the production of ROS [7], resulting in collagen degradation and the appearance of coarse wrinkling, a characteristic of photoaging [8]. The application of high sun-protection factor (SPF) broad-spectrum sunscreens is considered an integral component of photoprotection for exposed skin [9].

The photobiological response to UVR depends on the energy associated with the incident photon flux and the relative effectiveness of photon energy to produce a given biological effect. This effectiveness is determined by the absorption spectrum of each skin chromophore (DNA, melanin etc.) which depends on its specific electronic configuration [10]. Action spectrum, a fundamental tool in medicine and photobiology, describes the relative effectiveness (used as a weighting function) of UVA and UVB wavelengths in the induction of health effects (i.e., DNA damage, skin cancer and erythema) usually expressed on a log scale.

Currently, the erythema (UVB-mediated skin injury) action spectrum is used for the in vitro SPF determinations, and Persistent Pigment Darkening (PPD) action spectrum for the UVA protection factor (UVA-PF). The European Union recommends both a critical wavelength of more than 370 nm and a UVA–PF of at least one third of the labelled SPF as the criterion for labelling as either UVA or broad-spectrum protection (ISO 24443:2012) [11]. However, other acute damages and most of the chronic ones are mediated by other wavelengths in the UV range, with known action spectra which could be used for complementary evaluations of sunscreen testing and labelling of broad-spectrum photoprotective capability in vitro. Especially, it may help to differentiate the effectiveness of sunscreen formulations with similar SPF in the future. Some of these action spectra are DNA damage [12], photocarcinogenesis non melanoma skin cancer (NMSC) [13], systemic immunosuppression of contact hypersensitivity (CHS) [14], cis-photoisomerization of urocanic acid [15], formation of oxygen radicals such as singlet oxygen [16] and photoaging [17], all related to UVB and UVA radiation exposure-induced skin damage.

The safety of sunscreen filters is being widely studied since there is evidence that synthetic organic filters are associated with allergic reactions or photo-toxicity [18–20], endocrine disruption [21], skin penetration [22], low photo-stability and biodegradability and a lack of effectiveness in skin protection [23,24]. Dibenzoilmethane, benzophenone, para-aminobenzoic acid (PABA) and their derivatives have been implicated as the cause of photoallergic dermatitis and the generation of oxygen radicals after solar exposition [25,26]. In addition, camphor derivatives showed skin permeation that permitted them to reach blood vessels located in deeper skin cell layers and thus entering the systemic circulation [27]. After long term exposure to UV, octocrylene produces ROS that accumulate in the body in measurable amounts, ultimately leading to cell mutations. Inorganic filters like TiO_2 and ZnO offer broad spectrum protection but exposure to micro and nanoparticles of these filters could produce toxic effects [28]. In addition, commercial particulate UV filters, both inorganic and organic, are accumulating in coastal and continental waters [29,30], inducing a rapid and complete bleaching of hard corals even at extremely low concentrations [31]. UV filters have been found in invertebrates and fishes [32–35]. In addition, inorganic oxide nanoparticles containing UV filters such as TiO_2 produce hydrogen peroxide, a major oxidizing agent entering coastal waters in touristic areas with direct ecological consequences to ecosystems [36].

There is a worldwide trend toward natural cosmetics and to the development of high UV protection sunscreens using low concentrations of chemical filters. The use of natural compounds in combination with synthetic agents may provide an effective strategy for preventing the harmful effects of UV radiation. Among the natural UV-absorbing molecules proposed in several studies as an alternative to synthetic filters, are flavonoids like quercetin and rutin (polyphenolic compounds) present in strawberries, grape fruits, apples, vegetables, tea, and red wine with multiple functions in photoprotection by suppressing the UV-induced damage in keratinocites [37]. In addition, some isoflavones like genistein and daidzein also block UVB induced skin burns in humans and show anti-photocarcinogenic and anti-photoaging effects [38]. Mycosporine-like amino acids have a good position since they are filters obtained from natural resources with no reported toxicity, high photo-stability and antioxidant properties [39–43]. Many studies suggest the use of MAAs as UV screen [44–47] and some extracts and formulations containing these compounds have been patented for the treatment of actinic erythema [48,49] as well as to avoid the oxidation of cosmetic and pharmaceutical products [50–53].

In this study, porphyra-334 (P-334), shinorine (SH) and asterina-330 (AS-330), with absorption maxima between 330–334 nm, mycosporine-serinol (M-Ser (OH)) with an absorption maximum at 310 nm and palythine (PNE) with an absorption maximum at 320 nm, were isolated in high purity grade and their thermo-stabilities at different pH and temperature conditions were evaluated. P-334 (+ SH), as a natural UVA sunscreen, and M-Ser (OH), as a natural UVB sunscreen, were brought together in the same topical formula as well as separately and SPFs and other Biological Effective Protection Factors (BEPFs) were calculated according to the Diffey method [48]. A reference sunscreen containing butylmethoxydibenzoylmethane (BMDM) and octylmethoxycinnamate (OMC), synthetic UV filters used in photoprotection by Cosmetics Europe [54–56], was formulated with the same percentage as that of the MAAs combination sunscreen and used as a control.

2. Results

2.1. Isolation and Purification of MAAs

Four different aqueous extracts containing MAAs with a high grade of purity were obtained. After HPLC and ESI-MS analysis, a combination of P-334 plus SH (88:12), AS-330 plus PNE (88:12), M-Ser (OH) plus an unknown UV absorbing compound with a similar absorption maximum (84:16), and SH as a unique MAA were identified and quantified (Figure 1). P-334 (+SH) and AS-330 (+PNE) results are expressed as percentages of each MAA with respect to total MAAs concentration, i.e., considering total MAAs the 100%. For M-Ser (OH) is referred to as the ratio of the chromatographic area of these two peaks. The ESI-MS analysis of purified MAAs showed a prominent ion peak of protonated molecules ([M + H]+) at m/z which is consistent with the MS analysis of MAAs derived from algae [57] (Table 1). Based on their on-line UV–visible absorption spectra and mass spectrometry, the MAAs were identified as porphyra-334 (UV λ_{max} 334 nm, m/z 347.1460) plus shinorine (UV λ_{max} 334 nm, m/z 333.130), mycosporine-serinol (UV λ_{max} 310 nm, m/z 262.1294), shinorine (UV λ_{max} 334 nm, m/z 333.130 and asterina-330 (UV λ_{max} 331 nm, m/z 289.1398) plus palythine (UV λ_{max} 320 nm, m/z 245.1135). In the case of the unknown molecule present in M-Ser (OH) extract, no concordance was found after checking 13 Mono-Substituted MAAs (Aminocyclohexenona-Type MAAs) with absorption maxima between 309-311 nm [58], neither the selected glycosylated derivatives of porphyra-334 or shinorine in the extracts of P-334 (+SH) and SH.

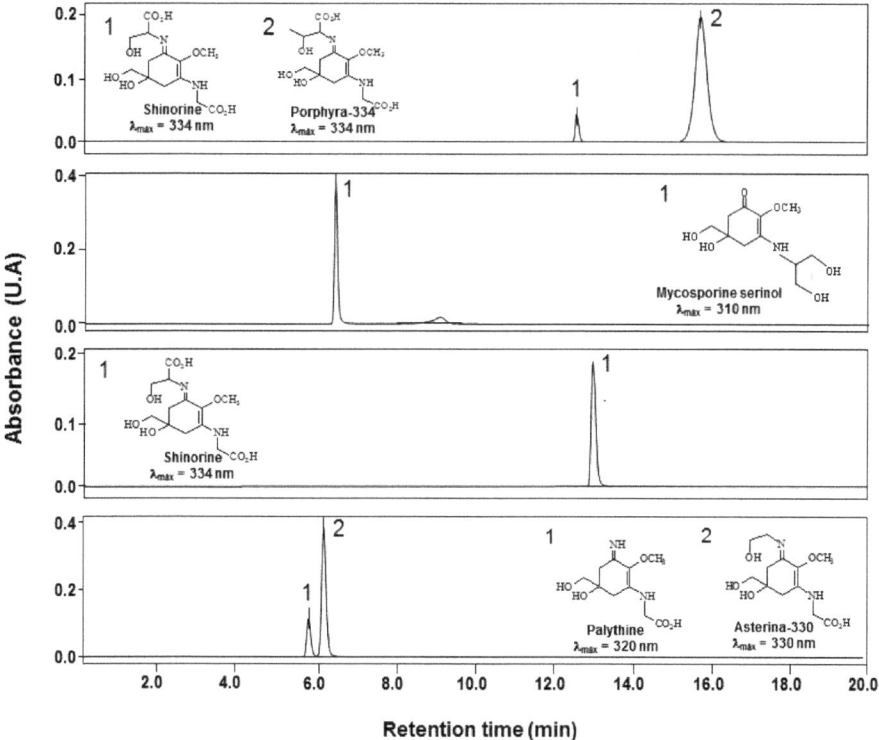

Figure 1. HPLC chromatograms of MAAs extracts after the Dowex chromatography purification process measured at the maximum absorption wavelength of the main MAA in each extract. The mobile phase was 1.5% aqueous methanol (v/v) plus 0.15% acetic acid (v/v) in water run isocratically at 0.5 mL min^{-1}. Analyses were performed at 20 °C using a C8 chromatographic column.

Table 1. ESI-MS results of MAA extracts in high grade of purity.

Fraction	MAAs	Mol.formula	UV λ$_{max}$ (nm)	Exact (ppm)	m/z [M + H]$^+$ Parent Ion	Theoretical
P-334 (+SH)	Porphyra-334	$C_{14}H_{22}N_2O_8$	334	3.1	347.1460	347.1449
	Shinorine	$C_{13}H_{20}N_2O_8$	334	2.5	333.1301	333.1292
M-Ser (OH)	Mycosporine-serinol	$C_{11}H_{19}NO_6$	310	3.4	262.1294	262.1285
SH	Shinorine	$C_{13}H_{20}N_2O_8$	334	3.0	333.1302	333.1292
AS-330 (+PNE)	Asterina-330	$C_{12}H_{20}N_2O_6$	331	1.3	289.1398	289.1394
	Palythine	$C_{10}H_{16}N_2O_5$	320	1.3	245.1135	245.1132

2.2. Influence of pH and Temperature on MAAs Stability

MAAs extracts incubated for 1 h at different pH conditions at room temperature (25 °C) did not show significant differences ($p > 0.05$) in concentration and absorption spectra. However, significant absorption decreases of MAAs ($p < 0.05$), except M-Ser (OH), were registered after 24 h of incubation at pH 10.5 (Figure 2). Initial absorbance of P-334 (+SH), SH, AS-330 (+PNE) decreased 18.4 ± 0.05%, 19.6 ± 0.04 and 13.8 ± 0.05 respectively.

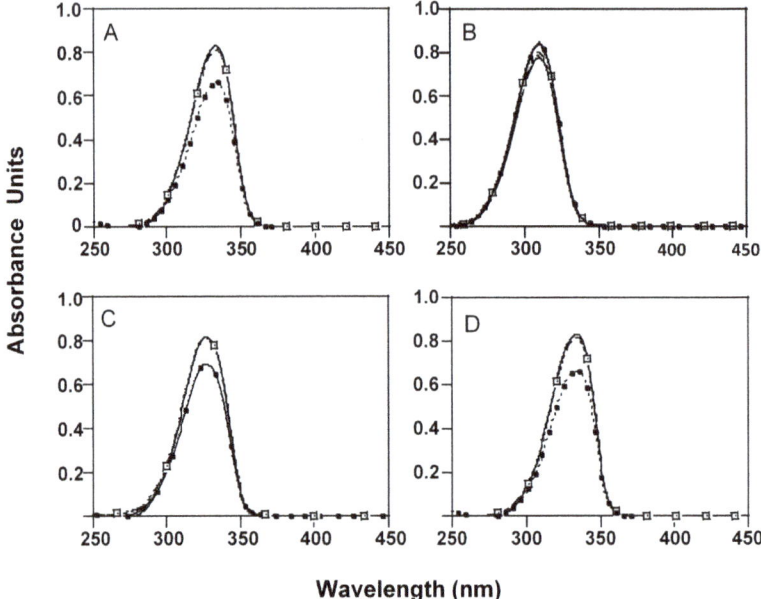

Figure 2. Absorption spectra of MAAs extracts after 24 h of incubation in 50 mM phosphate buffer pH 4 (····), 7.5 (— · —), 8.5 (· ▫ ·) or 10.5 (··■··) at room temperature (25 °C). Initial absorbance (——). (**A**) P-334 (+SH), (**B**) M-Ser (OH), (**C**) AS-330 (+PNE) and (**D**) SH.

When the effects of pH and temperature on the stability of MAAs were analyzed, all MAAs were stable at 50 °C in buffer solutions with pH ≤ 8.5 (Figure 3) while their concentrations decreased in a time-dependent manner at pH 10.5, except M-Ser (OH), which remained stable (Figure 3B). After 1.5 h of incubation, AS-300 (+PNE) concentration decreased 33.3 ± 0.56%, SH 29.9 ± 0.63% and P-334 (+SH) 38.9 ± 0.45%. After 6 h, the concentrations decreased over 75% for all MAAs (Figure 3). In these conditions, UV-absorption maxima of AS-330 and P-334 (+SH) showed hypsochromic shifts from 330 nm to 334 and 334 to 333 nm respectively.

At 85 °C MAAs stability decreased with increasing the alkalinity of the medium (Table 2). In pH 4 solutions, P-334 (+SH), M-Ser (OH) and AS-330 (+PNE) registered decreases in absorbance of 17-18% ($p > 0.05$), while SH was smaller ($p < 0.05$). At pH 7.5, MAAs showed strong absorbance declines of up to 40% during the first 1.5 h of incubation while M-Ser (OH) was completely stable ($p > 0.05$). At pH 8.5, P-334 (+SH) and SH registered falls in absorbance of up to 90% after 1.5 h of incubation and their absorption maxima were 332 and 331 nm respectively. AS-330 (+PNE) resulted highly unstable, showing a single absorption peak at 304 nm unlike M-Ser (OH), the most stable MAA. All MAAs, except M-Ser (OH), were highly unstable at 85 °C and pH 10.5. Only small absorption peaks around 298–302 nm were measured during the first 1.5 h of incubation, indicating the presence of degraded products. M-Ser (OH) was also fairly unstable, but only after 3 h of incubation (Table 2).

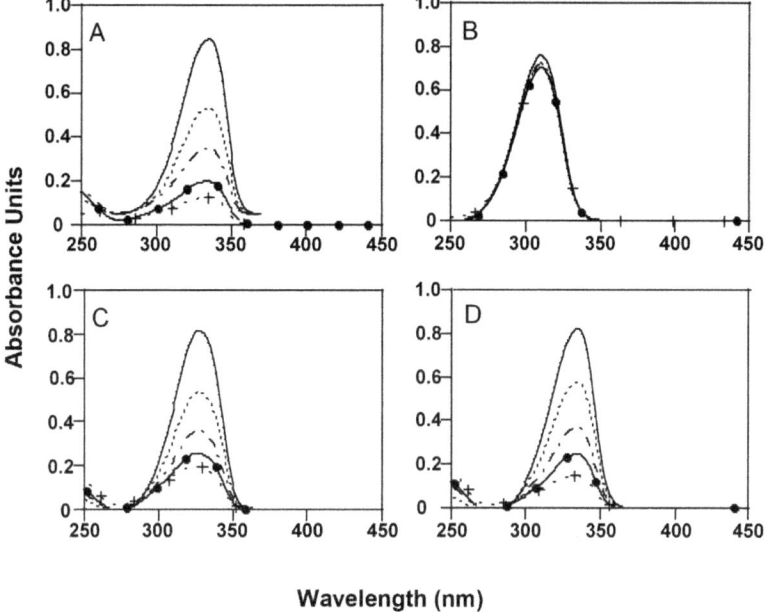

Figure 3. Absorption spectra of MAAs extracts after 1.5 (- - - -), 3 (· – · ·), 4.5 (—●—) and 6 (· + ·) hours of incubation in 50 mM phosphate buffer at pH 10.5 and 50 °C. Initial absorbance (———). (**A**) P-334 (+SH), (**B**) M-Ser (OH), (**C**) AS-330 (+PNE) and (**D**) SH.

Table 2. Absorbance decreases (%) of different MAAs at 85 °C and different pH conditions for 4.5 h of incubation. The values are expressed as mean ± SD ($n = 4$). Different letters indicate significant differences ($p < 0.05$) between values for each MAAs and pH condition.

MAAs Extract	pH	Time (Hours)		
		1.5	3	4.5
P-334 (+SH)	4	6.9 ± 0.04 [a]	11.2 ± 0.04 [b]	18.3 ± 0.05 [c]
	7.5	41.8 ± 1.19 [a]	67.6 ± 1.62 [b]	80.4 ± 1.12 [c]
	8.5	93.5 ± 0.07 [a]	100 [b]	
	10.5	100		
M-Ser (OH)	4	7.4 ± 1.03 [a]	14.7 ± 1.92 [b]	17.4 ± 2.03 [b]
	7.5	-	6.4 ± 0.08 [a]	10.0 ± 0.08 [b]
	8.5	17.2 ± 0.03 [a]	20.7 ± 0.04 [b]	25.1 ± 0.04 [c]
	10.5	69.5 ± 0.06 [a]	100 [b]	
AS-330 (+PNE)	4	-	-	12.6 ± 0.05
	7.5	54.9 ± 1.23 [a]	77.6 ± 1.56 [b]	86.7 ± 0.08 [c]
	8.5	100		
	10.5	100		
SH	4	-	12.8 ± 0.03 [a]	17.6 ± 0.03 [b]
	7.5	50.6 ± 2.03 [a]	74.6 ± 1.87 [b]	85.4 ± 1.23 [c]
	8.5	89.8 ± 0.08 [a]	100 [b]	-
	10.5	100		

In high basic solution (pH 10.5) and high temperatures (50–85 °C), both absorption maxima and extinction coefficients of the studied MAAs decreased in a time-dependent manner, registering the minimum values at 85 °C before 1.5 h of incubation for AS (+PNE) and after 3 h for M-Ser (OH).

2.3. Galenic Formula

After the preparation of topical emulsions, chemically stable and resistant to photo-degradation formulations were obtained. These creams were easily absorbed by the skin and able to create continuous and uniform films. The pH values of MAAs formulations were very homogeneous (6.2 ± 0.5). The sunscreens containing P-334 (+ SH) and M-Ser (OH) showed spectral absorption maxima at 334 (UVA) and 308 nm (UVB) respectively, corresponding to the absorption maxima of previous highly purified MAAs aqueous extracts (Figure 4). However, the absorption maximum of the sunscreen containing the mixture of these MAAs was 329 nm (UVA). The reference sunscreen, containing a combination of OMC and BMDM, showed two absorbance peaks at 310 and 360 nm, corresponding to λ maxima of each component (Figure 4).

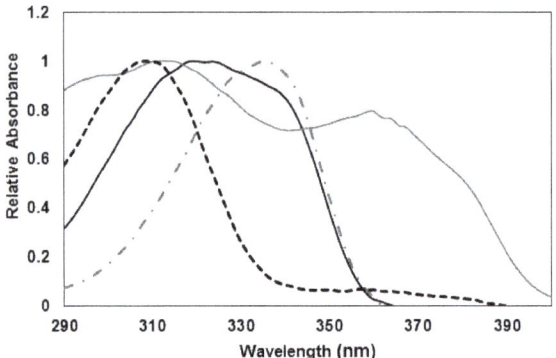

Figure 4. UV relative absorption spectra of different sunscreens studied: P-334 (+SH) plus M-Ser (OH) (——) reference (OMC Y BMDM) (——), P-334 (+SH) (— · -) and M-Ser (OH) (- - -).

2.4. SPF and BEPFs Determinations

SPF and BEPF values of the different sunscreens are presented in Table 3. The formulations containing P-334 (+SH) as a UVA absorbing filter or M-Ser (OH) as a UVB sunscreen presented similar SPFs (among 4-6) ($p > 0.05$), while the SPF of the formula containing the combination of these MAAs increased significantly up to 8.37 ± 2.12 ($p < 0.05$) and showed a similar values to those of the reference formula (9.54 ± 1.53). The λ critical values for P-334 (+SH), M-Ser (OH) and the MAAs combination sunscreens were 353.5 ± 3.0, 332 ± 1.5 and 343.6 ± 1.4 nm respectively. The reference were 374.4 ± 0.5 nm, being considered a broad-spectrum sunscreen.

Table 3. SPF and BEPFs values for tested formulations : P-334 (+SH) at 5.6%, M-Ser (OH) at 5.1%, P-334 +(SH) at 4.1% plus M-Ser (OH) at 2.9% and the reference containing BMDM at 4.5% and OMC at 2.6% (w/w). The values are expressed as mean ± SD ($n = 4$). Different letters indicate significant differences ($p < 0.05$) between different purified MAAs extracts for a UV-mediated effect (BEPF).

UV-mediated Effects	P-334 (+SH)	M-Ser (OH)	MAA Combination	Reference
Erythema (SPF)	4.53 ± 1.58 [a]	6.47 ± 1 [ab]	8.37 ± 2.12 [bc]	9.54 ± 1.53 [c]
DNA Damage	4.17 ± 1.55 [a]	9.27 ± 1.98 [b]	10.18 ± 2.99 [b]	9.71 ± 1.58 [b]
Photocarcinogenesis (NMSC)	4.60 ± 1.63 [a]	7.55 ± 1.31 [b]	8.74 ± 2.24 [b]	9.50 ± 1.49 [b]
Systemic Immunosuppression (CHS)	5.63 ± 2.23 [a]	9.73 ± 2.17 [b]	10.72 ± 2.99 [b]	10.41 ± 1.68 [b]
Urocanic acid photoisomerization	7.22 ± 3.21 [a]	9.21 ± 2.37 [a]	10.90 ± 2.95 [a]	11.00 ± 2.38 [a]
Formation of singlet oxygen radicals	6.51 ± 2.25 [b]	2.62 ± 0.18 [a]	6.45 ± 1.69 [b]	9.74 ± 1.89 [c]
Photoaging	4.81 ± 1.72 [b]	2.16 ± 0.10 [a]	4.37 ± 0.94 [b]	10.63 ± 2.63 [c]

In relation to UVB-BEPFs, P334 (+SH) sunscreen registered the lowest values in photoprotection against DNA damage, photocarcinogenesis (NMSC), and systemic immunosuppression. For the formation of singlet oxygen radicals and photoaging effects, M-Ser (OH) formula showed the lowest photoprotection. When BEPF values of separated MAAs (formulated at 5.6% for P-334 (+SH) and 5.1% for M-Ser (OH)) were compared with the MAAs combination emulsion (formulated at 4.5 and 2.6% respectively), the last one presented similar BEPF-UVB values to M-Ser (OH) ($p < 0.05$) and similar BEPF-UVA values to P-334 (+SH). Therefore, an additive effect was found when these MAAs were formulated together.

The MAAs combination sunscreen presented similar BEPF-UVB compared with the reference formula ($p > 0.05$). Photoprotection capabilities against the formation of singlet oxygen radicals and photoaging were significantly lower ($p > 0.05$).

3. Discussion

In recent years, mycosporine-like amino acids have gained considerable attention as highly active photoprotective candidates for the prevention of harmful effects of UVR on human skin, due to their physico-chemical characteristics. Many studies suggest the use of MAAs in topical creams [45,46,59]. High molar extinction coefficients (ε) or strong absorption in UVA and UVB regions allow to reduce the concentration of UV filters in sunscreens; ε values up to 20,000 $M^{-1} \cdot cm^{-1}$ are considered effective for commercial sunscreens [60]. MAAs with molar extinction coefficients up to 50000 $M^{-1}\,cm^{-1}$ are considered very effective UV filters, even more than other synthetic UVA absorber filters, such as BMDM (ε: 31000 $M^{-1}\,cm^{-1}$). Their strong photo-stability in both aqueous solution [39–41,61] and seawater, as well as in the presence of abiotic stressors and strong photosensitizing agents and antioxidant properties, makes them considered safety sunscreens [42,52]. In fact, it was recently found that palythine showed only 3% degradation after an exposure of 40 standard erythema doses of solar simulated radiation [62]. However, the stability of these MAAs in a wide pH-temperature range have not been well studied, although it is very important to guarantee their stability both during and after they are added to cosmetic formulations.

Most synthetic UV filters, i.e., OMC and BMDM, present photo-stability problems. OMC degrades into photoproducts when it is exposed to sunlight for a short period of time, losing its efficiency in UV absorption [63]. BMDM has also been shown to be photo-labile after one hour of exposure to sunlight; this photo-decomposition not only reduces its photoprotective capacity by 50–60%, but also favors the generation of free radicals which causes ruptures in DNA plasmids and modifications in some proteins [64]. Some authors have even described the pro-oxidant nature of this filter in lipid peroxidation reactions [65]. The stability of both filters does not improve when they are formulated together, since irreversible photochemical reactions of cyclo-addition occur which lead to the loss of their photoprotective capacity [66]. To increase the stability of both filters, it is common to combine them with other substances (micronized ZnO/TiO_2, salicylates, tinosorbs, etc.) [67,68].

In this study, we have demonstrated that P-334 (+SH), SH and AS-330 (+PNE) were very stable over a wide pH range (4.5–10.5) at room temperature in 24 hour experiments, registering slight absorbance decreases in alkaline solutions (pH 10.5), while M-Ser (OH) remained stable throughout all pH conditions. These results are in accordance with a previous work [69] in which porphyra-334 was found to be stable in solutions with pH from 1 to 11 up to 24 h at room temperature and rapidly degraded at extremely high pH 12 and 13. Mycosporine glycine, a MAA analogous to M-Ser (OH), showed high resistance to various pH conditions for up to 24 h [70,71]. The absorption maxima in the UV region of this MAA and shinorine were practically unaffected over the wide range of pH 4−10, being then the 3-aminocyclohexenone as well as the 1-amino-3-iminocyclohexene moieties, protonated at a wide range of pH, responsible for their UV-protective abilities in aqueous solution [72]. Combining high temperature and pH, MAAs absorbance decreased in a time-dependent manner and degradation products appeared; MAAs showed instability in alkaline buffer at 50 °C, and progressive disappearances were observed for MAAs through the studied pH range at 85 °C. In alkaline conditions, their degradation were much faster.

The stability of porphyra-334 in solutions of different pH and temperatures was previously reported [73]. Only high acidic conditions, (pH below 3) and high alkaline conditions (pH over 12), as well as temperatures higher than 60 °C promotes its decomposition. A dehydrated sub-product of porphyra 334 with λ maxima at 226 nm was discovered at pH 7 and 120 °C [74]. Rastogi and Incharoensakdi [75] showed very high stability of partially purified extracts of palythine and asterina-330 from a cyanobacterium at 60 °C after 1 hour assay. In our study, degraded products of P-334 (+SH) and AS-330 (+PNE) were only detected at 50 °C and pH 10.5 after 6 h of incubation, in accordance with Rastogi and Incharoensakdi [75] and Korbee et al. [76]. MAAs showed the minimum concentration values at 85 °C and pH 4-10.5 before 1.5 h of incubation for AS-330 (+PNE) and after 3 h for M-Ser (OH).

Among the pH-temperature conditions studied, M-Ser (OH) and P-334 (+SH) were found to be the most stable MAAs and asterina-330 the most labile one. According to these results, M-Ser (OH) was selected as natural UVB filter and P-334 (+SH) as natural UVA filter to be added to different topical galenic emulsions and evaluating their photoprotective capabilities in vitro. Different MAAs sunscreens were obtained according with the safety pH-temperature range defined in this work: pH 6 and 60 °C.

Although the need to prevent acute (erythema) and chronic skin damage (cancer and photoaging) resulting from exposure to ultraviolet radiation (UVB and UVA) is well understood, the safest and most effective way to achieve this protection still presents a number of challenges, specifically in the practical implementation of photoprotective measures. SPF only provides information regarding the photoprotective capacity of topical sunscreen products against the erythematic action of ultraviolet radiation. It does not provide data regarding the level of protection against other UV- mediated biological effects. In this context, this study proposes a novel method for the evaluation of the in vitro photoprotection capacity of topical formulations for the main UV-induced skin injuries (acute and chronic disorders) using their action spectra and transmission measurements. Thus, the photoprotection capacity of the studied formulations based on MAAs purified extracts has been established for a total of 7 UV-mediated biological effects with action spectra referenced in the Photobiology literature (Table 4). BEPF can be understood as the number of times a person can be exposed to the sun compared to an unprotected person before this person suffers the biological injury in question.

Table 4. Absorption maxima, UVB/UVA relative effectiveness (%) and experimental model for the selected UV-mediated biological injuries.

Biological Effects	λ_{max} (nm)	UVB/UVA	Experimental Model
Erythema	250–298	99/1	Human skin [77]
DNA damage	270	100/0	Function [12]
Photocarcinogenesis (NMSC)	298	99/1	SCUP-h (human) [13]
Inmunosuppression CHS	270	100/0	Balb/c mouse [14]
Photoisomerization of urocanic acid	303–309	86/14	Human skin [15]
Formation of Singlet oxygen	342–343	4/96	In vitro [16]
Photo-aging	340	4/96	SKHR-1 H mouse [17]

In this study, we demonstrated that two galenic emulsions containing purified MAAs (P-334 (+SH) or M-Ser (OH)) in similar percentages as natural UVA and UVB filters (5.6 or 5.1%, respectively) showed similar SPF values, providing similar photoprotection against erythema. The extinction molar coefficient of P-334 (+SH) is much higher than M-Ser (OH) in spite of its UVA maximum absorption. Both MAAs sunscreens registered λ critical values below 370 nm, indicating they are not broad-spectrum sunscreens. According to these results, both MAAs could be used indiscriminately as sunscreens against erythema, with P334 (+SH) being the best candidate to provide even greater protection against UVA (λ critical higher). When P334 (+SH) and M-Ser (OH) were included in lower concentrations in the same formula, the SPF of this sunscreen was significantly similar to the SPF of M-Ser (OH), denoting a possible synergistic effect between them due to both broadband covering of UV solar spectrum and high extinction molar coefficients. When these results were compared with the reference sunscreen which contains the same percentage of UVA+UVB synthetic filters, we found similar SPF for both formulas. These results confirm that these MAAs provide great photoprotection in vitro against erythema and their potentiality for possible substitutions of synthetic UV filters. From an economic point of view and regarding our experience with these compounds, a high quantity of fresh material is necessary in order to get the required amount of purified MAAs. Purification yields of 40–50% were obtained for the MAAs studied. For this reason, the manufacturing of sunscreens with P-334 (+SH) as unique UV filter with high SPF (30–50) is not easy to achieve as large amounts of biomass would be necessary. Furthermore, due to the regulation of the individual filters in sunscreen formulas, in this case, the combination of different filters would be necessary. MAAs could be good candidates to be used together with other commercial filters. In the case of cosmetics with 100% natural filters, commercial viability could be reached with a low SPF formula (as hydration creams).

There is a lot of research that supports the relationship between the photoprotective role against UVA and UVB harmful diseases of porphyra334 (and shinorine) in vitro and in vivo experiments. Our research group [78] studied the in vivo UV-protective properties of purified porphyra-334 and shinorine isolated from *P. rosengurttii*. Results showed that the galenic formulation containing P-334 (+SH) included at 2% (w/w) with SPF 3.71 and critical wavelength 357–358 nm, applied topically at a concentration of 4 mg·cm^{-2} on the dorsal skin of SkhR-1 H hairless mice and irradiated with a single UV radiation dose of 3.87 J·cm^{-2} (3.6 MEDs for a human phototype of skin III/5.1 MEDs for a phototype IV) prevented UV-induced clinical and histopathological skin alterations observed in non-UV-protected biopsies. The expression of the heat shock protein Hsp70, a potential biomarker of acute UV damage, and the antioxidant defense enzymes also were preserved. In addition, Porphyra-334 protected cell viability in vitro studies with keratinocytes (human HaCat) and reduced the DNA damage in fibroblasts (IMR-90) and dimers formation [79,80]. Regarding UVA-mediated injuries, Porphyra-334 suppressed ROS production and the expression of matrix metalloproteinase following UVA irradiation, while increasing levels of procollagen, type I collagen and elastin [81,82].

Erythema is the end point of the main index of sunscreen efficacy, SPF, which is mainly, but not exclusively, an index of UVB protection. The time-point for evaluating erythema and the erythematic doses for each human phototype of skin are fully standardized parameters, but for most of the biological effects shown in Table 4, these circumstances do not occur, and some of them begin to develop at sub-erythematic doses [83]. Additionally, high-SPF products tend to lull users into staying in the sun longer and overexposing themselves to both UVA and UVB rays. In view of this perspective, to provide more useful information to consumers, more studies are necessary to study the biologically effective doses for each biological effect in order to find safe UV-exposure limits that may be equivalent to minutes of sun exposure (immediate or long-term photobiological and degenerative skin changes). Nevertheless, high UVA-BEPF values for a galenic sunscreen formula are correlated to high UVA range protection as UVB-BEPF values to high UVB protection in this study.

When the photoprotective capability of these different sunscreens were analyzed against other UV-mediated injuries, M-Ser (OH) showed higher UVB-BEPFs values than P-334 (+SH), although their SPF were similar, unlike for UVA-BEPFs. Although the formation of singlet oxygen radicals and photoaging process are both mediated mainly by UVA radiation (96%) and both present the maxima effectiveness at 340 nm, the solar effective irradiance between 350-380 nm is higher for the photoaging response than formation of singlet oxygen. Therefore the protective capability of P-334 (+SH) is higher for this injury. The combination of MAAS sunscreen showed similar UVB-BEPFs to those of M-Ser (OH) and the reference formula, indicating an additive photoprotective effect between P-334 (+SH) and M-Ser (OH) for these UVB injuries and a similar effectiveness to that of synthetic UV filters. The combination of MAAs sunscreen (λ critical 343.6 nm) presented similar UVA-BEPFs values to P-334 (+SH) one (λ critical 353.5 nm) and very close to the reference formula (λ critical 374.4) nm. However, these formulas could be enriched with other natural UVA-absorbing substances like scytonemin (λ_{max} 384 nm) to increase λ critical rate and then, broad spectrum absorption.

Therefore it is demonstrated that topical sunscreens containing a combination of MAAs P-334 (+SH) and M-Ser (OH) provide excellent photo-protective in vitro capabilities against the main UV-mediated injuries compared to chemical UV filters. For UVB mediated process, an additive photoprotection effect is observed when these MAAs are used together, unlike many associations of synthetic UV filters used in commercial sunscreens. This effect is smaller for UVA injuries. Currently, BEPFs indicators could be useful tools to compare the UVA+UVB protection given by different commercial sunscreen products beyond their SPF and λ critical values.

Due to a greater understanding of the effects of visible light and infrared radiation, it is now clear that available organic (chemical) UV filters are not sufficient to protect the skin. Only optically opaque filters such as non-micronized form of zinc oxide, titanium dioxide and iron oxide are able to block visible light, but these galenic forms are unacceptable to many users [84]. In addition, photoprotection long after UV exposure is being demanded since the generation of DNA damage and the synthesis of cyclobutane pyrimidine dimers (CPDs) are believed to occur hours after UV exposure. The so-called dark CPDs are mediated by ROS and the use of systemic or topical antioxidants could prevent their synthesis [85]. Natural compounds with broad biological activities are important in the manufacturing of sunscreen products due to their modulation of several signaling pathways in reducing the deleterious effects of UV radiation on the skin. Antioxidants topically applied and their oral and subcutaneous topical forms of photoprotection are ongoing and the protective effect of β-carotene topically applied [86] and *Polypodium leucotomos* extracts [87] have been proven. In addition, the antioxidant properties of MAAs have been widely studied [58,71,88], specifically the purified MAAs tested in this study, in terms of scavenging hydrosoluble radicals (ABTS assay), inhibition of β-carotene oxidation, and superoxide radical scavenging [42] describing moderate activity of P-334 (+SH) and high activity of Mycosporine glycine (analogous to M-Ser (OH)) and AS-330 (+PNE) relative to ascorbic acid and vitamin E.

4. Materials and Methods

4.1. Isolation, Identification and Characterization of MAAs

Three red macroalgae (*Porphyra rosengurttii*, *Gelidium corneum* and *Ahnfeltiopsis devoniensis*) and one marine lichen (*Lichina pygmaea*) were selected for this study, considering their high contents in P-334 (4.85 ± 0.31 mg/g DW), AS-330+PNE (0.57 ± 0.03 mg/g DW), SH (0.8 ± 0.17 mg/g DW) and M-Ser (OH) (1.1 ± 0.23 mg/g DW) respectively. The extraction and isolation of these MAAs in high purification grade was carried out by adsorption and ionic exchange chromatography based on published protocols [59,89] modified by De la Coba et al. [42]. MAAs were identified both by HPLC according to Korbee-Peinado et al. [90] and by using Electrospray Ionization Mass Spectrometry (ESI-MS). For HPLC analysis, a Waters 600 HPLC System (Waters Cromatografía S.L., Barcelona, Spain) was used with a mobile phase of 1.5% aqueous methanol (v/v) plus 0.15% acetic acid (v/v) in water, run isocratically at 0.5 mL min^{-1}. Sample volumes of 10 μl (μg/mL MAAs concentrations) were injected into a C8 chromatographic column (4 μm average particle size, 250 × 4.6 mm; Luna, Phenomenex, Aschaffenburg, Germany) with a guard column (C8, Octyl, MOS, Phenomenex). Autosample temperature was maintained at 20 °C. MAAs were detected online with a Waters Photodiode Array Detector 996 (Waters Cromatografía S.L., Barcelona, Spain), and absorption spectra (290–400 nm) were recorded each second directly on the HPLC-separated peaks. Mycosporine-like amino acids were also analyzed by mass spectrometry (ESI-MS) with a high-resolution mass spectrometer (model Orbitrap Q-Exactive, Thermo Scientific, Bremen, Germany) provided with an electrospray ionization-heated probe (HESI-II), in the premises of the Central Service for Research Support (SCAI, University of Málaga, Málaga, Spain). This technique ionizes molecules while preserving their structures, unlike low resolution techniques that involves the breakdown of analytes. The identification of MAAs was according to comparing their protonated theoretical molecular masses m/z [M + H]⁺ with the parent ions detected, with an allowed approximation of 4 decimals. The samples were dissolved in 100% methanol in order to µg/L MAAs concentrations. Mass calibration for Orbitrap was performed once a week, in both positive and negative modes, to ensure a working mass accuracy lower than or equal to 5 ppm. The HESI parameters were optimized as follows: sheath gas flow rate 12 arbitrary unit; auxiliary gas flow rate 0 arbitrary unit; capillary temperature 320 °C; heater temperature 50 °C; spray voltage 4.0 KV and S lens RF level 50. Full scan data in positive polarity mode were acquired at a resolving power of 140,000 FWHM (full width half maximum) at m/z 200, and a scan range of m/z 100–700 was chosen. The AGC (Automatic gain control) target was set to 10^6, with a maximum injection time of 30 ms.

MAAs were identified firstly by HPLC by comparing absorption spectra, retention times and by co-chromatography using high purified grade MAAs extracts provided from the Unit of Photobiology of the Central Service for Research Support (SCAI, University of Málaga, Málaga, Spain). Their molecular structures were confirmed by High- resolution Electrospray Ionization Mass Spectrometry (ESI-MS) using their protonated molecular masses with an accuracy to the fourth decimal. Molecular structures of glycosylated derivatives of porphyra 334 (478–508 Da) and shinorine (464 Da) described by Nazifi et al. [91] with absorption maxima at 334–335 nm were also checked in ESI-MS spectra of P-334 (+SH) and SH extracts. Quantification was carried out using published extinction coefficients [89,92–95] extracting chromatographic peak areas of each MAA at its maximum absorption wavelength.

4.2. pH MAAs Stability Determination

The different aqueous purified extracts were diluted in a final volume of 1 ml phosphate buffer (50 mM) at different pH conditions (4.5, 7.5, 8.5 and 10.5) with an initial absorbance of 0.8 ± 0.05 in each MAA solution. Absorbance spectra (from 250 to 450 nm) were measured after 1 and 24 h of incubation using a UV-Vis spectrophotometer Shimadzu 1603 (Shimadzu Co., Kyoto, Japan). All determinations were carried out in triplicate at room temperature (25 °C).

4.3. Temperature and pH MAAs Stability Determination

In order to evaluate the combined effect to different temperature and pH conditions, purified MAA extracts were incubated at 50 °C and 85 °C during 6 h using screw cap tubes to avoid volume loss. After that time, in a final volume of 1 ml, the different aqueous purified extracts were diluted in phosphate buffer (50 mM) at different pH values (4.5, 7.5, 8.5 and 10.5) to an initial absorbance of 0.8 ± 0.05 in each MAA solution. Absorbance spectra (from 250 to 450 nm) were measured 1.5, 3, 4.5 and 6 h post-incubation. All determinations were carried out in triplicate.

4.4. Galenic Formulations

In order to analyze the MAAs photoprotection capabilities in vitro, different oil/water emulsions were formulated containing a mixture of Neo PCL self-emulsifying base (Acofarma, Barcelona, Spain) and propylene glycol in water as the base formula. This formulation presented pH 5.8. Different aqueous filters were added to the propylene glycol-water phase prior to mixing with Neo PCL. The ratio of these three components was 4:1:14 (expressed in w/v for Neo PCL and v/v for propylene glycol and water extracts) and 19.6% w/v, 4.9% v/v and 68.6% v/v in the final formula respectively. The galenic compositions were formulated at 60 °C (the safety range for MAAs according to this study). New pH measurements of MAAs sunscreens were taken once they were tempered. Absorbance spectra were measured at a rate of 2 mg · cm^{-2} of the different sunscreens on 3M Transpore self-standing substrates. The products were distributed uniformly in a circular motion with a finger equipped with a rubber thimble for about 30 s. The preparations were allowed to dry for 15 minutes and then were irradiated using a double band UV spectrophotometer Shimadzu UV-1800 (Shimadzu Co., Kyoto, Japan) between 290–400 nm wavelengths. Transpore substrate with base formula was used as a baseline.

Four emulsions were formulated: P- 334 (+ SH) at 5.6% (w/w); M-Ser (OH) at 5.1% (w/w); a combination of these MAAs where P-334 (+ SH) were the majority MAAs (4.1 vs. 2.9 %); and finally, a reference cream containing a combination of UVA and UVB-absorbing reference filters: BMDM, UVA1 filter (λ_{max} between 355–359 nm) (Fagrón Ibérica S.A., Barcelona, Spain) and OMC, UVB filter (λ_{max} 311 nm) (Fagrón Ibérica S.A., Barcelona, Spain) with similar rate to the MAAs combination one (4.5 and 2.6% respectively).

4.5. In vitro Sun Protection Factor (SPF) Determination

SPF was characterized according to the Diffey method [96] with some modifications, and protection in the UVA band was calculated by the critical wavelength [97,98]. The UVA/UVB ratio defines the performance of a sunscreen in the UVA range (320–400 nm) in relation to its performance in the UVB range (290–320 nm), while the critical wavelength is given as the upper limit of the spectral range from 290 nm on, within which 90% of the area under the extinction curve of the whole UV range between 290 and 400 nm is covered. When the critical wavelength is 370 nm or greater, the product is considered broad spectrum, which denotes balanced protection throughout the UVB and UVA ranges.

Transmittance measurements were performed on 3M surgical Transpore self-standing substrate, a material chosen to simulate the roughness of human skin with better correlation between in vitro and in vivo SPF measurements when the test is not pre-irradiated [99]. Transpore tape was stuck onto a light-diffusing double- ground quartz plate and placed on an analytical balance. The sunscreens were plotted onto the tape from a pre-weighted syringe at a rate of 2 mg·cm^{-2} along the selected surface (4 cm^2) and spread evenly with a gloved finger for about 30 s. The preparation was allowed to dry for 15 min and then, was irradiated using a double band UV spectrophotometer (Shimadzu UV-1800) between 290–400 nm wavelengths, collecting the resulting transmittance spectrum. A Transpore substrate with base formula was used as a baseline.

The sun protection factor (SPF) was calculated from transmission measurements according to:

$$SPF = \sum_{290}^{400} E(\lambda) \cdot S(\lambda) / \sum_{290}^{400} E(\lambda) \cdot S(\lambda) \cdot T(\lambda)$$

where

$E\lambda$ = CIE standard Skin reference erythema action spectrum [77].
$T\lambda$ = Transmitance values (0–1).
$S\lambda$ = Spectral irradiance of a midday clear sky of summer, terrestrial sunlight in Spain (22 June at 36.71° N, −4.47° W).

Sunlight was measured by using a portable double monochromator spectrorradiometer Bentham IDR300-PSL (Bentham Co., Reading, UK) which takes measurements in W m^{-2}·s^{-1} between 200 to 500 nm (Device located at Unit of Photobiology of the Central Service for Research Support, SCAI, University of Malaga, Malaga, Spain).

4.6. Biological Effective Protection Factors (BEPFs)

BEPF calculation for a determined UV-mediated skin response was obtained through transmission measurements according to the Diffey method using the relative action spectrum for this biological effect (Table 4). BEPF can be understood as an indicator given to sunscreen consumers, informing them about the number of times a photoprotected person can be exposed versus a person with unprotected skin before this process begins to develop.

In this study, the level of UV photoprotection for the different formulated emulsions was determined for a total of seven UV-biological mediated processes with a well-known action spectra associated with human skin. Some of them have maximum effect on UVB (UVB-BEPFs) and others in the UVA wavelengths (UVA-BEPFs) (Table 4). Data for erythema, DNA damage, and photocarcinogenesis of non-melanoma skin cancers (NMSC- SCUP-h) spectra were available in the literature [12–14]. For the other action spectra selected, cubic splinic interpolation between the data points of the respective action spectrum has been employed to provide values of 1 nm increments and the integral in the Equation (1) replaced by a summation in 1 nm step. Splinic interpolation was done by means of the software Table curve 2D 5.0.1. (Systat Software Inc., San Jose, CA, USA). The error in the interpolation and summation in 1 nm step is estimated to be lower than 5% (Figure 5).

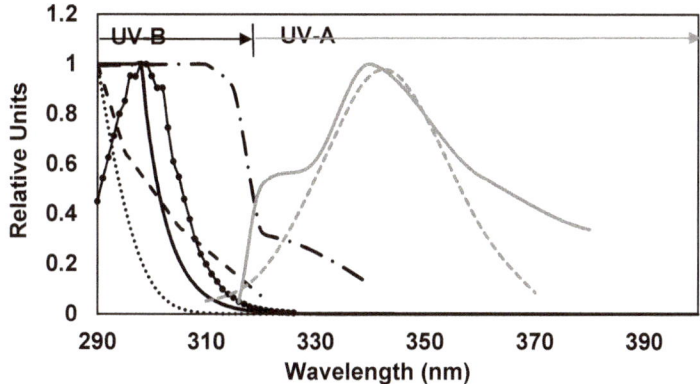

Figure 5. Normalized Action Spectra (290–400 nm) for different UVB and UVA mediated harmful biological effects used in this study: DNA Damage (······), erythema (———), photocarcinogenesis (NMSC) (—•—), induction of systemic suppression of CHS (— — —), photoisomerization of urocanic acid (— · -), formation of singlet oxygen (- - - - -) and photoaging (———).

4.7. Statistical Analysis

The results are presented as the mean value ± standard deviation of at least 4 samples. The statistical significance of the means was contrasted by one-factor Analysis of Variance (ANOVA) followed by Tukey's multiple comparison test [100]. A fixed level of significance of 95% ($p < 0.05$) was used in all cases.

5. Conclusions

The high stability of MAAs over a wide range of temperature and pH, together with their antioxidant properties in aqueous and lipid solutions and photoprotective capabilities against adverse effects of UVB and UVA solar radiation (patented), make them excellent cosmeceutical compounds, which have grown exponentially over the years and have become feasible substitutes of active products used in some medical treatments. The discovery of new active agents, such as those of marine origin, is currently the focus of intense research. We have also proposed new complementary in vitro tests to evaluate the efficacy of commercial sunscreens that we recommend to be included in the information given to consumers.

6. Patents

Part of the results obtained in this research were registered in the patent "López-Figueroa, F.; Aguilera Arjona, J.; de la Coba-Luque, F.; Korbee Peinado, N. Composición para protección solar a base de extractos de algas y líquenes. ES Patent 2,317,741, A1, 16 April 2009".

Author Contributions: Conceptualization, J.A., M.V.d.G., F.L.F. and F.d.l.C. ; Data curation, J.A. and F.d.l.C. ; Formal analysis, F.d.l.C., J.A. and N.K.; Funding acquisition, F.L.F; Investigation, F.d.l.C., J.A., N.K., M.V.d.G., E.H-C and F.L.F.; Methodology, F.d.l.C., J.A. and N.K; Project administration, F.L.F.; Resources, F.L.F and E.H-C; Software, F.d.l.C., J.A. and F.A-G; Supervision, J.A. and F.L.F.; Validation, F.d.l.C and J.A.; Visualization, F.d.l.C., J.A. and F.L.F.; Writing—original draft, F.d.l.C.; Writing—review & editing, F.d.l.C. and N.K.

Funding: This research was funded by the Ministry of Education and Science of Spain (AGL 2005–02655) and Junta de Andalucía to the research group "Photobiology and Biotechnology of aquatic organisms (RNM-295)".

Conflicts of Interest: The authors declare no conflict of interest.

References

1. Young, A.R. Acute effects of UVR on human eyes and skin. *Prog. Biophys. Mol. Biol.* **2006**, *92*, 80–85. [CrossRef] [PubMed]
2. Matsumura, Y.; Ananthaswamy, H.N. Short-term and long-term cellular and molecular events following UV irradiation of skin: Implications for molecular medicine. *Expert Rev. Mol. Med.* **2002**, *4*, 1–22. [CrossRef] [PubMed]
3. Liu, D.; Fernandez, B.O.; Hamilton, A.; Lang, N.N.; Gallagher, J.M.C.; Newby, D.E.; Feelisch, M.; Weller, R.B. UVA irradiation of human skin vasodilates arterial vasculature and lowers blood pressure independently of nitric oxide synthase. *J. Investig. Dermatol.* **2014**, *134*, 1839–1846. [CrossRef]
4. Johnson, R.S.; Titze, J.; Weller, R. Cutaneous control of blood pressure. *Curr. Opin. Nephrol. Hypertens.* **2016**, *25*, 11–15. [CrossRef] [PubMed]
5. Randhawa, M.; Seo, I.; Liebel, F.; Southall, M.D.; Kollias, N.; Ruvolo, E. Visible light induces melanogenesis in human skin through a photoadaptive response. *PLoS ONE* **2015**, *10*, e0130949. [CrossRef] [PubMed]
6. Sklar, L.R.; Almutawa, F.; Lim, H.W.; Hamzvi, I. Effects of ultraviolet radiation, visible light, and infrared radiation on erythema and pigmentation: A review. *Photochem. Photobiol. Sci.* **2013**, *12*, 54–64. [CrossRef] [PubMed]
7. Liebel, F.; Kaur, S.; Ruvolo, E.; Kollias, N.; Southall, M.D. Irradiation of skin with visible light induces reactive oxygen species and matrix-degrading enzymes. *J. Investig. Dermatol.* **2012**, *132*, 1901–1907. [CrossRef] [PubMed]
8. Schroeder, P.; Lademann, J.; Darvin, M.E.; Stege, H.; Marks, C.; Bruhnke, S.; Krutmann, J. Infrared radiation-induced matrix metalloproteinase in human skin: Implications for protection. *J. Investig. Dermatol.* **2008**, *128*, 2491–2497. [CrossRef]
9. Lim, H.W.; Arellano-Mendoza, M.-I.; Stengel, F. Current challenges in photoprotection. *J. Am. Acad. Dermatol.* **2017**, *76*, S91–S99. [CrossRef]
10. Rundel, R.D. Action spectra and estimation of biologically effective UV radiation. *Physiol. Plant.* **1983**, *58*, 360–366. [CrossRef]
11. International Organization for Standardization. *ISO 2443: 2012—Determination of Sunscreen UVA Photoprotection In Vitro*; ISO: Geneva, Switzerland, 2012.
12. Setlow, R.B. The wavelengths in sunlight effective in producing skin cancer: A theoretical analysis. *Proc. Natl. Acad. Sci. USA* **1974**, *71*, 3363–3366. [CrossRef] [PubMed]
13. De Gruijl, F.R.; Van der Leun, J.C. Estimate of the wavelength dependency of ultraviolet carcinogenesis in humans and its relevance to the risk assessment of a stratospheric ozone depletion. *Health Phys.* **1994**, *67*, 319–325. [CrossRef] [PubMed]
14. De Fabo, E.; Noonan, F. Mechanism of immune suppression by ultraviolet irradiation in vivo. I. Evidence for the existence of a unique photoreceptor in skin and its role in photoimmunology. *J. Exp. Med.* **1983**, *158*, 84–98. [CrossRef] [PubMed]
15. McLoone, P.; Simics, E.; Barton, A.; Norval, M.; Gibbs, N.K. An action spectrum for the production of cis-urocanic acid in human skin in vivo. *J. Investig. Dermatol.* **2005**, *124*, 1071–1074. [CrossRef] [PubMed]
16. Hanson, K.M.; Simon, J.D. Epidermal trans-urocanic acid and the UV-A-induced photoaging of the skin. *Proc. Natl. Acad. Sci. USA* **1998**, *95*, 10576–10578. [CrossRef] [PubMed]
17. Bissett, D.L.; Hannon, D.P.; Orr, T.V. Wavelength dependence of histological, physical, and visible changes in chronically UV-irradiated hairless mouse skin. *Photochem. Photobiol.* **1989**, *50*, 763–769. [CrossRef] [PubMed]
18. Gaspar, L.R.; Campos, P.M. Evaluation of the photostability of different UV filter combinations in a sunscreen. *Int. J. Pharm.* **2006**, *307*, 123–128. [CrossRef] [PubMed]
19. Gaspar, L.R.; Camargo, F.B.; Gianeti, M.D.; Campos, P.M. Evaluation of dermatological effects of cosmetic formulations containing *Saccharomyces cerevisiae* extract and vitamins. *Food Chem. Toxicol.* **2008**, *46*, 3493–3500. [CrossRef]
20. Kawakami, C.M.; Gaspar, L.R. Mangiferin and naringenin affect the photostability and phototoxicity of sunscreens containing avobenzone. *J. Photochem. Photobiol. B Biol.* **2015**, *151*, 239–247. [CrossRef]

21. Krause, M.; Klit, A.; Blomberg Jensen, M.; Søeborg, T.; Frederiksen, H.; Schlumpf, M.; Lichtensteiger, W.; Skakkebaek, N.E.; Drzewiecki, K.T. Sunscreens: Are they beneficial for health? An overview of endocrine disrupting properties of UV-filters. *Int. J. Androl.* **2012**, *35*, 424–436. [CrossRef]
22. Sarveiya, V.; Risk, S.; Benson, H.A.E. Liquid chromatographic assay for common sunscreen agents: Application to in vivo assessment of skin penetration and systemic absorption in human volunteers. *J. Chromatogr. B* **2004**, *803*, 225–231. [CrossRef] [PubMed]
23. Kockler, J.; Oelgemöller, M.; Robertson, S.; Glass, B.D. Photostability of sunscreens. *J. Photochem. Photobiol. C Photochem. Rev.* **2012**, *13*, 91–110. [CrossRef]
24. Morabito, K.; Shapley, N.C.; Steeley, K.G.; Tripathi, A. Review of sunscreen and the emergence of non-conventional absorbers and their applications in ultraviolet protection. *Int. J. Cosmet. Sci.* **2011**, *33*, 385–390. [CrossRef]
25. Schauder, S.; Ippen, H. Contact and photocontact sensitivity to sunscreens: Review of a 15-year experience and of the literature. *Contact Dermatitis* **1997**, *37*, 221–232. [CrossRef] [PubMed]
26. Greenspoon, J.; Ahluwalia, R.; Juma, N.; Rosen, C.F. Allergic and photoallergic contact dermatitis: A 10-year experience. *Dermatitis* **2013**, *24*, 29–32. [CrossRef] [PubMed]
27. Navarro, N.; Figueroa, F.L.; Korbee, N.; Bonomi, J.; Álvarez-Gómez, F.; De la Coba, F. Mycosporine-Like Amino Acids from Red Algae to Develop Natural UV Sunscreens. In *Sunscreens: Source, Formulations, Efficacy and Recommendations*; Ragesh, P.R., Ed.; Nova Science Publishers Inc.: Hauppauge, NY, USA, 2018; pp. 99–129. ISBN 9781631172557.
28. Pan, Z.; Lee, W.; Slutsky, L.; Clark, R.A.F.; Pernodet, N.; Rafailovich, M.H. Adverse effects of titanium dioxide nanoparticles on human dermal fibroblasts and how to protect cells. *Small* **2009**, *5*, 511–520. [CrossRef] [PubMed]
29. Zenker, A.; Schmutz, H.; Fent, K. Simultaneous trace determination of nine organic UV-absorbing compounds (UV filters) in environmental samples. *J. Chromatogr. A* **2008**, *1202*, 64–74. [CrossRef]
30. Fent, K.; Zenker, A.; Rapp, M. Widespread occurrence of estrogenic UV-filters in aquatic ecosystems in Switzerland. *Environ. Pollut.* **2010**, *158*, 1817–1824. [CrossRef]
31. Danovaro, R.; Bongiorni, L.; Corinaldesi, C.; Giovannelli, D.; Damiani, E.; Astolfi, P.; Greci, L.; Pusceddu, A. Sunscreens cause coral bleaching by promoting viral infections. *Environ. Health Perspect.* **2008**, *116*, 441. [CrossRef]
32. Balmer, M.E.; Buser, H.-R.; Müller, M.D.; Poiger, T. Occurrence of some organic UV filters in wastewater, in surface waters, and in fish from Swiss lakes. *Environ. Sci. Technol.* **2005**, *39*, 953–962. [CrossRef]
33. Buser, H.-R.; Balmer, M.E.; Schmid, P.; Kohler, M. Occurrence of UV filters 4-methylbenzylidene camphor and octocrylene in fish from various Swiss rivers with inputs from wastewater treatment plants. *Environ. Sci. Technol.* **2006**, *40*, 1427–1431. [CrossRef] [PubMed]
34. Gago-Ferrero, P.; Alonso, M.B.; Bertozzi, C.P.; Marigo, J.; Barbosa, L.; Cremer, M.; Secchi, E.R.; Azevedo, A.; Lailson-Brito, J., Jr.; Torres, J.P.M. First determination of UV filters in marine mammals. Octocrylene levels in Franciscana dolphins. *Environ. Sci. Technol.* **2013**, *47*, 5619–5625. [CrossRef] [PubMed]
35. Kaiser, D.; Sieratowicz, A.; Zielke, H.; Oetken, M.; Hollert, H.; Oehlmann, J. Ecotoxicological effect characterisation of widely used organic UV filters. *Environ. Pollut.* **2012**, *163*, 84–90. [CrossRef] [PubMed]
36. Sánchez-Quiles, D.; Tovar-Sánchez, A. Sunscreens as a source of hydrogen peroxide production in coastal waters. *Environ. Sci. Technol.* **2014**, *48*, 9037–9042. [CrossRef] [PubMed]
37. Park, J.M.; Cho, J.-K.; Mok, J.Y.; Jeon, I.H.; Kim, H.S.; Kang, H.J.; Jang, S. Il Protective effect of astragalin and quercetin on ultraviolet (UV)-irradiated damage in HaCaT cells and Balb/c mice. *J. Korean Soc. Appl. Biol. Chem.* **2012**, *55*, 443–446. [CrossRef]
38. Wei, H.; Saladi, R.; Lu, Y.; Wang, Y.; Palep, S.R.; Moore, J.; Phelps, R.; Shyong, E.; Lebwohl, M.G. Isoflavone genistein: Photoprotection and clinical implications in dermatology. *J. Nutr.* **2003**, *133*, 3811S–3819S. [CrossRef]
39. Conde, F.R.; Churio, M.S.; Previtali, C.M. The photoprotector mechanism of mycosporine-like amino acids. Excited-state properties and photostability of porphyra-334 in aqueous solution. *J. Photochem. Photobiol. B Biol.* **2000**, *56*, 139–144. [CrossRef]
40. Conde, F.R.; Churio, M.S.; Previtali, C.M.; Sandra, C.M.; Carlos, M.P. The deactivation pathways of the excited-states of the mycosporine-like amino acids shinorine and porphyra-334 in aqueous solution. *Photochem. Photobiol. Sci.* **2004**, *3*, 960–967. [CrossRef]

41. Fernandes, S.C.M.; Alonso-Varona, A.; Palomares, T.; Zubillaga, V.; Labidi, J.; Bulone, V. Exploiting mycosporines as natural molecular sunscreens for the fabrication of UV-absorbing green materials. *ACS Appl. Mater. Interfaces* **2015**, *7*, 16558–16564. [CrossRef]
42. De La Coba, F.; Aguilera, J.; Figueroa, F.L.; De Gálvez, M.V.; Herrera, E. Antioxidant activity of mycosporine-like amino acids isolated from three red macroalgae and one marine lichen. *J. Appl. Phycol.* **2009**, *21*, 161–169. [CrossRef]
43. Dunlap, W.C.; Yamamoto, Y. Small-molecule antioxidants in marine organisms: Antioxidant activity of mycosporine-glycine. *Comp. Biochem. Physiol. Part B Biochem. Mol. Biol.* **1995**, *112*, 105–114. [CrossRef]
44. De la Coba, F. *Evaluación de la capacidad fotoprotectora y antioxidante de aminoácidos tipo micosporina. Aplicaciones biotecnológicas*; Universidad de Málaga. Servicio de publicaciones: Málaga, Spain, 2007.
45. Torres, A.; Enk, C.D.; Hochberg, M.; Srebnik, M. Porphyra-334, a potential natural source for UVA protective sunscreens. *Photochem. Photobiol. Sci.* **2006**, *5*, 432–435. [CrossRef] [PubMed]
46. Cardozo, K.H.M.; Guaratini, T.; Barros, M.P.; Falcão, V.R.; Tonon, A.P.; Lopes, N.P.; Campos, S.; Torres, M.A.; Souza, A.O.; Colepicolo, P. Metabolites from algae with economical impact. *Comp. Biochem. Physiol. Part C Toxicol. Pharmacol.* **2007**, *146*, 60–78. [CrossRef] [PubMed]
47. Chrapusta, E.; Kaminski, A.; Duchnik, K.; Bober, B.; Adamski, M.; Bialczyk, J. Mycosporine-Like Amino Acids: Potential Health and Beauty Ingredients. *Mar. Drugs* **2017**, *15*, 326. [CrossRef] [PubMed]
48. De la Coba-Luque, F.; Aguilera-Arjona, J.; López-Figueroa, F. Uso de Aminoácido Tipo Micosporina (porfira 334) en Productos Para Prevención y Tratamiento de Eritema Actínico, Fotocarcinogénesis y Fotoenvejecimiento. ES Patent 2,301,435 B1, 4 April 2009.
49. De la Coba-Luque, F.; Aguilera-Arjona, J.; López-Figueroa, F. Uso de una Mezcla Purificada de Aminoácidos Tipo Micosporina (Asterina 330 + Palitina) en Productos para Prevención y Tratamiento de Eritema actínico, Fotocarcinogénesis y Fotoenvejecimiento. ES Patent 2,303,487 B1, 7 May 2009.
50. De la Coba-Luque, F.; Aguilera-Arjona, J.; López-Figueroa, F. Uso de una Mezcla Purificada de Aminoácidos Tipos Micosporina (Asterina 330 + Palitina) en la Prevención de la Oxidación de Productos Cosméticos y Farmacéuticos 2009. ES Patent 2,307,438 B1, 18 August 2009.
51. De la Coba-Luque, F.; Aguilera-Arjona, J.; López-Figueroa, F. Uso de Aminoácido Tipos Micosporina (Porfira 334) en la Prevención de la Oxidación de Productos Cosméticos y Farmacéuticos 2009. ES Patent 2,301,437 B1, 15 April 2009.
52. De la Coba-Luque, F.; Aguilera-Arjona, J.; López-Figueroa, F. Uso de Aminoácido Tipo Micosporina (Shinorine) en la Prevención de la Oxidación de Productos Cosméticos y Farmacéuticos 2009. ES Patent 2,301,428 B1, 15 April 2009.
53. López-Figueroa, F.; Aguilera Arjona, J.; de la Coba-Luque, F.; Korbee Peinado, N. Composición para Protección solar a Base de Extractos de Algas y Líquenes. ES Patent 2,317,741 A1, 16 April 2009.
54. Diffey, B.L.; Tanner, P.R.; Matts, P.J.; Nash, J.F. In vitro assessment of the broad-spectrum ultraviolet protection of sunscreen products. *J. Am. Acad. Dermatol.* **2000**, *43*, 1024–1035. [CrossRef] [PubMed]
55. COLIPA. *Guideline for the Colorimetric Determination of Skin Colour Typing and Prediction of the Minimal Erythemal Dose (MED) without UV Exposure*; The European Cosmetic and Perfumery Association: Brussels, Belgium, 2007.
56. COLIPA. *In Vitro Method for the Determination of the UVA Protection Factor and "Critical Wavelength" Values of Sunscreen Products*; The European Cosmetic and Perfumery Association: Brussels, Belgium, 2011.
57. Barceló-Villalobos, M.; Figueroa, F.L.; Korbee, N.; Álvarez-Gómez, F.; Abreu, M.H. Production of Mycosporine-Like Amino Acids from *Gracilaria vermiculophylla* (Rhodophyta) Cultured Through One Year in an Integrated Multi-trophic Aquaculture (IMTA) System. *Mar. Biotechnol.* **2017**, *19*, 246–254. [CrossRef] [PubMed]
58. Wada, N.; Sakamoto, T.; Matsugo, S. Mycosporine-Like Amino Acids and Their Derivatives as Natural Antioxidants. *Antioxidants* **2015**, *4*, 603–646. [CrossRef]
59. Bandaranayake, W.M. Mycosporines: Are they nature's sunscreens? *Nat. Prod. Rep.* **1998**, *15*, 159–172. [CrossRef]
60. Wolf, R.; Tüzün, B.; Tüzün, Y. Sunscreens. In *Dermatologic Therapy*; Wiley Online Library: Hoboken, NJ, USA, 2001; pp. 208–2014.
61. Schmid, D.; Schürch, C.; Zülli, F. Mycosporine-like amino acids from red algae protect against premature skin-aging. *Eur. Cosmet.* **2006**, *9*, 1–4.

62. Lawrence, K.P.; Long, P.F.; Young, A.R. Mycosporine-like Amino Acids for Skin Photoprotection. *Curr. Med. Chem.* **2017**. [CrossRef] [PubMed]
63. Kullavanijaya, P.; Lim, H.W. Photoprotection. *J. Am. Acad. Dermatol.* **2005**, *52*, 937–958. [CrossRef] [PubMed]
64. Damiani, E.; Greci, L.; Parsons, R.; Knowland, J. Nitroxide radicals protect DNA from damage when illuminated in vitro in the presence of dibenzoylmethane and a common sunscreen ingredient. *Free Radic. Biol. Med.* **1999**, *26*, 809–816. [CrossRef]
65. Armeni, T.; Damiani, E.; Battino, M.; Greci, L.; Principato, G. Lack of in vitro protection by a common sunscreen ingredient on UVA-induced cytotoxicity in keratinocytes. *Toxicology* **2004**, *203*, 165–178. [CrossRef] [PubMed]
66. Dondi, D.; Albini, A.; Serpone, N. Interactions between different solar UVB/UVA filters contained in commercial suncreams and consequent loss of UV protection. *Photochem. Photobiol. Sci.* **2006**, *5*, 835–843. [CrossRef] [PubMed]
67. Pathak, M.A. Sunscreens: Progress and perspectives on photoprotection of human skin against UVB and UVA radiation. *J. Dermatol.* **1996**, *23*, 783–800. [CrossRef]
68. Chatelain, E.; Gabard, B. Photostabilization of Butyl methoxydibenzoylmethane (Avobenzone) and Ethylhexyl methoxycinnamate by Bis-ethylhexyloxyphenol methoxyphenyl triazine (Tinosorb S), a New UV Broadband Filter. *Photochem. Photobiol.* **2001**, *74*, 401–406. [CrossRef]
69. Zhang, Z.; Tashiro, Y.; Matsukawa, S.; Ogawa, H. Influence of pH and temperature on the ultraviolet-absorbing properties of porphyra-334. *Fish. Sci.* **2005**, *71*, 1382–1384. [CrossRef]
70. Gröniger, A.; Häder, D.-P. Stability of mycosporine-like amino acids. *Recent Res. Dev. Photochem. Photobiol.* **2000**, 247–252.
71. Rastogi, R.P.; Incharoensakdi, A. Characterization of UV-screening compounds, mycosporine-like amino acids, and scytonemin in the cyanobacterium *Lyngbya* sp. CU2555. *FEMS Microbiol. Ecol.* **2014**, *87*, 244–256. [CrossRef]
72. Matsuyama, K.; Matsumoto, J.; Yamamoto, S.; Nagasaki, K.; Inoue, Y.; Nishijima, M.; Mori, T. pH-independent charge resonance mechanism for UV protective functions of shinorine and related mycosporine-like amino acids. *J. Phys. Chem. A* **2015**, *119*, 12722–12729. [CrossRef] [PubMed]
73. Zhang, Z.; Gao, X.; Yuri, T.; Shingo, M.; Hiroo, O. Researches on the stability of porphyra-334 solution and its influence factors. *J. Ocean Univ. China* **2004**, *3*, 166–170. [CrossRef]
74. Yoshiki, M.; Tsuge, K.; Tsuruta, Y.; Yoshimura, T.; Koganemaru, K.; Sumi, T.; Matsui, T.; Matsumoto, K. Production of new antioxidant compound from mycosporine-like amino acid, porphyra-334 by heat treatment. *Food Chem.* **2009**, *113*, 1127–1132. [CrossRef]
75. Rastogi, R.P.; Incharoensakdi, A. UV radiation-induced accumulation of photoprotective compounds in the green alga *Tetraspora* sp. CU2551. *Plant Physiol. Biochem.* **2013**, *70*, 7–13. [CrossRef]
76. Korbee-Peinado, N. *Fotorregulación y Efecto del Nitrógeno Inorgánico en la Acumulación de Aminoácidos Tipo Micosporina en Algas Rojas*; Universidad de Málaga, Servicio de Publicaciones: Málaga, Spain, 2003.
77. McKinlay, A.F.; Diffey, B.L. A reference action spectrum for ultraviolet induced erythema in human skin. *CIE J.* **1987**, *6*, 17–22.
78. de la Coba, F.; Aguilera, J.; De Galvez, M.V.; Alvarez, M.; Gallego, E.; Figueroa, F.L.; Herrera, E. Prevention of the ultraviolet effects on clinical and histopathological changes, as well as the heat shock protein-70 expression in mouse skin by topical application of algal UV-absorbing compounds. *J. Dermatol. Sci.* **2009**, *55*, 161–169. [CrossRef]
79. Misonou, T.; Saitoh, J.; Oshiba, S.; Tokitomo, Y.; Maegawa, M.; Inoue, Y.; Hori, H.; Sakurai, T. UV-absorbing substance in the red alga *Porphyra yezoensis* (Bangiales, Rhodophyta) block thymine photodimer production. *Mar. Biotechnol.* **2003**, *5*, 194–200. [CrossRef]
80. Schmid, D.; Schürch, C.; Zülli, F.; Nissen, H.-P.; Prieur, H. Mycosporine-like amino acids: Natural UV-screening compounds from red algae to protect the skin against photoaging. *SÖFW-J.* **2003**, *129*, 38–42.
81. Ryu, J.; Park, S.-J.; Kim, I.-H.; Choi, Y.; Nam, T.-J. Protective effect of porphyra-334 on UVA-induced photoaging in human skin fibroblasts. *Int. J. Mol. Med.* **2014**, 796–803. [CrossRef]
82. Suh, S.-S.; Hwang, J.; Park, M.; Seo, H.H.; Kim, H.-S.; Lee, J.H.; Moh, S.H.; Lee, T.-K. Anti-inflammation activities of mycosporine-like amino acids (MAAs) in response to UV radiation suggest potential anti-skin aging activity. *Mar. Drugs* **2014**, *12*, 5174–5187. [CrossRef]

83. Morliere, P.; Annie, M.; Isabelle, T. Action spectrum for UV-inducen lipid peroxidation in cultured human skin fibroblast. *Free Radic. Biol. Med.* **1995**, *19*, 365–371. [CrossRef]
84. Kaye, E.T.; Levin, J.A.; Blank, I.H.; Arndt, K.A.; Anderson, R.R. Efficiency of opaque photoprotective agents in the visible light range. *Arch. Dermatol.* **1991**, *127*, 351–355. [CrossRef] [PubMed]
85. Premi, S.; Wallisch, S.; Mano, C.M.; Weiner, A.B.; Bacchiocchi, A.; Wakamatsu, K.; Bechara, E.J.H.; Halaban, R.; Douki, T.; Brash, D.E. Chemiexcitation of melanin derivatives induces DNA photoproducts long after UV exposure. *Science* **2015**, *347*, 842–847. [CrossRef] [PubMed]
86. Darvin, M.E.; Sterry, W.; Lademann, J.; Vergou, T. The role of carotenoids in human skin. *Molecules* **2011**, *16*, 10491–10506. [CrossRef]
87. Gonzalez, S.; Pathak, M.A.; Cuevas, J.; Villarrubia, V.G.; Fitzpatrick, T.B. Topical or oral administration with an extract of *Polypodium leucotomos* prevents acute sunburn and psoralen-induced phototoxic reactions as well as depletion of Langerhans cells in human skin. *Photodermatol. Photoimmunol. Photomed.* **1997**, *13*, 50–60. [CrossRef] [PubMed]
88. Torres, P.; Santos, J.P.; Chow, F.; Ferreira, M.J.P.; dos Santos, D.Y.A.C. Comparative analysis of in vitro antioxidant capacities of mycosporine-like amino acids (MAAs). *Algal Res.* **2018**, *34*, 57–67. [CrossRef]
89. Tsujino, I.; Yabe, K.; Sekekawa, I. Isolation and structure of a new amino acid, shinorine, from the red alga *Chondrus yendoi. Bot. Mar.* **1980**, *23*, 65–68.
90. Korbee, N.; Abdala Díaz, R.T.; Figueroa, F.L.; Helbling, E.W.; Peinado, N.K.; Abdala Díaz, R.T.; Figueroa, F.L.; Helbling, E.W. Ammonium and UV radiation stimulate the accumulation of mycosporine-like amino acids in *Porphyra columbina* (Rhodophyta) from Patagonia, Argentina. *J. Phycol.* **2004**, *40*, 248–259.
91. Nazifi, E.; Wada, N.; Asano, T.; Nishiuchi, T.; Iwamuro, Y.; Chinaka, S.; Matsugo, S.; Sakamoto, T. Characterization of the chemical diversity of glycosylated mycosporine-like amino acids in the terrestrial cyanobacterium Nostoc commune. *J. Photochem. Photobiol. B Biol.* **2015**, *142*, 154–168. [CrossRef]
92. Takano, S.; Uemura, D.; Hirata, Y. Isolation and structure of two new amino acids, palythinol and palythene, from the zoanthid *Palythoa tuberculosa. Tetrahedron Lett.* **1978**, *26*, 4909–4912. [CrossRef]
93. Takano, S.; Daisuke, U.; Yoshimasa, H. Isolation and structure of a new amino acid, palythine, from the zoanthid Palythoa tuberculosa. *Tetrahedron Lett.* **1978**, *19*, 2229–2300.
94. Dunlap, W.C.; Chalker, B.E.; Oliver, J.K. Bathymetric adaptations of reef-building corals at Davies Reef, Great Barrier Reef, Australia. III. UV-B absorbing compounds. *J. Exp. Mar. Bio. Ecol.* **1986**, *104*, 239–248. [CrossRef]
95. Gleason, D.F. Differential effects of ultraviolet radiation on green and brown morphs of the Caribbean coral *Porites astreoides. Limnol. Oceanogr.* **1993**, *38*, 1452–1463. [CrossRef]
96. Diffey, B.L.; Robson, J. A new substrate to measure sunscreen protection factors throughout the ultraviolet spectrum. *J. Soc. Cosmet. Chem.* **1989**, *40*, 127–133.
97. Diffey, B.L. Indices of protection from in vitro assay of sunscreens. *Sunscreens Dev. Eval. Regul. Asp.* **1997**, 589–600.
98. Diffey, Bl. A method for broad spectrum classification of sunscreens. *Int. J. Cosmet. Sci.* **1994**, *16*, 47–52. [CrossRef]
99. Garoli, D.; Pelizzo, M.G.; Nicolosi, P.; Peserico, A.; Tonin, E.; Alaibac, M. Effectiveness of different substrate materials for in vitro sunscreen tests. *J. Dermatol. Sci.* **2009**, *56*, 89–98. [CrossRef]
100. Sokal, R.R.; Rohlf, F.J. *Introducción a la Bioestadística*; Reverté: Barcelona, Spain, 1986; Volume 5, ISBN 8429118624.

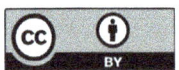

© 2019 by the authors. Licensee MDPI, Basel, Switzerland. This article is an open access article distributed under the terms and conditions of the Creative Commons Attribution (CC BY) license (http://creativecommons.org/licenses/by/4.0/).

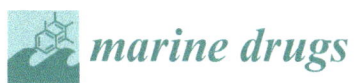

Article

Elicited ROS Scavenging Activity, Photoprotective, and Wound-Healing Properties of Collagen-Derived Peptides from the Marine Sponge *Chondrosia reniformis*

Marina Pozzolini [1,*], Enrico Millo [2,3], Caterina Oliveri [1], Serena Mirata [1], Annalisa Salis [2,3], Gianluca Damonte [2,3], Maria Arkel [2,3] and Sonia Scarfì [1,4]

1. Department of Earth, Environment and Life Sciences (DISTAV), University of Genova, Via Pastore 3, 16132 Genova, Italy; caterina.oliveri@unige.it (C.O.); serenamira94@gmail.com (S.M.); soniascarfi@unige.it (S.S.)
2. Department of Experimental Medicine (DIMES), Biochemistry Section, University of Genova, Viale Benedetto XV 1, 16132 Genova, Italy; enrico.millo@unige.it (E.M.); annalisa.salis@unige.it (A.S.); gianluca.damonte@unige.it (G.D.); mariaarkel27@gmail.com (M.A.)
3. Centre of Excellence for Biomedical Research (CEBR), University of Genova, Viale Benedetto XV 9, 16132 Genova, Italy
4. Inter-University Center for the Promotion of the 3Rs Principles in Teaching & Research (Centro 3R), 56122 Pisa, Italy
* Correspondence: marina.pozzolini@unige.it; Tel.: +39-010-3533-8227

Received: 11 October 2018; Accepted: 20 November 2018; Published: 23 November 2018

Abstract: Recently, the bioactive properties of marine collagen and marine collagen hydrolysates have been demonstrated. Although there is some literature assessing the general chemical features and biocompatibility of collagen extracts from marine sponges, no data are available on the biological effects of sponge collagen hydrolysates for biomedical and/or cosmetic purposes. Here, we studied the in vitro toxicity, antioxidant, wound-healing, and photoprotective properties of four HPLC-purified fractions of trypsin-digested collagen extracts—marine collagen hydrolysates (MCHs)—from the marine sponge *C. reniformis*. The results showed that the four MCHs have no degree of toxicity on the cell lines analyzed; conversely, they were able to stimulate cell growth. They showed a significant antioxidant activity both in cell-free assays as well as in H_2O_2 or quartz-stimulated macrophages, going from 23% to 60% of reactive oxygen species (ROS) scavenging activity for the four MCHs. Finally, an in vitro wound-healing test was performed with fibroblasts and keratinocytes, and the survival of both cells was evaluated after UV radiation. In both experiments, MCHs showed significant results, increasing the proliferation speed and protecting from UV-induced cell death. Overall, these data open the way to the use of *C. reniformis* MCHs in drug and cosmetic formulations for damaged or photoaged skin repair.

Keywords: marine collagen peptide; collagen hydrolysates; antioxidant; cosmetics; inflammation

1. Introduction

Collagens constitute a variegated family of structural proteins that are usually found in the extracellular matrix (ECM) of many tissues in multicellular organisms. Here, they participate in the formation of a complex glycosaminoglycan/protein network ensuing the structural support and physiological integrity of the tissues, mainly, but not exclusively, of mesodermal origin. Thanks to their low immunogenicity across the species and the remarkable mechanical and/or bioactive properties, their collagen extracts, derived gelatins, and peptide hydrolysates are frequently used in health-related sectors [1], cosmetics, and the food industry [2].

Collagen and collagen derivatives are mainly obtained from porcine and bovine skin and bones. Unfortunately, in the last years, the increased risk of BSE and TSE (bovine spongiform encephalopathy and transmissible spongiform encephalopathy, respectively) human infections from cows and pigs, as well as religious constraints on use of porcine derivatives, has led to the investigation of new possible animal sources of collagen. The most intriguing and promising ones come from the marine environment [3]. These collagens are mainly extracted and processed from the waste of fish and molluscs in the fishing industry [4,5], as well as from other invertebrates that are particularly abundant in the marine environment and rich in collagen, such as jellyfishes or sponges [6–8]. Indeed, the successful use of marine collagens from fish, echinoderms, molluscs, and jellyfish populations in human health-related applications such as the evaluation of biological compatibility and use in regenerative medicine, wound-healing, and cosmetics has been increasingly reported [9–13].

Over the years, several studies have also been performed to evaluate the biocompatibility and regenerative medicine potential of marine sponge-derived collagen extracts [8,14,15]. The phylum Porifera is the most ancient metazoan group still thriving on our planet. These are very simple, sessile animals, lacking any real tissue or organ, and formed only by few specialized cell types embedded in a complex ECM network that is very rich in collagen [16–18]. In particular, one of the most described collagens in this phylum derives from the demosponge *Chondrosia reniformis*; indeed, in this animal, it displays peculiar physicochemical characteristics and dynamic plasticity [19,20]. Quite recently, some collagen gene sequences, as well as that of a collagen maturation enzyme, have been uncovered in this animal [21–23]. Furthermore, *C. reniformis* collagen has also demonstrated its utility as a carrier in form of nanoparticles and as a coating for drug preparations, and its lack of toxicity on human skin has been assessed [24–26]. Recently, also, the possibility of using it in the form of thin biocompatible membranes for tissue engineering and regenerative medicine purposes has been evaluated [7].

Overall, the high biotechnological potential of sponges has been clearly recognized in the last years due also to the noteworthy production of bioactive secondary metabolites [27]. Indeed, these molecules have arisen the interest of the pharmacological industry. Thus, in order to obtain commercial quantities of the compounds of interest, various mariculture systems [28,29] have been developed for the full exploitation of the pharmacological potential of these organisms. In this view, bioactive compound extraction from sponge aquacultures would lead to the waste of sponge biomass by-products that could be further employed for the extraction of marine collagen. Furthermore, the great biodiversity in the phylum Porifera may give rise, depending on the species exploited, to a wide variety of different sponge biomasses suitable for different applications, alternatively privileging collagen and/or silica-producing sponges [30].

In addition to the pharmacological and cosmetic use of marine collagens and gelatins from various animal sources per se, also, the employ of bioactive peptides derived from controlled collagen enzymatic hydrolysis has been increasingly reported. Indeed, the potentialities both in the nutraceutical field as well as in vitro, in vivo, and eventually in clinical studies have been evaluated, demonstrating the significant positive effects of collagen hydrolysates both in physiological conditions as well as in ill health [31].

Indeed, a plethora of biological activities have been ascertained by the use of marine collagen-derived peptides such as antimicrobial, antihypertensive, antidiabetic, opioid, calciotropic, secretagogue, joint and bone-regenerative, antioxidant, wound-healing, UV-protective, and antityrosinase activities, both in vitro and/or in vivo, alternatively administered orally or systemically or even in topical concoctions [11,31]. In the years, particular attention has been given to the antioxidant properties of these peptides, since excess of intracellular reactive oxygen species (ROS) has been linked to the development and chronicization of many pathological conditions such as cardiovascular, neurodegenerative, inflammatory, cancer, and age-related illnesses [32–34]. Thus, the search for new molecules with antioxidant activity, especially from natural sources, is continuously pursued as potential drugs for many pathological conditions. In this regard, a significant antioxidant activity has been demonstrated in collagen hydrolysates from different invertebrates such squid and jellyfishes [35,36], as well as from many fishes, such as cod, cobia, Nile tilapia, tuna, and sole skin [35,37–40] to cite a few. Another important field of studies where marine collagen hydrolysates have proven valuable results is related to skin repair, regeneration, and aging [11]. Skin is a physical and chemical barrier of the body against harmful foreign events and pollutants. Indeed, environmental attacks under the form of chemicals, ultraviolet (UV) light, mechanical injuries, and temperature changes may cause serious damage to this important natural barrier [41]. In recent years, a considerable amount of attention has been given to the use of marine collagen hydrolysates as skin repairing/regenerating agents in nutraceutical, pharmacological, and cosmetic formulations in different pre-clinical and clinical studies. Collagen hydrolysates from various sources have demonstrated good biocompatibility, penetration ability, and skin-protective properties in different experimental contexts. As a few examples, in pre-clinical studies, collagen hydrolysates from jellyfish, salmon, and Pacific cod skin have proven significant protective effects on photoaging in vivo [42–44], while collagen peptides from Nile tilapia and Chum salmon skin have demonstrated wound-healing properties [40,45]. Last but not least, clinical studies have also shown improved skin aging parameters after the oral administration of fish collagen peptides [46], definitely indicating the plausibility of exploiting the bioactive properties of marine collagen hydrolysates in many physiopathological conditions of the skin.

Although the bioactive properties of several natural peptides extracted from various sponges have already been reported [47], to date, no information is available on the antioxidant and skin-healing properties of collagen hydrolysates derived from sponges. Indeed, the only available data are on the cosmetic use of *C. reniformis* (non-digested) collagen extracts in cosmetic formulations to assess their biocompatibility and use in substitution to conventional collagens from mammals, which proved successful [24]. Thus, starting from the above-mentioned observations of *C. reniformis* collagen biocompatibility in vivo, the aim of the present work was to produce trypsin-derived *C. reniformis* collagen hydrolysates and explore their performance as antioxidant, UV-protecting, and wound-healing molecules. To this purpose, four fractions of marine collagen hydrolysates (MCHs) from *C. reniformis* were obtained by the enzymatic digestion of sponge collagen extracts followed by reverse-phase HPLC purification, and subsequently their ROS scavenging activity in cell-free tests as well as in an in vitro macrophage model of cell inflammation was investigated. Conversely, the ability to stimulate collagen production in a fibroblast cell line and protect from UV-induced cell damage both in a fibroblast and in a keratinocyte cell line was assessed; the wound-healing properties were also demonstrated by the well-known in vitro "scratch test".

2. Results and Discussion

2.1. Marine Collagen Hydrolysate (MCHs) Purification Yield and Chemical Features

Initially, the yield of total protein content in the *C. reniformis* sponge collagen suspension (before the enzymatic digestion to obtain MCHs) was evaluated, giving a value of 1.2 g $\pm$ 0.17 of proteins from 25 g of wet sponge tissue (starting material). Following 18 h of trypsin digestion at 37 °C, the viscous collagen suspension that resulted was only partially solubilized. After enzyme inactivation and sample centrifugation, the supernatant containing the MCH solution mixture had the aspect of a clear, dark-colored solution. An initial characterization of the MCH clear solution mixture was obtained by evaluating the hydrolysis degree (HD) after the trypsin digestion procedure. The value was calculated as the percentage of the amino acid content of the MCH clear solution mixture with respect to the amino acid content of the undigested suspension, and resulted in 53.5 $\pm$ 7.1% protein total digestion. Then, to obtain a raw evaluation of the peptide sizes in the MCH solution mixture, an SDS gel electrophoresis was performed on the undigested, and trypsin-digested, collagen suspensions (Figure 1A). In particular, the electrophoretic analysis of a 7.5% polyacrylamide gel of the undigested collagen suspension (lane 3) revealed the presence of two bands of about 100 kDa corresponding to α1-fibrillar and α2-fibrillar collagen chains, and one band at 70 kDa that likely could correspond to the non-fibrillar collagen, which was identified, characterized, and obtained in recombinant form by some of us [21–23,48]. Conversely, in the trypsin-digested MCH solution mixture (lane 1 and lane 2, two different digestions), no protein bands were observable, indicating that in the established enzymatic conditions, a good degree of collagen digestion, and release of peptides with a molecular average size lower than 40 kDa, was obtained. The trypsin-digested collagen solution was then purified by preparative reversed phase high-performance liquid chromatography to obtain different fractions of MCHs. The Figure 2B shows a comparative analysis of the RP-HPLC profile at λ = 220 and 254 nm of the MCH mixture. The fractions were collected every two minutes starting from minute seven until minute 21; then, the fractions deriving from three different HPLC runs were concentrated under vacuum and repeatedly lyophilized to remove formic acid before suspension in water. In preliminary experiments (not shown), all of the fractions were analyzed for their cytotoxicity and their antioxidant activity by the DPPH assay, but only four fractions, which were indicated as M3, M4, M5, and M6 in Figure 1B, showed activity. As such, only these four fractions were used to perform all of the following experiments to evaluate the biological activity of the *C. reniformis* MCHs. The characterization experiments throughout the paper are the mean of two different extractions from different sponges. HPLC spectra were very similar from one preparation to the other (not shown); thus, we can say that the extraction procedure and the enzymatic digestion giving the MCH mixture were quite reproducible.

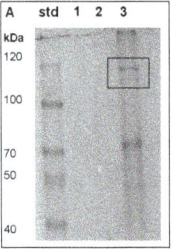

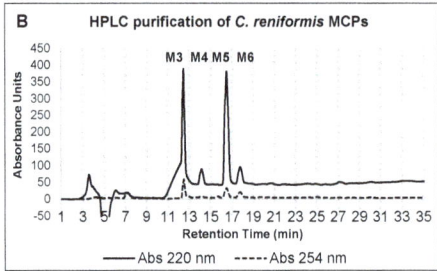

Figure 1. Characterization and purification of *C. reniformis* marine collagen hydrolysates (MCHs). (**A**) SDS-PAGE analysis of undigested and digested sponge collagen. *C. reniformis* trypsin-digested collagen solutions, two different preparations (lane 1 and 2), and undigested collagen suspension (lane 3) were analyzed on 7.5% SDS polyacrylamide gel and Coomassie blue stained. std = standard molecular weight markers. In lane 3, highlighted in the box, α1-chain and α2-chain of fibrillar collagen. (**B**) RP-HPLC (reversed phase high-performance liquid chromatography) profile of the *C. reniformis* trypsin-digested collagen solution in the chromatography used to obtain the MCH fractions. During the purification, fractions were collected every two minutes, as indicated by the vertical dotted grey lines on the chromatogram. The fractions of interest are indicated by the abbreviations M3, M4, M5, and M6, respectively. The analytical conditions are reported in the Materials and Methods (Section 4.4). The continuous line indicates the chromatogram registered at 220 nm, while the dotted line indicates the chromatogram of the same run at 254 nm.

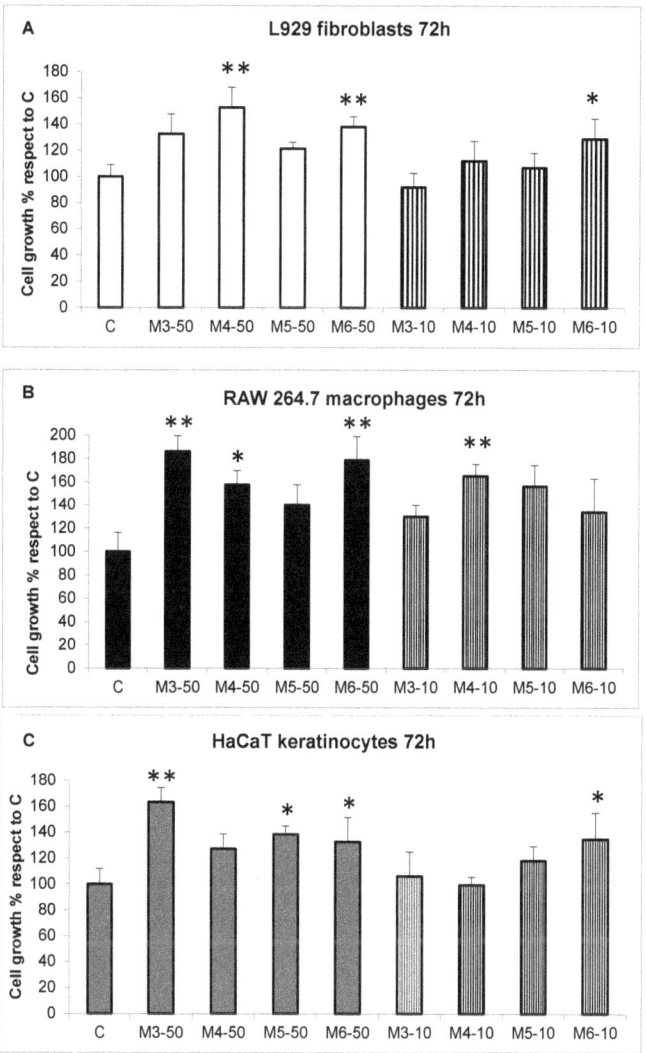

Figure 2. Cell toxicity evaluation. (**A**) L929 fibroblast cell growth quantitative evaluation, by the cell viability MTT test at 72 h, in the presence or absence of the four different MCHs (M3–M6) at the concentration of 50 g/mL (white bars) and 10 g/mL (striped bars). Results are expressed as cell percentages with respect to controls, and are the mean ± S.D. of three experiments performed in quadruplicate. Asterisks indicate the significance in a paired Tukey test (ANOVA, $p < 0.0005$; Tukey vs. C: * $p < 0.05$, ** $p < 0.005$, respectively). (**B**) RAW 264.7 macrophages cell growth quantitative evaluation, in the same conditions as (A). Black bars: MCH fractions 50 g/mL, striped bars: MCH fractions 10 g/mL. Results are expressed as cell percentages with respect to controls, and are the mean ± S.D. of three experiments performed in quadruplicate. Asterisks indicate significance in a paired Tukey test (ANOVA, $p < 0.005$; Tukey vs. C: * $p < 0.05$, ** $p < 0.01$, respectively). (**C**) HaCaT keratinocytes cell growth quantitative evaluation, in the same conditions as (A). Grey bars: MCH fractions 50 g/mL, striped bars: MCH fractions 10 g/mL. Results are expressed as cell percentages with respect to controls, and are the mean ± S.D. of three experiments performed in quadruplicate. Asterisks indicate significance in paired Tukey test (ANOVA, $p < 0.00005$; Tukey vs. C: * $p < 0.05$, ** $p < 0.0005$, respectively).

A first attempt of the chemical characterization of the four MCH fractions by HPLC coupled to electrospray mass spectrometry has been made, giving us indications that the peptides obtained are not attributable to simple amino acid chains from which, by MS/MS (tandem Mass Spectrometry) analysis, it would be possible to reveal the sequences (data not shown). Preliminary MS/MS experiments did not obtain any conclusive data. This could be due to the presence of PTMs (post-translational modifications). It is well-known that collagen from sponges, and from C. reniformis in particular, undergoes significant glycosylation [49], which could impair a direct MS identification. In addition, the widespread presence in collagen of proline and lysine and their hydroxylated forms further complicates the enzymatic cleavage and subsequent characterization. Supplementary and more specific analyses will help us in the future shed light on the peptide composition of the most interesting MCH fractions.

Finally, to obtain a measure of the fractions of peptides solely deriving from the sponge collagen digestion and not from other extracellular matrix sponge proteins co-purified with collagen, the hydroxyproline content was evaluated by the chloramine-T method. Starting from one mg/mL of undigested collagen suspension, the amount of the cyclic amino acid was of 83.21 ± 12.3 µg/mL, while in the same amount of MCH clear solution mixture, it was of 109.99 ± 4.78 µg/mL. Thus, the percentage of this amino acid with respect to the total protein content is 8.3% and 10.9% for the two solutions respectively, and since its presence in marine collagen proteins is usually in the range of 10%, we can conclude that both the collagen suspension as well as the digested MCH solution are mostly composed of collagen or collagen derivatives. Finally, in the HPLC-purified MCH fractions, the concentration of hydroxyproline content ranged from a minimum of ≈7 µg/mL in an M3 fraction to a maximum of ≈37 µg/mL in an M5 fraction (Table 1). These data confirm the presence of collagen-derived peptides in all four MCH fractions, although they also indicate the presence of variable moieties of peptides directly deriving from the digestion of collagen domains containing the cyclic amino acid in the various fractions. In particular, the M4 and M5 fractions that resulted were particularly enriched in collagen-derived peptides containing hydroxylproline (≈ four and five times higher than the less performant M3 fraction, respectively), and were probably the most promising for the biological activities that were subsequently tested.

Table 1. Hydroxyproline content in the various samples before and after HPLC fractionation. Hydroxyproline content in µg/mL measured by the chloramine-T assay (see Methods (Section 4.6)) in the C. reniformis undigested collagen suspension (CS), in the trypsin-digested collagen solution (Total MCP), and in the four HPLC-purified hydrolysate fractions (M3–M6). Data are expressed as the mean ± S.D. of three independent experiments performed in duplicate.

	µg/mL Hyp
undigested CS	83.21 ± 12.3
Total MCPs	109.99 ± 4.78
M3	7.04 ± 0.32
M4	30.40 ± 6.72
M5	37.23 ± 3.56
M6	16.76 ± 4.51

2.2. Effect of the MCP Fractions on Cell Growth of Specific Cell Lines

The biocompatibility and lack of toxicity of collagen extracts from C. reniformis on human skin have already been demonstrated [24], as well as their use as biocompatible material/scaffold for cell adhesion/proliferation and regenerative medicine purposes [7]. This opens the door also to the possible use of C. reniformis collagen derivatives for human health purposes, although the utility and feasibility of the latter has to be demonstrated. In fact, to our knowledge, no studies on the biocompatibility and biological effects of collagen hydrolysates obtained from marine sponges have ever been performed. Thus, the four MCH fractions obtained by the HPLC separation of C. reniformis collagen suspensions were initially analyzed in vitro on different cell types for their effects on cell growth and toxicity. The immortalized cell lines were chosen for the further evaluation of the specific biological activities of the MCH fractions on each cell line, namely the stimulation of collagen production and release in fibroblasts, ROS scavenging activity in activated macrophages, and photoprotective and wound-healing properties in keratinocytes and fibroblasts. Thus, the cell lines that were utilized in our experiments were the collagen-producing L929 murine fibroblasts, the activated-ROS producing RAW 264.7 murine macrophages, and the photosensitive HaCaT human keratinocytes. Cells were treated for 72 h with the four MCH fractions (M3 to M6) at the final concentrations of 50 µg/mL and 10 µg/mL (Figure 2, panels A–C, full colored bars and striped bars, respectively), and then analyzed by the MTT (3-(4,5-dimethylthiazol-2-yl)-2,5-diphenyltetrazolium bromide) cytotoxicity test. At both concentrations, no cytotoxicity was ever observable for all of the MCH fractions that were used, nor in the three cell lines tested, with respect to untreated cells (C). Surprisingly, a slight cell growth stimulation was measured in all of the cell lines, even if with different MCH fractions. In particular, in L929 fibroblasts (panel A), a slight but significant increase of cell number after 72 h was observed with M4 and M6 MCH fractions (1.52 ± 0.155 fold increase for M4-50; 1.38 ± 0.077 and 1.29 ± 0.015 fold increase for M6-50 and M6-10, respectively, compared to control). On the other hand, in RAW 264.7 macrophages, cell growth was stimulated by M3, M4, and M6 fractions (1.86 ± 0.136-fold increase for M3-50; 1.57 ± 0.122 and 1.65 ± 0.179 for M4-50 and M4-10, respectively, and 1.78 ± 0.021 for M6-50, compared to control). Finally, in HaCaT keratinocytes, a slight cell proliferation was observed in the presence of M3, M5, and M6 MCH fractions (1.63 ± 0.112 fold increase for M3-50; 1.38 ± 0.063 for M5-50; and 1.32 ± 0.019 and 1.35 ± 0.020 for M6-50 and M6-10, respectively, compared to control). These data clearly indicate for the first time, that not only are the marine sponge-derived MCHs biocompatible with mammalian cells and do not cause direct toxicity, but also that the positive effects on proliferation could be exploited for cosmetic or regenerative medicine purposes.

2.3. Radical Scavenging Activity of MCH Fractions

Since the antioxidant properties of marine collagen peptides both from invertebrate and vertebrate sources have been well-documented in the last decade [36,42,50–55], we also decided to assess the radical scavenging activity of the four MCH fractions, both in cell-free and cellular in vitro tests to evaluate their potential as antioxidant drugs/supplements. In particular, for the cell-free measurements, two spectrophotometric tests were employed: the DPPH radical scavenging activity test for generic reactive oxygen species (ROS), and the Nitro Blue Tetrazolium (NBT)/riboflavin test measuring superoxide anion scavenging activity (Figure 3). All four MCH fractions showed generic ROS scavenging activity by the DPPH test that was 23% higher than the negative control at concentrations of 50 µg/mL and 100 µg/mL (Panel A, striped bars and black bars, respectively). In particular, the fractions with the lowest activity were M3 and M4, whose values ranged from 31.3% to 37.9% for M3, and from 23.6% to 33.2% for M4, at 50 and 100 µg/mL, respectively. Conversely, the most effective fractions were M5 and M6, which showed an increase in scavenging activity of 39.5% and 37.3% at 50 µg/mL concentration (striped bars) for M5, and 59.6% and 47.2% at 100 µg/mL for M6, respectively (black bars). Similar chemical behavior was also observed in the NBT/riboflavin test, where the ability to scavenge the superoxide anion was measured again for the MCP fractions at concentrations of 50 µg/mL and 100 µg/mL (Panel B, pointed bars and black bars, respectively). Also, in this case, M3 and M4 fractions showed the lowest scavenging activity, especially at 50 µg/mL concentration, which was slightly below 10% for both (dotted bars); while at 100 µg/mL, the increases were 22.2% for M3, and 19.9% for M4 (black bars). Again, M5 and M6 showed the highest scavenging values, ranging from 19.1% to 29.7% for M5, and from 29.2% to 35.5% for M6, at 50 and 100 µg/mL concentrations, respectively. Our results regarding the ROS scavenging activity analyzed by spectrophotometric tests often showed a higher performance with respect to a number of papers analyzing the scavenging activity by the very same analytical tests in marine collagen peptides from fishes [51–55], molluscs [50], and jellyfishes [36,42]. Indeed, in these papers, percentages of scavenging activity in the same range of our results are observable (≈20–70% scavenging activity). In some cases, peptide concentrations were similar to ours [50,52], with a DPPH scavenging activity in the range of 10–25% for squid-derived peptides [50] and 10–40% for crocein croaker-derived peptides [52]. However, significantly much higher peptide concentrations were used in other cases (from 500 µg/mL to 1 mg/mL), and obtained lower performances with respect to ours by DPPH scavenging assay [53,55]. One example is the case of peptides from shark collagen, which demonstrated a scavenging activity of 19–22% at a concentration of 500 µg/mL [53], or for peptides from Nile Tilapia [55], resulting in a scavenging activity of 10–25% at a concentration of one mg/mL. Thus, these data indicate a much better performance of the MCH fractions from *C. reniformis* with respect to other marine sources in the antioxidant activity. Since it has been demonstrated that *C. reniformis* collagen is significantly more glycosylated by post-translational modifications [49] with respect to the other collagens in the Metazoa, the presence of sugar moieties on the peptides deriving from the enzymatic hydrolysis could enhance the antioxidant activity with respect to collagen hydrolysates from other marine sources.

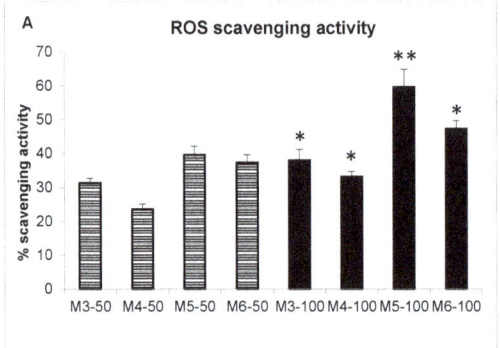

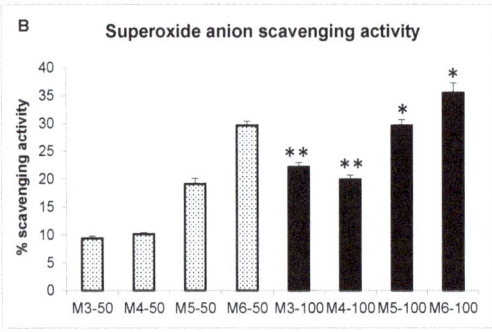

Figure 3. Antioxidant activity of *C. reniformis* MCHs in spectrophotometric tests. (**A**) MCH reactive oxygen species (ROS) scavenging activity by DPPH assay. Data are the mean ± S.D. of three experiments performed in duplicate, and are expressed as a percentage of antioxidant activity with respect to the absorbance of the negative control (calculated as specified in Methods (Section 4.6)). Striped bars: MCH concentration 50 g/mL; black bars: MCH concentration 100 g/mL. Asterisks indicate significance in a paired Tukey test between the same MCH fraction at 100 g/mL and at 50 g/mL concentration (* $p < 0.05$, ** $p < 0.005$, respectively). (**B**) MCH superoxide scavenging activity by Nitro Blue Tetrazolium (NBT)/riboflavin assay. Data are the mean ± S.D. of three experiments performed in duplicate, and are expressed as a percentage of antioxidant activity with respect to the absorbance of the negative control (calculated as specified in the Methods (Section 4.7)). Dotted bars: MCH concentration 50 g/mL; black bars: MCH concentration 100 g/mL. Asterisks indicate significance in a paired Tukey test between the same MCH fraction at 100 g/mL and at 50 g/mL concentration (* $p < 0.05$, ** $p < 0.005$, respectively).

The choice of the DPPH assay was done because is the most used method to measure the ROS scavenging activity of collagen hydrolysates [50–55], which allowed us to compare our results to those of other papers in the field. Notwithstanding, there are some drawbacks in this method, i.e., it does not enable discriminating between hydrogen atom transfer and single electron transfer mechanisms, and could fail in measuring peroxyl radical scavenging ability [56]. Thus, to overcome these limits, and in order to assess the antioxidant activity in a more physiological setting, we measured the intracellular scavenging activity of the four MCP fractions also in an activated macrophage cellular model by use of the 2′,7′-dichlorodihydrofluorescein diacetate (H_2DCF-dA) fluorescent probe. Indeed, this is the same probe used in the fluorimetric cell-free ORAC (Oxygen Radical Absorbance Capacity) test, which is considered an accurate and physiologically relevant method for measuring the antioxidant capacity. In detail, the inhibition of ROS production was measured in stimulated RAW 264.7 murine macrophages by the use of an H_2DCF-dA in vitro assay. Cells were challenged with 200 µM of hydrogen peroxide or with 100 µg/mL crystalline silica (quartz, mean microparticle size below five µm) in the presence or absence of the four MCH fractions (50 µg/mL and 10 µg/mL). After two hours of incubation, the intracellular ROS production was quantified by the use of the ROS-sensitive fluorescent probe (Figure 4). Both stimuli significantly enhanced ROS production in RAW macrophages by 334 ± 28.1% in the case of hydrogen peroxide and by 201 ± 39.5% in the case of quartz with respect to untreated cells. The inhibition of ROS production by the different MCH fractions was then expressed as the percentage with respect to the two positive controls, hydrogen peroxide (H_2O_2, panel A) and quartz (Quartz, panel B). All of the MCH fractions were able to inhibit, even if by different degrees of efficiency, both hydrogen peroxide and quartz-induced ROS in RAW macrophages. In particular, in the hydrogen peroxide-stimulated samples (Figure 4A), all of the MCH fractions significantly inhibited ROS production both at the concentration of 10 µg/mL (striped bars, 63.5% inhibition for M3, 48.4% for M4, 24.7% for M5, and 37% for M6, respectively, compared to H_2O_2), as well as at 50 µg/mL (black bars, 32%, 28.7%, 26.9%, and 46.2% inhibition for M3, M4, M5, and M6, respectively, compared to H_2O_2). For what concerns the quartz stimulation, the significant inhibition of ROS production was obtained by the use of M4 and M6 MCH fractions at the concentration of 50 µg/mL (Panel B, white bars, 29.6% and 30.6% inhibition, respectively, compared to quartz) and by M3, M4, and M5 MCH fractions at 10 µg/mL (striped bars, 37.8%, 32.5% and 29% inhibition, respectively, compared to quartz). Since the ROS that were measured in these experiments are indeed intracellular species produced in activated cells, the antioxidant activity demonstrated by the C. reniformis MCH fractions is even more significant. In fact, it means that these peptides are able to be at least partially internalized by cells, and are able to act directly in the cell cytoplasm, with the result of quenching the potentially dangerous respiratory burst in the activated cells of the immune system. Overall, these results open the possibility of using C. reniformis MCH fractions as antioxidant drugs through systemic, oral, or cosmetic supplementations.

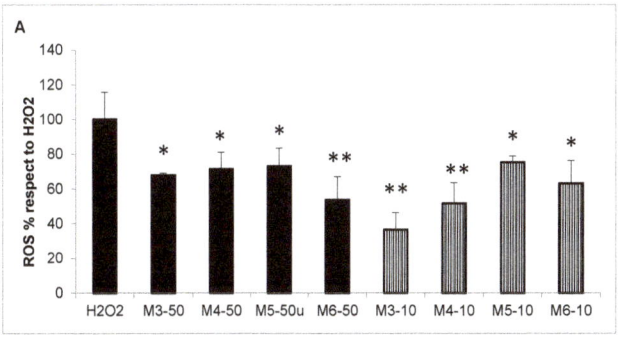

Figure 4. Cont.

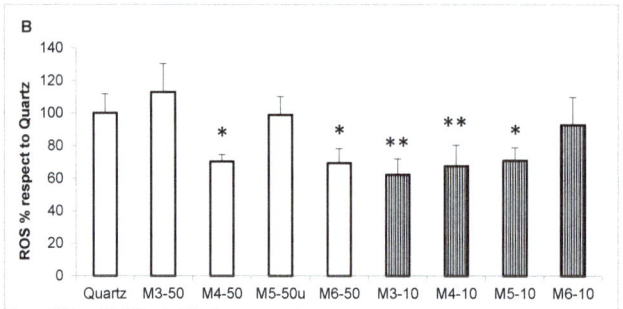

Figure 4. *C. reniformis* MCH ROS scavenging activity in in vitro assays. (**A**) Intracellular ROS production measured by H2DCF-dA (2′,7′-dichlorodihydrofluorescein diacetate) fluorimetric analysis in RAW 264.7 murine macrophages incubated for two hours with 200 µM of H_2O_2 (positive control) in the presence or absence of 50 µg/mL (black bars) or 10 µg/mL (striped bars) of MCH fractions. Results are expressed as percentages of ROS production with respect to the positive control (H_2O_2), and are the mean ± SD of three experiments performed in quadruplicate. Asterisks indicate significance in Tukey test (ANOVA $p < 0.0001$; Tukey vs. H_2O_2, * $p < 0.05$, ** $p < 0.005$, respectively). (**B**) Intracellular ROS production in RAW 264.7 cells incubated for two hours with 100 µg/mL of quartz (positive control) in the presence or absence of 50 µg/mL (white bars) or 10 µg/mL (striped bars) MCH fractions. Results are expressed as percentages of ROS production with respect to the positive control (quartz), and are the mean ± SD of three experiments performed in quadruplicate. Asterisks indicate significance in Tukey test (ANOVA $p < 0.005$; Tukey vs. quartz, * $p < 0.05$, ** $p < 0.01$, respectively).

2.4. Effect of MCH Fractions on Fibroblast Collagen Expression and Release

Quite recently, it has been reported that collagen and/or collagen hydrolysates from various marine sources are able to stimulate collagen deposition in higher organisms [11,42,45,46]. Thus, we tested in vitro, by molecular studies, the hypothesis regarding whether the MCH fractions obtained from *C. reniformis* were able to stimulate collagen deposition in fibroblasts. In synthesis, the four peptide fractions were added to L929 murine fibroblasts for 24 h to evaluate their effect on collagen 1A (Col1A) expression and release. Indeed, all MCH fractions (100 µg/mL concentration) significantly enhanced Col1A mRNA expression and protein release in the cell medium (Figure 5). By qPCR analysis, it was possible to observe an mRNA expression fold increase of 1.74 ± 0.18, 2.64 ± 0.42, 1.91 ± 0.294, and 1.82 ± 0.22 for the M3, M4, M5, and M6 fractions, respectively, compared to the control (Panel A). Similarly, the protein release in the cell medium was quantified by Sircol assay, and the results of collagen production (Panel B) parallel the qPCR analysis. In detail, the fold increase of collagen release in the fibroblast cell medium was of 3.3 ± 0.68, 4.1 ± 1.12, 3.8 ± 1.08, and 3.4 ± 0.97 for the M3, M4, M5, and M6 fractions, respectively, compared to control. From these results, we can infer that the M4 fraction seems to be the most efficient.

We can conclude that in the fibroblast cellular model, the *C. reniformis* MCHs are not only able to promote cell proliferation (Figure 2), but also stimulate collagen deposition with a regulation of the gene at the transcriptional level. These characteristics, together with the significant antioxidant activity (Figure 4) of these peptides, could be very well employed in cosmetic formulations for anti-aging treatments. Since it is quite uncommon to have single molecular species with such heterogeneous and exploitable biological activities, as in the case of *C. reniformis* MCHs, and on the contrary, cosmetic formulations usually are a concoction of many different compounds, the possibility of using a single component that exerted all the necessary actions on aged and wrinkled skin would be an added value in those formulations. Indeed, in vivo results from a cosmetic formulation containing *C. reniformis* (non-digested) collagen extracts have already demonstrated their usability on human skin [24], obtaining results comparable to conventional mammalian collagen formulations by the evaluation of classical skin parameters (pH, hydration, sebum production). Starting from our promising in vitro results, hopefully, we will perform similar experiments in the future in an in vivo setting with the possibility of comparing the two *C. reniformis* collagen formulations (i.e., non-digested and digested) and definitely assessing the advantages and disadvantages of each.

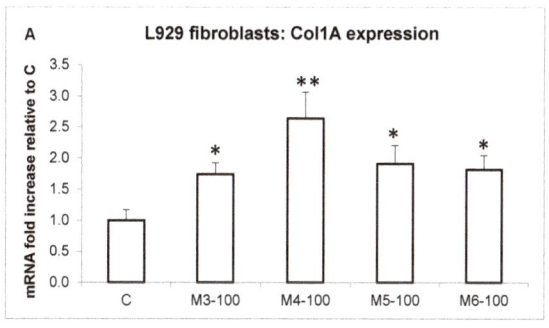

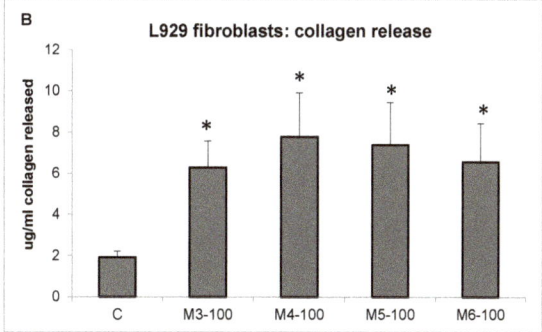

Figure 5. MCH-stimulated collagen gene expression and release. (**A**) L929 fibroblast gene expression measured by qPCR analysis of collagen 1A after 24 h of incubation with 100 μg/mL of the four MCH fractions. Data are normalized on the ubiquitin housekeeping gene, and expressed as an mRNA fold increase compared to control cells. Results are the mean ± SD of three experiments performed in triplicate. Asterisks indicate significance in Tukey test (ANOVA $p < 0.0001$, Tukey vs. C, * $p < 0.05$, ** $p < 0.005$, respectively). (**B**) Colorimetric collagen quantification by Sircol assay in the cell medium of L929 fibroblasts incubated in the same conditions as (A). Results are the mean ± SD of three experiments performed in duplicate. Asterisks indicate significance in Tukey test (ANOVA $p < 0.001$, Tukey vs. C, * $p < 0.05$).

2.5. Effect of MCP Fractions on UV-Induced Cell Death and Gene Expression

Another recently investigated property of collagen and collagen hydrolysates from marine sources is their photoprotective effect on UV-damaged skin cells, which has already shown some promising in vivo results [42,57,58]. Thus, also for our sponge collagen hydrolysate fractions, the effect in favoring cell survival was evaluated in UV-challenged fibroblasts and keratinocytes in order to assess their potential use as photoprotective agents in cosmetic assets (Figure 6). L929 fibroblasts (panels A–B) and HaCaT keratinocytes (panels C–D) were flashed with a UV bulb light for two minutes and five minutes (corresponding to total radiation doses of 90 mJ/cm^2 and 227 mJ cm^2) in the presence or absence of 50 μg/mL MCP fractions, and cell viability was then measured after 24 h or 72 h by the MTT test (panels A/C, and panels B/D, respectively). Results are expressed as percentages of cell survival with respect to untreated, control cells (black bars, C sample) both at 24-h and 72-h end points. At 24 h (panel A), L929 fibroblasts showed a slight but significant increase in cell number in untreated, not-UV flashed cells, after incubation with M3, M4, and M6 fractions (black bars, 15.5%, 15.3%, and 29.3% cell number increase compared to C, respectively). In the same panel, after the two UV doses, an increased cell survival was also observed in the cells incubated with the four MCHs, even if at different rates. In particular, at the lowest UV dose (grey bars, UV 2′) a higher and significant cell survival was guaranteed by all four MCH fractions with respect to the control cells (13.1%, 17.4%, 19.1%, and 21.2% cell number increase for the M3–M6 fraction, respectively), while at the highest UV dose (striped bars, UV 5′), only the M3 and M4 fractions were still able to slightly increase cell survival compared to the control (8.1% and 10.2% cell increase, respectively). On the other hand, at 72 h (panel B), since the control, which were untreated cells (black bars) in these conditions, had reached confluence, it was not possible to observe any cell number increase after incubation with the four MCH fractions alone without UV treatment. Conversely, all four fractions were able to ensure a greater cell number survival after the two UV-dose treatments. In particular, at the lowest UV dose (grey bars, UV 2′), the increased rates of survival, compared to the control, were 22.0%, 34.6%, 40.8%, and 30.9% for M3–M6 fraction, respectively; while at the highest UV dose (striped bars, UV 5′), the increased cell survival rates were 8.4%, 17.5%, 24.0%, and 17.9% for M3–M6 fractions compared to the control, respectively.

The positive effect on cell survival after UV treatment was also observed in HaCaT keratinocytes in the presence of the four MCH fractions both at 24-h and 72-h end points (panels C and D, respectively). In particular, at 24 h (panel C), a significant increase in cell number was observed even in untreated, not-UV flashed cells (black bars) incubated with the M6 fraction, compared to the control (33.3% cell number increase). On the other hand, in the same panel, all four MCH fractions were able to enhance cell survival after the two UV-dose treatments. In particular, at the lowest UV dose (grey bars, UV 2′), the increased rates of survival were of 18.9%, 25.4%, 26.2%, and 14.6% for M3–M6 compared to the control, respectively; while at the highest UV dose (striped bars, UV 5′), the increased cell number percentage was of 32.1%, 16.3%, 16.8%, and 19.4% for M3–M6 compared to the control, respectively. Similarly, at the 72-h end point (panel D), the increased survival rates at the lowest UV-dose (grey bars, UV 2′) were 13.4% 17.4%, 27.9%, and 20.3% for M3–M6 compared to the control, while for the highest UV dose (striped bars, UV 5′), the enhanced cell number percentage was 10.3%, 8.1%, 13.0%, and 12.1% for M3–M6 treated cells compared to the control, respectively. As observed in L929 cells, as well as for HaCaT keratinocytes at the 72-h end point, it was not possible to observe any increase in the number of cells incubated with the four MCHs alone without UV treatment (black bars), which was again due to all the samples reaching confluence in these conditions.

Overall, these results demonstrate a clear beneficial effect regarding the cell survival of all four *C. reniformis* MCH fractions in UV-damaged skin cell cultures, with the M4 and M5 fractions showing the most performing features. From the data collected until now, we can infer that the rescuing abilities are probably due to a combination of effects between the antioxidant properties of the sponge collagen peptides together with the cell growth-promoting abilities that have been demonstrated in this paper (Figures 2–4).

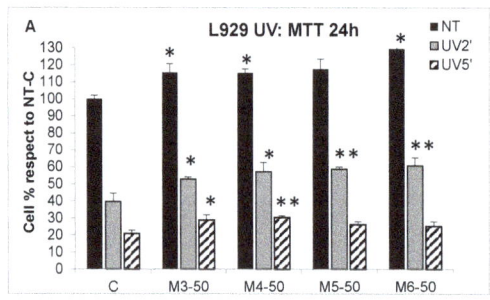

Figure 6. *Cont.*

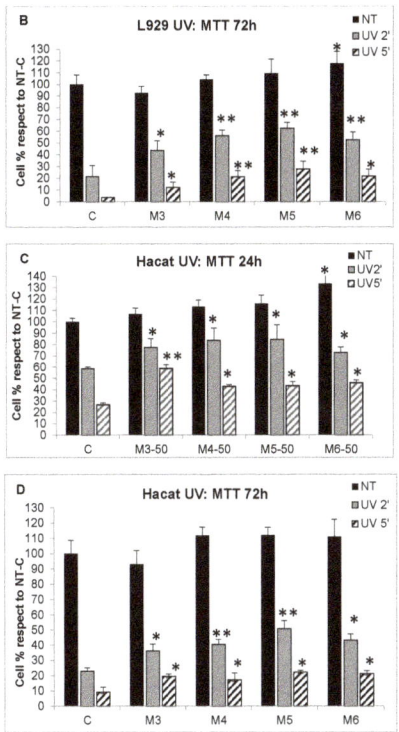

Figure 6. MCH cell death rescue after UV radiation. (**A**) Cell death evaluation by the MTT test at 24 h in L929 fibroblasts after UV radiation for two minutes and five minutes (corresponding to total radiation doses of 90 mJ/cm^2 and 227 mJ cm^2, respectively) in the presence or absence of 50 µg/mL MCH fractions. Black bars, untreated cells; grey bars, cells irradiated for two minutes; striped bars, cells irradiated for five minutes. Results are expressed as cell percentage compared to control cells (NT-C bar), and are the mean ± SD of three experiments performed in quadruplicate. Asterisks indicate significance in Tukey test (ANOVA $p < 0.001$, Tukey vs. the respective C, * $p < 0.05$, ** $p < 0.01$). (**B**) L929 in the same conditions as (A) evaluated at 72 h. Asterisks indicate significance in Tukey test (ANOVA $p < 0.0001$, Tukey vs. the respective C, * $p < 0.05$, ** $p < 0.01$). (**C**) Cell death evaluation by the MTT test at 24 h in HaCaT keratinocytes after UV radiation for two minutes and five minutes in the presence or absence of 50 µg/mL MCH fractions. Black bars, untreated cells; grey bars, cells irradiated for two minutes; striped bars, cells irradiated for five minutes. Results are expressed as cell percentage compared to control cells (NT-C bar), and are the mean ± SD of three experiments performed in quadruplicate. Asterisks indicate significance in Tukey test (ANOVA $p < 0.01$, Tukey vs. the respective C, * $p < 0.05$, ** $p < 0.01$). (**D**) HaCaT cells in the same conditions as (C) evaluated at 72 h. Asterisks indicate significance in Tukey test (ANOVA $p < 0.01$, Tukey vs. the respective C, * $p < 0.05$, ** $p < 0.01$).

Finally, the gene expression profile of two important genes that are highly overexpressed in UV-stressed keratinocytes and are responsible for skin thickening and loss of elasticity [59], namely keratin 1 and 10 (KRT1 and KRT10), were analyzed by qPCR in HaCaT cells. The results are displayed in Figure 7, and show the expression profile at 24 h of the two keratin genes (KRT1 in panel A and KRT10 in panel B, respectively) in cells incubated with the four MCHs alone (black bars) or after a two-minute UV treatment (corresponding to a 90 mJ/cm^2 total radiation dose, white bars). M3, M4, and M6 fractions were able to inhibit both KRT1 and 10 mRNA expression already in untreated, not-UV challenged cells compared to the control (black bars, both panels). In particular, the KRT1 gene (panel A) underwent mRNA decreases of 43%, 47%, and 44% in the presence of M3, M4, and M6 fractions, respectively, compared to the control (C-untreated); meanwhile, the mRNA of the KRT10 gene (panel B) diminished by 40%, 41%, and 32% in the presence of M3, M4, and M6, respectively. On the other hand, after UV challenging, all of the MCH fractions were able to inhibit KRT1 and 10 mRNA overexpression (white bars, both panels). In detail, KRT1 showed a 4.75 ± 0.174 mRNA fold increase after UV treatment compared to the untreated control (white C-UV bar, versus black C-untreated bar, panel A), while in the same conditions, KRT10 mRNA increased by 6.88 ± 0.504-fold compared to the untreated control (white C-UV bar, versus black C-untreated bar, panel B). This significant mRNA increase of the two genes after HaCaT UV-flashing was partially inhibited by the treatment with the MCH fractions. In particular, KRT1 overexpression was inhibited by M5 and M6 fractions alone (Panel A, white bars, 1.44 and 1.73-fold decrease compared to C-untreated, respectively), while KRT10 overexpression was inhibited by all of the MCH fractions, even if with different rates (Panel B, white bars, 1.52, 1.92, 2.21, and 2.28-fold decreases for M3–M6 compared to C-untreated, respectively). Overall, these data indicate a real therapeutic effect of the four MCH fractions on UV-stressed skin cells. Indeed, *C. reniformis* MCHs, through their properties, can act on the skin in different ways by (i) promoting a partial rescue from UV-induced cell death (Figure 7), which is likely thanks to the ROS scavenging activity (Figures 3 and 4) and the cell growth stimulation (Figure 2), (ii) reducing the inflammatory response of immune cells recruited in the damaged skin, again by its ROS scavenging activity, and (iii) by counterbalancing the stress molecular responses of keratinocytes to UV radiation such as the increase of keratin production and deposition that contribute to photoaging through loss of elasticity and skin thickening. Finally, if we add to these already important effects also the stimulation of collagen production in fibroblasts (Figure 5), we can conclude that indeed, cosmetic and pharmacological formulations for aged and photodamaged skin repair could really benefit from the presence of *C. reniformis*-derived MCHs to enhance their efficacy.

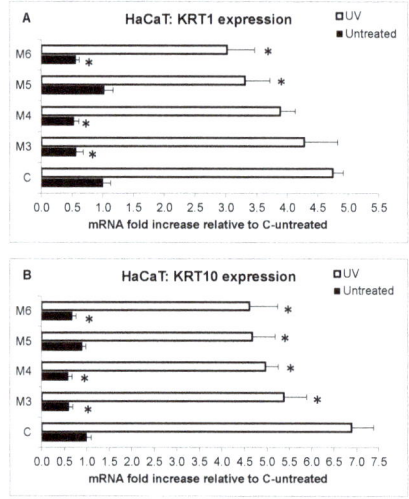

Figure 7. Gene expression of keratins in UV-radiated HaCaT keratinocytes. (**A**) Keratin 1 (KRT1) gene expression after 24 h measured by qPCR analysis in HaCaT keratinocytes irradiated (white bars) or not (black bars) by UV for two minutes in the presence or absence of 50 g/mL MCH fractions. Data are normalized on the ubiquitin housekeeping gene and expressed as an mRNA fold increase compared to the control, which was untreated cells (C, black bar), and are the mean $\pm$ SD of three experiments performed in triplicate. Asterisks indicate significance in Tukey test (ANOVA $p < 0.00001$, Tukey vs. the respective C, * $p < 0.05$). (**B**) Keratin 10 (KRT10) gene expression in HaCaT keratinocytes in the same conditions as (A). Asterisks indicate significance in Tukey test (ANOVA $p < 0.00001$, Tukey vs. the respective C, * $p < 0.05$).

2.6. Effect of MCP Fractions on Wound Healing

The use of marine collagen in composite biomaterials as wound dressing to enhance healing has sporadically been reported [60,61], as well as the use of marine collagen peptides alone or in combined biomaterials demonstrating wound-healing properties in vivo [40,45,62,63]. Thus, the four MCH fractions were also tested for their wound-healing properties both in HaCaT keratinocytes and in L929 fibroblasts. Cell migration/proliferation was performed by the "scratch" assay, which is an in vitro test that is widely used for these purposes [40,63,64], and is described in detail in the Materials and Methods section. The assay was performed in the presence or absence of the different MCH fractions at a concentration of 50 µg/mL. Cells were photographed at 0 h, 6 h, 24 h, and 30 h; pictures were analyzed and quantified as described in Materials and Methods, and the results are displayed in Figures 8 and 9. In particular, from a qualitative point of view, in HaCaT keratinocytes (Figure 8, panels A–O) after the scratch at time = 0 (panels in the first column), it was possible to observe a progressive closure of the scratch in all of both the MCH-treated and untreated samples (panels in the second and third column corresponding to time = 24 h and = 30 h, respectively). The behavior of HaCaT cells indicates a cell proliferation by the sides of the wound gradually filling the gap that is significantly accelerated both at 6 h and 24 h by M5 treatment and at 24 h by M4 treatment with respect to the controls (CT) at the same time points, as quantified in Figure 8P (dotted bars and white bars versus black bars, respectively). In particular, for M5 treatment, the percentage of wound extension at 6 h and at 24 h was 22.7% and 15.7% less than its control, respectively (panels J–L and dotted bar in panel P), while in the case of M4 treatment, the percentage of wound extension at 24 h was 22.6% less than the control (panels G–I and white bars in panel P). Conversely, in L929 fibroblasts after the scratch at time = 0 (Figure 9, panels in the first column), it was possible to observe a progressive migration and colonization of the scratch by cells in all of the both MCH-treated and untreated samples (panels in the second and third column corresponding to time = 24 h and 30 h, respectively). The behavior of L929 fibroblasts in this case indicates first a migration of cells into the gap, and afterwards a proliferation, since it is possible to observe single cells scattered all over the scratch, even in its center, already at 24 h, while the sides of the wound are no more clearly visible, as it was indeed possible in HaCaT cells. This being the case, a qualitative wound-healing score was assigned based on the observation on increasing cell density into the scratches instead of a quantification of wound restriction, as in HaCaT analysis. Anyway, also in L929 cells, the qualitative wound-healing score assigned in blind (Table 2) revealed an increased cell migration/density in M4 and M5-treated cells both at 24 h and 30 h (second and third column, respectively) compared to the controls (CT) at the same time points. The results from both cell lines are quite comparable to those obtained by Hu et al. [40] and Ouyang et al. [63] on the same cell lines, HaCaT and L929, respectively, in both papers treated with marine collagen peptides from Nile Tilapia, with [63] and without [40] the concomitant use of chitosan. In both cases, a similar increase of wound closure was obtained at the same time and at the same concentration of peptides used by us in the two cell lines tested.

Table 2. Wound-healing score in L929 cells, in the presence or absence of MCHs, obtained by a qualitative visual method to quantify the increase of cell density in the scratches of each sample during time. Photographs at the various end points were scored in blind from + to +++, indicating the increasing cell density in the area of the scratches. Data are the mean of two experiments performed in quadruplicate.

P	Wound Healing Score in L929 Fibroblasts	
	24 h	30 h
CT	+	++
M3	++	++
M4	++	+++
M5	+++	+++
M6	+	++

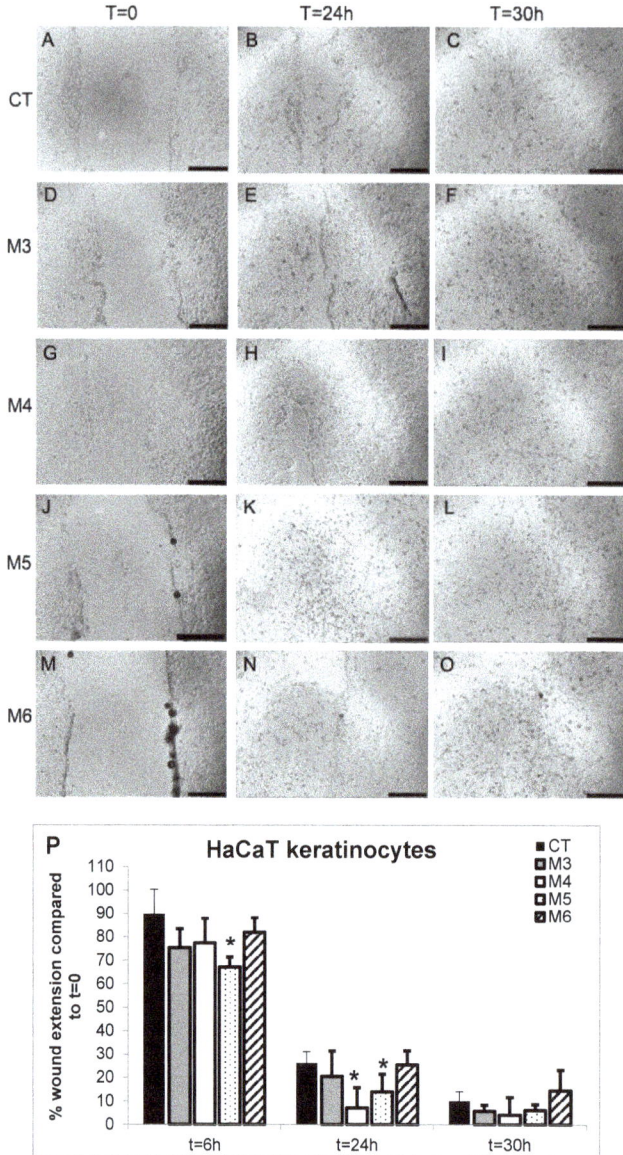

Figure 8. Wound-healing assay in MCH-treated HaCaT keratinocytes. (**A–O**) Microphotographs taken at 0 h, 24 h, and 30 h with a 4× objective of HaCaT keratinocyte monolayers during the wound-healing assay in the presence or absence of 50 µg/mL MCH fractions, in the area of the scratch made at time = 0. A–C control cells, D–F M3-treated cells, G–I M4-treated cells, J–L M5-treated cells, and M–O M6-treated cells. Black bars span 50 µm. (**P**) Quantitative evaluation of the wound-healing degree of HaCaT cells over time. To determine the degree of wound healing, the closing distance of the scratch was measured two times in each photograph by using the ImageJ program free software (http://imagej.nih.gov/ij/). Data are expressed as percentages of the closing distance of each sample with respect to the same sample at time = 0. Experiments were repeated twice in quadruplicate, and data are the mean ± SD. Asterisks indicate significance in Tukey test (ANOVA $p < 0.00001$, Tukey vs. the same sample at t = 0, * $p < 0.05$).

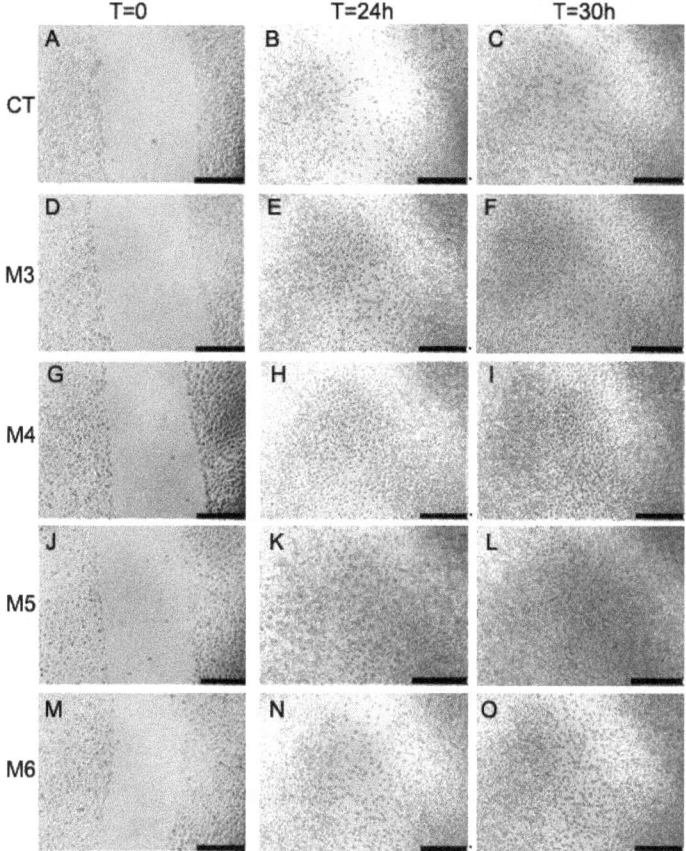

Figure 9. Wound-healing assay in MCH-treated L929 fibroblasts. (**A–O**) Microphotographs taken at 0 h, 24 h, and 30 h with a 4× objective of L929 fibroblast monolayers during the wound-healing assay in the presence or absence of 50 µg/mL MCH fractions, in the area of the scratch made at time = 0. A–C control cells, D–F M3-treated cells, G–I M4-treated cells, J–L M5-treated cells, and M–O M6-treated cells. Black bars span 50 µm.

We can conclude that in both cell types, keratinocytes and fibroblasts, the M4 and M5 fractions from *C. reniformis* MCHs demonstrated promising wound-healing properties, facilitating either cell migration or proliferation at the site of the wound of epidermal and dermal cells. These fractions could be used for the treatment of such injuries, with effects comparable to those of well-known MCHs from other sources.

3. Conclusions

The scientific literature on the bioactive properties of MCHs from several invertebrate and vertebrate sources, as well as their use for the treatment of different types of skin injuries or in regenerative medicine assets, has been constantly growing in the last decade. This actually demonstrates the safety, as well as, in many cases, the efficacy of pharmacological, nutraceutical, and cosmetic formulations of marine collagen-derived peptides in human health issues. To date, no information about the very same bioactive properties of collagen-derived peptides in the most primitive Metazoa, namely sponges, were available. Thus, we undertook our study by choosing a marine sponge that was particularly enriched in collagen, whose chemical and bioactive properties have already been in part documented as in the case of *C. reniformis*. The collagen of this demosponge already holds promising features for its use in the production of biomaterials that are suitable for tissue engineering and regenerative medicine purposes, as has been recently demonstrated by our group. Now, with the current study, also the successful employ of peptide mixture solutions derived from its enzymatic digestion have been ascertained in different cellular models, with a particular emphasis on the antioxidant and proliferative properties that seem particularly beneficial in relieving symptoms of various skin injuries derived from UV radiation or wounding. This opens a way to the use of *C. reniformis* MCHs in drug and cosmetic formulations in in vivo studies and in humans to definitely confirm their usability. Anyway, some further studies would be necessary for that to happen, such as for example a more precise description and chemical characterization of the peptide mixtures obtained by the enzymatic digestion of the sponge collagen suspensions, possibly concentrating on the most bioactive fractions as M4 and M5 seem to be, and last but not least, a serious study on the real performances of the aquaculture systems of this marine sponge in terms of growth rates, biomass yields, and the feasibility of this type of farming to really bring such a promising product to the market.

4. Materials and Methods

All reagents were acquired from SIGMA-ALDRICH (Milan, Italy), unless otherwise stated.

4.1. Preparation of MCHs

MCHs were obtained by trypsin digestion of a collagen fibril suspension isolated from *C. reniformis*, as previously described in Pozzolini et al. 2018 [7]. Briefly, 25 g of frozen sponge tissue was minced in five volumes of 100 mM of ammonium bicarbonate, pH 8.5, and incubated overnight at 37 °C on a horizontal shaker in presence of 0.1% trypsin. Afterwards, the fluid was removed by filtration with a metallic strainer, and the solid material was suspended in three volumes of deionized water and incubated at 5 °C for three days in a rotary disk shaker. The dark and viscous suspension was then filtered with a metallic strainer, and the remained solid material was subjected to a second round of three days of water extraction. The viscous fluid was pooled and centrifuged at $1200\times g$ for 10 min at 4 °C. The supernatant fluid containing the collagen suspension was then centrifuged at $12{,}000\times g$ for 30 min at 4 °C, and finally suspended in 100 mM of ammonium bicarbonate, pH 8.5. Total protein content was evaluated by BCA (Bicinchoninic Acid assay) assay as described in Pozzolini et al. 2018 [7]. MCHs from the fibrillar collagen extract were then obtained as follows: the collagen extract was heated at 90 °C for one hour; then, it was cooled on ice, and finally trypsin digested for 18 h at 37 °C, with a 1:20 (w/w) ratio of enzyme to substrate. Subsequently, the peptide mixture was heated at 70 °C for 10 min to inactivate the enzyme, and centrifuged. The supernatant containing the MCHs was frozen and stored at −20 °C for further high performance liquid chromatography (HPLC) purification. The procedure was repeated twice.

4.2. SDS-Page Analysis

In order to evaluate the digestion activity of trypsin on the purified fibrillar collagen extract, MCHs were analyzed by SDS-PAGE and compared with the undigested collagen suspension; 30 µL of 1 mg/mL of each sample was mixed with 4× loading buffer (60 mM of Tris-HCl, pH 8.0, containing 25% glycerol, 2% SDS, and 0.1% bromophenol blue); then, it was boiled for 10 min and loaded on a 7.5% SDS polyacrylamide gel. The electrophoresis was carried out for two hours at 70 mA. After electrophoresis, the gel was fixed in 10% acetic acid for 30 min, and then stained for three hours with 0.05% (w/v) Coomassie blue R-250 in 15% (v/v) methanol and 5% (v/v) acetic acid. The gel was finally destained with 30% (v/v) methanol and 10% (v/v) acetic acid prior to imaging.

4.3. Degree of Hydrolysis (DH) Evaluation

DH was calculated as the ratio between the total amino acid content in the MCHs and the amino acid content in the undigested collagen suspension. To determine the amino acid content, the samples were previously hydrolyzed with 2 N of NaOH by autoclaving at 120 °C for 20 min. Then, they were neutralized by adding one volume of 2 N HCl and diluted 10-fold in 50 mM of NaH_2PO_4, pH 8. Total amino acid content was finally evaluated by adding 0.25 volumes of 8% ninhydrin solution and incubating for 10 min at 80 °C. Absorbance of each sample was read at 570 nm using a Beckman spectrophotometer (DU 640), in comparison to a L-lysine standard curve. The procedure was carried out in duplicate.

4.4. HPLC MCP Purification

The trypsin-digested collagen suspensions, deriving from two different extractions/digestions, were purified by preparative reversed phase high-performance liquid chromatography (RP-HPLC) to obtain the MCH fractions. A Phenomenex C18 Luna (21.2 × 250 mm) column on an Agilent series 1260 Infinity preparative HPLC separation system (Agilent Technologies Italia SpA, Milan, Italy) was used. Before the preparative purification, an analytical reversed phase HPLC was performed using a similar C18 column to establish the best gradient for the following purification. Solvent A was 0.1% formic acid in water, and solvent B was 0.1% formic acid in acetonitrile. The gradient was 0–65% B from five to 35 min, the flow rate was set to 15 mL/min, and two-minute fractions were collected monitoring the chromatogram at the two different wavelengths of 220 nm and 254 nm. All of the fractions were then concentrated under vacuum and lyophilized to remove the formic acid. The fractions were suspended at a concentration of 10 mg/mL in water to obtain the starting MCH solutions for the biological assays.

4.5. Hydroxyproline Content Evaluation

The hydroxyproline content was estimated by a modified method based on the chloramine-T reaction [65]. First, 0.2 mL of 1 mg/mL solution of undigested collagen fibril suspension, trypsin-digested MCP mixture, and each of the four HPLC-purified fractions were hydrolyzed with two N of NaOH by autoclaving at 120 °C for 20 min. Samples were neutralized by adding one volume of two N of HCl and then, they were diluted fourfold in deionized water. The hydroxyproline concentration evaluation was obtained by adding chloramine-T and Ehrlich's reagent, as already described. Absorbance of each sample was read at 550 nm using a Beckman spectrophotometer (DU 640), in comparison to a cis-4–hydroxy-L-proline standard curve. The procedure was carried out in duplicate.

4.6. DPPH Radical Scavenging Activity

The total radical scavenging activity was evaluated by the DPPH method on each MCH fraction. The DPPH test solution, 1 mL/sample, was prepared with different amounts of the four MCH fractions (50 µg/mL and 100 µg/mL final dilution) put in 250 µL of deionized water and added to 500 µL of methanol and 250 µL of 0.2 mM of DPPH dissolved in methanol (2,2-diphenyl-1-picrylhydrazyl, Calbiochem®, Millipore SpA, Milan, Italy). A negative control sample containing only the DPPH test solution and a positive control sample with DPPH and 500 µg/mL ascorbic acid were prepared as well. All of the samples were incubated for 30 min at room temperature (RT) in the dark. Then, the samples were read at 517 nm using a Beckman spectrophotometer (DU 640). In the blank sample, the DPPH solution was substituted with methanol. The antioxidant activity of the MCH fractions was evaluated by the quenching of the DPPH radical using the following equation:

$$\text{DPPH radical scavenging activity (\%)} = (A0 - A)/A0 \times 100\%$$

where A was the sample absorbance rate; and A0 was the absorbance of the negative control. The procedure was carried out in duplicate.

4.7. NBT Superoxide Anion Scavenging Activity

The superoxide anion scavenging activity of the MCH fractions was evaluated by the NBT/riboflavin test. Briefly, the NBT/riboflavin test solution, 1 mL/sample, was prepared with or without different amounts the four MCH fractions in duplicate (100 µg/mL and 200 µg/mL final dilution). The composition of the NBT/riboflavin test solution was the following: 15 µM of riboflavin, 500 µM of Nitro Blue Tetrazolium (NBT), 10 mM of D-L methionine, 0.025% Triton x-100, and 50 mM of phosphate buffer, pH 7.8. The blank sample was prepared as follows: 500 µM of NBT in 50 mM of phosphate buffer, pH 7.8. The samples were transferred to 3.5-cm plastic petri dishes (without cover), and then flashed for two minutes under a UV lamp (Sanikyo Denki G20T10) at a 20-cm distance (90 mJ/cm^2 total radiation dose). Samples were then read in a Beckman spectrophotometer (DU640) at 560 nm against the blank sample. The scavenging activity (quenching of the blue color) was calculated by the same algorithm that was used for the DPPH scavenging activity.

4.8. Cell Cultures

The mouse macrophage cell line RAW 264.7 and the mouse fibroblast L929 cell line were obtained from the American Type Culture Collection (LGC Standards srl, Milan, Italy). The human keratinocyte HaCaT cell line (CLS Cell Lines Service, 300493) was obtained by the Cell Lines Service (GmbH, Eppelheim, Germany). Cells were cultured at 37 °C in a humidified, 5% CO_2 atmosphere in high glucose Dulbecco's modified Eagle's medium (DMEM) with glutamine (Microtech srl, Naples, Italy), and supplemented with 10% fetal bovine serum (Microtech) with penicillin/streptomycin as antibiotics.

4.8.1. Cell Viability

Experiments were performed in quadruplicate on 96-well plates. RAW 264.7 macrophages, L929 fibroblasts, and HaCaT keratinocytes were seeded at 5000 cells/well, and allowed to adhere overnight. Then, the four different MCH fractions (10 µg/mL and 50 µg/mL final dilutions) were added to each well, and the plates were incubated for three days at 37 °C. At the end of the experiments, cell viability was assayed by MTT test (0.5 mg/mL final concentration), as already reported [64]. Data are the means ± SD of three independent experiments performed in quadruplicate.

4.8.2. ROS Detection in RAW 264.7 Cells

Experiments were performed in quadruplicate on 96-well plates as described in Scarfi et al. [66]. Briefly, RAW 264.7 macrophages were plated at a density of 25,000 cells/well, and allowed to adhere overnight. Cells were then washed once with Hank's balanced salt solution (HBSS) and incubated for 40 min at 37 °C with 10 µM of 2′,7′-dichloro-dihydro-fluorescein diacetate (H_2DCF-dA) dye (Life Technologies, Milan, Italy). Cell stimulation was obtained either by using 200 µM of H_2O_2 or 100 µg/mL of sterilized quartz particles (Q) (MIN-U-SIL 5: US Silica, Berkeley Spring Plant, SSA$_{BET}$ = 5.2 m^2/g) prepared as described in Scarfi et al. [67] in the presence or absence of 10 µg/mL and 50 µg/mL of the four MCHs. Enhanced ROS concentration on the Q surface was obtained by ultrasound irradiation of a 10 mg/mL sterile quartz solution (three cycles of 10 pulses each at 50 Hz) prior to addition to the cell cultures.

After incubation with the dye, cells were washed with HBSS, incubated at 37 °C for 15 min, and then challenged with 100 µg/mL of Q particles or 200 µM of H_2O_2 for 2 h. The plates were finally read on a Fluostar Optima BMG using 485/520 excitation/emission wavelengths. Data are the means ± SD of three independent experiments performed in quadruplicate.

4.8.3. Collagen Quantification in the L929 Fibroblast Cell Medium

Collagen production by L929 fibroblasts was quantified in the cell medium by the SIRCOL™ Soluble Collagen Assay (Biocolor Ltd., Carrickfergus, Northern Ireland, UK). Fibroblasts were seeded in tissue culture six-well plates at a density of 5×10^5 cells/well in complete medium and allowed to adhere overnight. Then, cells were incubated for 24 h in the presence or absence of 100 µg/mL of the four MCH fractions. At the end of the incubation cell culture, media were collected, and the SIRCOL assay was performed according to the manufacturer's instructions. Data are the means ± S.D. of three independent experiments performed in duplicate.

4.8.4. UV Treatment

To evaluate cell death prevention from UV treatment by the four MCH fractions, both L929 fibroblasts and HaCaT keratinocytes were seeded in quadruplicate in 96-well plates. Both cell lines were plated at a density of 20,000 cells/well for the 24-h viability assay and at 10,000 cells/well for the 72-h assay, and allowed to adhere overnight. The four MCH fractions, at a final dilution of 50 µg/mL, were added to the wells, and then the plates were illuminated for two minutes and five minutes under an UV lamp (Sanikyo Denki G20T10) at a 20-cm distance (90 mJ/cm^2 and 227 mJ cm^2 total radiation dose, respectively). Cell viability was evaluated by the MTT test at 24 h and 72 h of incubation after the UV radiation, and compared to control non-irradiated samples cultured in the same conditions. Data are the mean ± SD of two independent experiments performed in quadruplicate.

4.8.5. Wound-Healing Assay

To evaluate the effect of the four MCHs on cell growth/migration, the wound-healing (WH) assay was performed on HaCaT and L929 cell lines as already reported [40,63,64]. Briefly, cells were seeded on 12-well tissue culture plates at a concentration of 140,000 cells/well and incubated in complete medium for 24 h or until confluence was reached. Before plating cells, with the help of a ruler, five dots were drawn with a permanent marker on the back of the plate with correspondence to the diameter in the center of each well. The cell monolayer in each well was then scraped with a p100 pipet tip, making a straight line to create a "scratch" with the help of a ruler, and following the five black dots drawn on the back of the well. Cells were washed with PBS (Phosphate Buffered Saline) to remove detached cells and debris, and fresh medium was added in the absence or presence of the four MCH fractions at the concentration of 50 µg/mL. Then, the straight scratch line in each well was photographed in four different fixed points to the microscope at 4× objective at times: 0 h, 6 h, 24 h, and 30 h. Photos were then taken always in the same points during the time course thanks to the five dots. In fact, in each well, there were four fixed areas in between two dots. Thus, each experiment is the mean of the results of four areas in each well made in duplicate.

To determine the degree of wound healing in HaCaT cells, the closing distance of the scratch was measured two times in each photograph by using the ImageJ program free software (http://imagej.nih.gov/ij/). Data are expressed as percentages of the closing distance of each sample with respect to the same sample at time = 0. A decrease of the percentage of the closing distance indicates an increase in the growth/migration of cells. Conversely, to determine the wound-healing degree in L929 cells, a qualitative visual method was used to score the increase of cell density in the scratches of each sample over time. Photographs at the various end points were scored in blind from + to +++, indicating the increasing cell density in the area of the scratches. Data are the mean of three independent experiments performed in duplicate.

4.8.6. RNA Extraction, cDNA Synthesis, and qPCR Analyses

L929 fibroblasts (5×10^5), seeded the day before in complete medium in six-well plates, were incubated with 100 µg/mL of the four different MCH fractions for 24 h, and then, expression of collagen 1A (Col1A) was quantified by qPCR respect to control, untreated cells. HaCaT keratinocytes (5×10^5) that were seeded the day before in complete medium in six-well plates, were challenged with 50 µg/mL of the four different MCH fractions, UV-irradiated for two minutes as already described, and then, the expression of Keratin 1 (KRT-1) and Keratin 10 (KRT-10) was quantified by qPCR after 24 h with respect to control untreated cells. Total RNA was extracted using the RNeasy Mini Kit (Qiagen, Milan, Italy) according to the manufacturer's instructions. The quality and quantity of RNA was analyzed using a NanoDrop spectrophotometer (Nanodrop Technologies, Wilmington, DE, USA). The cDNA (1 µg per sample for the L929 cells and 500 ng for the HaCaT cells) was synthesized by using an iScript cDNA Synthesis Kit (Bio-Rad Laboratories, Milan, Italy). Each PCR reaction was performed in 10 µL containing: 1× master mix iQ SYBR®Green (Bio-Rad), 0.2 µM of each primers, and 5 ng of synthesized cDNA. All of the samples were analyzed in triplicate. The following thermal conditions were used: initial denaturation at 95 °C for three minutes, followed by 45 cycles with denaturation at 95 °C for 15 s, and annealing and elongation at 60 °C for 60 s. The fluorescence was measured at the end of each elongation step. Values were normalized to ubiquitin (reference gene) mRNA expression both for L929 mouse fibroblasts and HaCaT human keratinocytes. All of the primers (Table 3) were designed using the Beacon Designer 7.0 software (Premier Biosoft International, Palo Alto, CA, USA) and obtained from TibMolBiol (Genova, Italy). Data analyses were obtained using the DNA Engine Opticon® 3 Real-Time Detection System Software program (3.03 version), and in order to calculate the relative gene expression compared to an untreated (control) calibrator sample, the comparative threshold Ct method [68] was used within the Gene Expression Analysis for iCycler iQ Real Time Detection System software (Bio-Rad) [69]. Data are means ± SD of two independent experiments performed in triplicate.

Table 3. Primer sequences used in the qPCR analyses. Primer pairs used for the qPCR experiments in gene expression quantification of murine collagen 1A (Col 1A MM), murine, and human ubiquitin (ubiquitin MM and HS, respectively), human Keratin 1 and 10 (keratin 1 HS and 10 HS, respectively).

GENE	GenBank	Forward	Reverse
Col1A MM	NM_007742.4	5'-CTgCTggTCCTgCTggTC-3'	5'-CCTTgTTCgCCTgTCTCAC-3'
Ubiquitin MM	NM_019639	5'-GACAGGCAAGACCATCAC-3'	5'-TCTGAGGCGAAGGACTAAG-3'
Keratin 1 HS	NM_006121.3	5'AAgCCACACCACCATCAg-3'	5'CACCTCCAgAgCCATAgC-3'
Keratin 10 HS	NM_000421.3	5'-CCgAgTgCCAgAATACTgAATACC-3'	5'-TAgCCgCCgCCgAAACTTC-3'
Ubiquitin HS	NM_021009.6	5'-ATTTgggTCgCAgTTCTTg-3'	5'TgCCTTgACATTCTCgATggT-3'

4.9. Statistical Analysis

Statistical analysis was performed using one-way ANOVA plus Tukey's post-test (GraphPad Software, Inc., San Diego, CA, USA). P values < 0.05 were considered significant.

Author Contributions: Conceptualization, M.P. and S.S.; Methodology, M.P., S.S. and E.M.; Investigation, M.P., S.S., E.M., A.S., S.M., C.O., G.D., M.A.; Data Curation M.P. and S.S.; Writing M.P., E.M. and S.S.; Review & Editing, S.S.; Supervision, S.S.; Funding Acquisition, M.P., G.D., E.M. and S.S.

Funding: This research was funded by University of Genova local funding to SS, EM and GD and by MIUR (Italian Ministry of University and Research) to MP (grant acronym: FFABR).

Conflicts of Interest: The authors declare no conflict of interest.

References

1. Meena, C.; Mengi, S.; Deshpande, S. Biomedical and industrial applications of collagen. *J. Chem. Sci.* **1999**, *111*, 319–329.
2. Nur Hanani, Z.A.; Roos, Y.H.; Kerry, J.P. Use and application of gelatin as potential biodegradable packaging materials for food products. *Int. J. Biol. Macromol.* **2014**, *71*, 94–102. [CrossRef] [PubMed]
3. Silva, T.; Moreira-Silva, J.; Marques, A.; Domingues, A.; Bayon, Y.; Reis, R. Marine origin collagens and its potential applications. *Mar. Drugs* **2014**, *12*, 5881–5901. [CrossRef] [PubMed]
4. Pati, F.; Adhikar, B.; Dhara, S. Isolation and characterization of fish scale collagen of higher thermal stability. *Bioresour. Technol.* **2010**, *101*, 3737–3742. [CrossRef] [PubMed]
5. Jridi, M.; Bardaa, S.; Moalla, D.; Rebaii, T.; Souissi, N.; Sahnoun, Z.; Nasri, M. Microstructure, rheological and wound healing properties of collagen-based gel from cuttlefish skin. *Int. J. Biol. Macromol.* **2015**, *77*, 369–374. [CrossRef] [PubMed]
6. Boero, F.; Bouillon, J.; Gravili, C.; Miglietta, M.P.; Parsons, T.; Piraino, S. Gelatinous plankton: Irregularities rule the world (sometimes). *Mar. Ecol. Prog. Ser.* **2008**, *356*, 299–310. [CrossRef]

7. Pozzolini, M.; Scarfì, S.; Gallus, L.; Castellano, M.; Vicini, S.; Cortese, K.; Gagliani, M.C.; Bertolino, M.; Costa, G.; Giovine, M. Production, Characterization and Biocompatibility Evaluation of Collagen Membranes Derived from Marine Sponge *Chondrosia reniformis* Nardo, 1847. *Mar. Drugs* **2018**, *16*, 111. [CrossRef] [PubMed]
8. Kim, M.M.; Mendis, E.; Rajapakse, N.; Lee, S.H.; Kim, S.K. Effect of spongin derived from *Hymeniacidon sinapium* on bone mineralization. *J. Biomed. Mater. Res. B Appl. Biomater.* **2009**, *90*, 540–546. [CrossRef] [PubMed]
9. Hayashi, Y.; Yamada, S.; Ikeda, T.; Yanagiguchi, K. Fish collagen and tissue repair. In *Marine Cosmeceuticals: Trends and Prospects*; Kim, S.K., Ed.; CRC Press-Taylor & Francis Group: Boca Raton, FL, USA, 2011; pp. 133–141.
10. Elangoa, J.; Zhanga, J.; Baoa, B.; Palaniyandib, K.; Wang, S.; Wua, W.; Robinson, J.S. Rheological, biocompatibility and osteogenesis assessment of fish collagen scaffolds for bone tissue engineering. *Int. J. Biol. Macromol.* **2016**, *91*, 51–59. [CrossRef] [PubMed]
11. Venkatesan, J.; Anil, S.; Kim, S.K.; Shim, M.S. Marine Fish Proteins and Peptides for Cosmeceuticals: A Review. *Mar. Drugs* **2017**, *15*, 143. [CrossRef] [PubMed]
12. Goh, K.L.; Holmes, D.F. Collagenous Extracellular Matrix Biomaterials for Tissue Engineering: Lessons from the Common Sea Urchin Tissue. *Int. J. Mol. Sci.* **2017**, *18*, 901. [CrossRef] [PubMed]
13. Addad, S.; Exposito, J.Y.; Faye, C.; Ricard-Blum, S.; Lethias, C. Isolation, Characterization and Biological Evaluation of Jellyfish Collagen for Use in Biomedical Applications. *Mar. Drugs* **2011**, *9*, 967–983. [CrossRef] [PubMed]
14. Nandi, S.K.; Kundu, B.; Mahato, A.; Thakur, N.L.; Joardard, S.N.; Mandale, B.B. In vitro and in vivo evaluation of the marine sponge skeleton as a bone mimicking biomaterial. *Integr. Biol.* **2015**, *7*, 250–262. [CrossRef] [PubMed]
15. Green, D.; Howard, D.; Yang, X.; Kelly, M.; Oreffo, R.O. Natural marine sponge fiber skeleton: A biomimetic scaffold for human osteoprogenitor cell attachment, growth, and differentiation. *Tissue Eng.* **2003**, *9*, 1159–1166. [CrossRef] [PubMed]
16. Simpson, T.L. Collagen fibrils, spongin, matrix substances. In *The Cell Biology of Sponges*; Springer: New York, NY, USA, 1984; ISBN1 978-1-4612-5214-6, ISBN2 978-1-4612-9740-6.
17. Garrone, R. *Phylogenesis of Connective Tissue. Morphological Aspects and Biosynthesis of Sponge Intercellular Matrix*; Karger, S., Ed.; S. Karger AG: Basel, Switzerland, 1978; pp. 1–250, ISBN 978-3-8055-2767-5.
18. Junqua, S.; Robert, L.; Garrone, R.; Pavans de Ceccatty, M.; Vacelet, J. Biochemical and morphological studies on collagens of horny sponges. Ircinia filaments compared to sponginse. *Connect. Tissue Res.* **1974**, *2*, 193–203. [CrossRef] [PubMed]
19. Wilkie, I.C.; Parma, L.; Bonasoro, F.; Bavestrello, G.; Cerrano, C.; Carnevali, M.D. Mechanical adaptability of a sponge extracellular matrix: Evidence for cellular control of mesohyl stiffness in *Chondrosia reniformis* Nardo. *J. Exp. Biol.* **2006**, *209*, 4436–4443. [CrossRef] [PubMed]
20. Fassini, D.; Parma, L.; Lembo, F.; Candia Carnevali, M.D.; Wilkie, I.C.; Bonasoro, F. The reaction of the sponge *Chondrosia reniformis* to mechanical stimulation is mediated by the outer epithelium and the release of stiffening factor(s). *Zoology (Jena)* **2014**, *117*, 282–291. [CrossRef] [PubMed]
21. Pozzolini, M.; Bruzzone, F.; Berilli, V.; Mussino, F.; Cerrano, C.; Benatti, U.; Giovine, M. Molecular characterization of a nonfibrillar collagen from the marine sponge *Chondrosia reniformis* Nardo 1847 and positive effects of soluble silicates on its expression. *Mar. Biotechnol. (NY)* **2012**, *14*, 281–293. [CrossRef] [PubMed]
22. Pozzolini, M.; Scarfì, S.; Mussino, F.; Ghignone, S.; Vezzulli, L.; Giovine, M. Molecular characterization and expression analysis of the first Porifera tumor necrosis factor superfamily member and of its putative receptor in the marine sponge *C. reniformis*. *Dev. Comp. Immunol.* **2016**, *57*, 88–98. [CrossRef] [PubMed]
23. Pozzolini, M.; Scarfì, S.; Mussino, F.; Ferrando, S.; Gallus, L.; Giovine, M. Molecular cloning, characterization, and expression analysis of a Prolyl 4-Hydroxylase from the marine sponge *Chondrosia reniformis*. *Mar. Biotechnol.* **2015**, *17*, 393–407. [CrossRef] [PubMed]
24. Swatschek, D.; Schatton, W.; Kellermann, J.; Muller, W.; Kreuter, J. Marine sponge collagen: Isolation, characterization and effects on the skin parameters surface-pH, moisture and sebum. *Eur. J. Pharm. Biopharm.* **2002**, *53*, 107–113. [CrossRef]

25. Nicklas, M.; Schatton, W.; Heinemann, S.; Hanke, T.; Kreuter, J. Enteric coating derived from marine sponge collagen. *Drug Dev. Ind. Pharm.* **2009**, *35*, 1384–1388. [CrossRef] [PubMed]
26. Kreuter, J.; Muller, W.; Swatschek, D.; Schatton, W.; Schatton, M. Method for Isolating Sponge Collagen and Producing Nanoparticulate Collagen, and the Use Thereof. Patent US20030032601 A1, 2003.
27. Mehbub, M.F.; Lei, J.; Franco, C.; Zhang, W. Marine Sponge Derived Natural Products between 2001 and 2010: Trends and Opportunities for Discovery of Bioactives. *Mar. Drugs* **2014**, *12*, 4539–4577. [CrossRef] [PubMed]
28. Sipkema, D.; Osinga, R.; Schatton, W.; Mendola, D.; Tramper, J.; Wijffels, R.H. Large-scale production of pharmaceuticals by marine sponges: Sea, cell, or synthesis? *Biotechnol. Bioeng.* **2005**, *90*, 201–222. [CrossRef] [PubMed]
29. Ruiz, C.; Valderrama, K.; Zea, S.; Castellanos, L. Mariculture and natural production of the antitumoural (+)-discodermolide by the Caribbean marine sponge *Discodermia dissoluta*. *Mar. Biotechnol. (NY)* **2013**, *15*, 571–583. [CrossRef] [PubMed]
30. Granito, R.N.; Custódio, M.R.; Rennó, A.C.M. Natural marine sponges for bone tissue engineering: The state of art and future perspectives. *J. Biomed. Mater. Res. B Appl. Biomater.* **2017**, *105*, 1717–1727. [CrossRef] [PubMed]
31. Aleman, A.; Martinez-Alvarez, O. Marine collagen as a source of bioactive molecules. A review. *Nat. Prod. J.* **2013**, *3*, 105–114. [CrossRef]
32. Temple, N.J. Antioxidant and disease: More questions than answers. *Nutr. Res.* **2000**, *20*, 449–459. [CrossRef]
33. Butterfield, D.A.; Castegna, A.; Pocernich, C.B.; Drake, J.; Scapagnini, G.; Calabrese, V. Nutritional approaches to combat oxidative stress in Alzheimer's disease. *J. Nutr. Biochem.* **2002**, *13*, 444–461. [CrossRef]
34. Correa, P.; Fontham, E.; Bravo, L.E.; Mera, R. Antioxidant supplements for prevention of gastrointestinal cancers. *Lancet* **2005**, *3*, 365–470. [CrossRef]
35. Giménez, B.; Alemán, A.; Montero, P.; Gómez-Guillén, M.C. Antioxidant and functional properties of gelatine hydrolysates obtained from skin of sole and squid. *Food Chem.* **2009**, *114*, 976–983. [CrossRef]
36. Leone, A.; Lecci, R.M.; Durante, M.; Meli, F.; Piraino, S. The bright side of gelatinous blooms: Nutraceutical value and antioxidant properties of three mediterranean jellyfish (Scyphozoa). *Mar. Drugs* **2015**, *13*, 4654–4681. [CrossRef] [PubMed]
37. Himaya, S.W.A.; Ngo, D.H.; Ryu, B.; Kim, S.K. An active peptide purified from gastrointestinal enzyme hydrolysate of Pacific cod skin gelatine attenuates angiotensin-1 converting enzyme (ACE) activity and cellular oxidative stress. *Food Chem.* **2012**, *132*, 1872–1882. [CrossRef]
38. Yang, J.I.; Ho, H.Y.; Chu, Y.J.; Chow, C.J. Characteristic and antioxidant activity of retorted gelatine hydrolysates from cobia (*Rachycentron canadum*) skin. *Food Chem.* **2008**, *110*, 128–136. [CrossRef] [PubMed]
39. Je, J.; Qian, Z.; Byun, H.; Kim, S. Purification and characterization of an antioxidant peptide obtained from tuna backbone protein by enzymatic hydrolysis. *Process. Biochem.* **2007**, *42*, 840–846. [CrossRef]
40. Hu, Z.; Yang, P.; Zhou, C.; Li, S.; Hong, P. Marine Collagen Peptides from the Skin of Nile Tilapia (*Oreochromis niloticus*): Characterization and Wound Healing Evaluation. *Mar. Drugs* **2017**, *15*, 102. [CrossRef] [PubMed]
41. Diffey, B.L. Solar ultraviolet radiation effects on biological systems. *Phys. Med. Biol.* **1991**, *36*, 299–328. [CrossRef] [PubMed]
42. Zhuang, Y.; Hou, H.; Zhao, X.; Zhang, Z.; Li, B. Effects of collagen and collagen hydrolysate from jellyfish (*Rhopilema esculentum*) on mice skin photoaging induced by UV irradiation. *J. Food Sci.* **2009**, *74*, H183–H188. [CrossRef] [PubMed]
43. Chen, T.; Hou, H. Protective effect of gelatin polypeptides from Pacific cod (*Gadus macrocephalus*) against UV irradiation-induced damages by inhibiting inflammation and improving transforming growth factor-β-Smad signaling pathway. *J. Photochem. Photobiol. B Biol.* **2016**, *162*, 633–640. [CrossRef] [PubMed]
44. Chen, T.; Hou, H.; Lu, J.; Zhang, K.; Li, B. Protective effect of gelatin and gelatin hydrolysate from salmon skin on UV irradiation-induced photoaging of mice skin. *J. Ocean Univ. China* **2016**, *15*, 711–718. [CrossRef]
45. Zhang, Z.; Wang, J.; Ding, Y.; Dai, X.; Li, Y. Oral administration of marine collagen peptides from Chum Salmon skin enhances cutaneous wound healing and angiogenesis in rats. *J. Sci. Food Agric.* **2011**, *91*, 2173–2179. [CrossRef] [PubMed]

46. De Luca, C.; Mikhal'chik, E.V.; Suprun, M.V.; Papacharalambous, M.; Truhanov, A.I.; Korkina, L.G. Skin Antiageing and Systemic Redox Effects of Supplementation with Marine Collagen Peptides and Plant-Derived Antioxidants: A Single-Blind Case-Control Clinical Study. *Oxid. Med. Cell. Longev.* **2016**, *2016*, 4389410. [CrossRef] [PubMed]
47. Blunt, J.W.; Carroll, A.R.; Copp, B.R.; Davis, R.A.; Keyzers, R.A.; Prinsep, M.R. Marine natural products. *Nat. Prod. Rep.* **2018**, *35*, 8–53. [CrossRef] [PubMed]
48. Pozzolini, M.; Scarfì, S.; Mussino, F.; Salis, A.; Damonte, G.; Benatti, U.; Giovine, M. Pichia pastoris production of a prolyl 4-hydroxylase derived from *Chondrosia reniformis* sponge: A new biotechnological tool for the recombinant production of marine collagen. *J. Biotechnol.* **2015**, *208*, 28–36. [CrossRef] [PubMed]
49. Garrone, R.; Huc, A.; Junqua, S. Fine structure and physiocochemical studies on the collagen of the marine sponge *Chondrosia reniformis* nardo. *J. Ultrastruct. Res.* **1975**, *52*, 261–275. [CrossRef]
50. Nam, K.A.; You, S.G.; Kim, S.M. Molecular and physical characteristics of squid (*Todarodes pacificus*) skin collagens and biological properties of their enzymatic hydrolysates. *J. Food Sci.* **2008**, *73*, C249–C255. [CrossRef] [PubMed]
51. Wu, R.; Chen, L.; Liu, D.; Huang, J.; Zhang, J.; Xiao, X.; Lei, M.; Chen, Y.; He, H. Preparation of Antioxidant Peptides from Salmon Byproducts with Bacterial Extracellular Proteases. *Mar. Drugs* **2017**, *15*, 4. [CrossRef] [PubMed]
52. Wang, B.; Wang, Y.M.; Chi, C.F.; Luo, H.Y.; Deng, S.G.; Ma, J.Y. Isolation and characterization of collagen and antioxidant collagen peptides from scales of croceine croaker (*Pseudosciaena crocea*). *Mar. Drugs* **2013**, *11*, 4641–4661. [CrossRef] [PubMed]
53. Jeevithan, E.; Bao, B.; Zhang, J.; Hong, S.; Wu, W. Purification, characterization and antioxidant properties of low molecular weight collagenous polypeptide (37 kDa) prepared from whale shark cartilage (*Rhincodon typus*). *J. Food Sci. Technol.* **2015**, *52*, 6312–6322. [CrossRef] [PubMed]
54. Sampath Kumar, N.S.; Nazeer, R.A.; Jaiganesh, R. Purification and identification of antioxidant peptides from the skin protein hydrolysate of two marine fishes, horse mackerel (*Magalaspis cordyla*) and croaker (*Otolithes ruber*). *Amino Acids* **2012**, *42*, 1641–1649. [CrossRef] [PubMed]
55. Zhang, Y.; Duan, X.; Zhuang, Y. Purification and characterization of novel antioxidant peptides from enzymatic hydrolysates of tilapia (*Oreochromis niloticus*) skin gelatin. *Peptides* **2012**, *38*, 13–21. [CrossRef] [PubMed]
56. Prior, R.L.; Wu, X.; Schaich, K. Standardized methods for the determination of antioxidant capacity and phenolics in foods and dietary supplements. *J. Agric. Food Chem.* **2005**, *53*, 4290–4302. [CrossRef] [PubMed]
57. Hou, H.; Li, B.; Zhang, Z.; Xue, C.; Yu, G.; Wang, J.; Bao, Y.; Bu, L.; Sun, J.; Peng, Z.; et al. Moisture absorption and retention properties, and activity in alleviating skin photodamage of collagen polypeptide from marine fish skin. *Food Chem.* **2012**, *135*, 1432–1439. [CrossRef] [PubMed]
58. Fan, J.; Zhuang, Y.; Li, B. Effects of collagen and collagen hydrolysate from jellyfish umbrella on histological and immunity changes of mice photoaging. *Nutrients* **2013**, *5*, 223–233. [CrossRef] [PubMed]
59. Moravcová, M.; Libra, A.; Dvořáková, J.; Víšková, A.; Muthný, T.; Velebný, V.; Kubala, L. Modulation of keratin 1, 10 and involucrin expression as part of the complex response of the human keratinocyte cell line HaCaT to ultraviolet radiation. *Interdiscip. Toxicol.* **2013**, *6*, 203–208. [CrossRef] [PubMed]
60. Shen, X.; Nagai, N.; Murata, M.; Nishimura, D.; Sugi, M.; Munekata, M. Development of salmon milt DNA/salmon collagen composite for wound dressing. *J. Mater. Sci. Mater. Med.* **2008**, *19*, 3473–3479. [CrossRef] [PubMed]
61. Ramasamy, P.; Shanmugam, A. Characterization and wound healing property of collagen-chitosan film from Sepia kobiensis (Hoyle, 1885). *Int. J. Biol. Macromol.* **2015**, *74*, 93–102. [CrossRef] [PubMed]
62. Vigneswari, S.; Murugaiyah, V.; Kaur, G.; Abdul Khalil, H.P.S.; Amirul, A.A. Simultaneous dual syringe electrospinning system using benign solvent to fabricate nanofibrous P(3HB-co-4HB)/collagen peptides construct as potential leave-on wound dressing. *Mater. Sci. Eng. C Mater. Biol. Appl.* **2016**, *66*, 147–155. [CrossRef] [PubMed]
63. Ouyang, Q.Q.; Hu, Z.; Lin, Z.P.; Quan, W.Y.; Deng, Y.F.; Li, S.D.; Li, P.W.; Chen, Y. Chitosan hydrogel in combination with marine peptides from tilapia for burns healing. *Int. J. Biol. Macromol.* **2018**, *112*, 1191–1198. [CrossRef] [PubMed]

64. Pozzolini, M.; Vergani, L.; Ragazzoni, M.; Delpiano, L.; Grasselli, E.; Voci, A.; Giovine, M.; Scarfì, S. Different reactivity of primary fibroblasts and endothelial cells towards crystalline silica: A surface radical matter. *Toxicology* **2016**, *361–362*, 12–23. [CrossRef] [PubMed]
65. Reddy, G.K.; Enwemeka, C.S. A simplified method for the analysis of hydroxyproline in biological tissues. *Clin. Biochem.* **1996**, *29*, 225–239. [CrossRef]
66. Scarfì, S.; Magnone, M.; Ferraris, C.; Pozzolini, M.; Benvenuto, F.; Giovine, M.; Benatti, U. Ascorbic Acid pre-treated quartz stimulates TNF-α release in RAW 264.7 murine macrophages through ROS production and membrane lipid peroxidation. *Respir. Res.* **2009**, *10*, 25–40. [CrossRef] [PubMed]
67. Scarfì, S.; Benatti, U.; Pozzolini, M.; Clavarino, E.; Ferraris, C.; Magnone, M.; Valisano, L.; Giovine, M. "Ascorbic acid pre-treated quartz enhances Cyclooxygenase-2 expression in RAW 264.7 murine macrophages". *FEBS J.* **2007**, *274*, 60–73. [CrossRef] [PubMed]
68. Aarskog, N.K.; Vedeler, C.A. Real-time quantitative polymerase chain reaction. A new method that detects both the peripheral myelin protein 22 duplication in Charcot-Marie-Tooth type 1A disease and the peripheral myelin protein 22 deletion in hereditary neuropathy with liability to pressure palsies. *Hum. Genet.* **2000**, *107*, 494–498. [PubMed]
69. Vandesompele, J.; De Preter, K.; Pattyn, F.; Poppe, B.; Van Roy, N.; De Paepe, A.; Speleman, F. Accurate normalization of real-time quantitative RT-PCR data by geometric averaging of multiple internal control genes. *Genome Biol* **2002**, *3*, RESEARCH0034. [CrossRef] [PubMed]

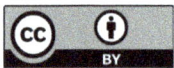

© 2018 by the authors. Licensee MDPI, Basel, Switzerland. This article is an open access article distributed under the terms and conditions of the Creative Commons Attribution (CC BY) license (http://creativecommons.org/licenses/by/4.0/).

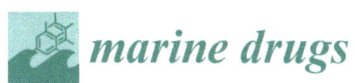

Article

Physicochemical and Antioxidant Properties of Acid- and Pepsin-Soluble Collagens from the Scales of Miiuy Croaker (*Miichthys Miiuy*)

Long-Yan Li [1], Yu-Qin Zhao [1], Yu He [1], Chang-Feng Chi [2,*] and Bin Wang [1,*]

1. Zhejiang Provincial Engineering Technology Research Center of Marine Biomedical Products, School of Food and Pharmacy, Zhejiang Ocean University, Zhoushan 316022, China; 15576494647@163.com (L.-Y.L.); zhaoy@hotmail.com (Y.-Q.Z.); heyu19950618@163.com (Y.H.)
2. National and Provincial Joint Laboratory of Exploration and Utilization of Marine Aquatic Genetic Resources, National Engineering Research Center of Marine Facilities Aquaculture, School of Marine Science and Technology, Zhejiang Ocean University, Zhoushan 316022, China
* Correspondence: chichangfeng@hotmail.com (C.-F.C.); wangbin4159@hotmail.com (B.W.); Tel.: +86-580-255-4818 (C.-F.C.); +86-580-255-4781 (B.W.); Fax: +86-580-255-4818 (C.-F.C.); +86-580-255-4781 (B.W.)

Received: 24 September 2018; Accepted: 18 October 2018; Published: 20 October 2018

Abstract: In this report, acid-soluble collagen (ASC-MC) and pepsin-soluble collagen (PSC-MC) were extracted from the scales of miiuy croaker (*Miichthys miiuy*) with yields of $0.64 \pm 0.07\%$ and $3.87 \pm 0.15\%$ of dry weight basis, respectively. ASC-MC and PSC-MC had glycine as the major amino acid with the contents of 341.8 ± 4.2 and 344.5 ± 3.2 residues/1000 residues, respectively. ASC-MC and PSC-MC had lower denaturation temperatures (32.2 °C and 29.0 °C for ASC-MC and PSC-MC, respectively) compared to mammalian collagen due to their low imino acid content (197.6 and 195.2 residues/1000 residues for ASC-MC and PSC-MC, respectively). ASC-MC and PSC-MC were mainly composed of type I collagen on the literatures and results of amino acid composition, SDS-PAGE pattern, ultraviolet (UV) and Fourier-transform infrared spectroscopy (FTIR) spectra. The maximum solubility of ASC-MC and PSC-MC was appeared at pH 1–3 and a sharp decrease in solubility was observed when the NaCl concentration was above 2%. Zeta potential studies indicated that ASC-MC and PSC-MC exhibited a net zero charge at pH 6.66 and 6.81, respectively. Furthermore, the scavenging capabilities on 1,1-diphenyl-2-picrylhydrazyl (DPPH) radical, hydroxyl radical, superoxide anion radical and 2,2′-azino-bis-3-ethylbenzothiazoline-6-sulfonic acid (ABTS) radical of ASC-MC and PSC-MC were positively correlated with their tested concentration ranged from 0 to 5 mg/mL and PSC-MC showed significantly higher activity than that of ASC-MC at most tested concentrations ($p < 0.05$). In addition, the scavenging capability of PSC-MC on hydroxyl radical and superoxide anion radical was higher than those of DPPH radical and ABTS radical, which suggested that ASC-SC and PSC-SC might be served as hydroxyl radical and superoxide anion radical scavenger in cosmeceutical products for protecting skins from photoaging and ultraviolet damage.

Keywords: miiuy croaker (*Miichthys miiuy*); scale; acid-soluble collagen (ASC); pepsin-soluble collagen (PSC); antioxidant activity; radical scavenging activity

---

1. Introduction

Collagen is the most abundant protein constituting nearly 30% of all proteins in the animal body and is a primary component of the extracellular matrix [1]. Collagen plays an important role in the formation of organs and maintenance of the structural integrity of cells [2]. Up to the present, genetically distinct 29 types of collagen (type I-XXIX) with right-handed triple helical conformation have been isolated from animal tissue that differ considerably in their amino acid composition, sequence, structural and functional properties [3,4]. Traditionally, collagens were mainly prepared from bovine tendon and porcine skins and have been extensively utilized as biomedical materials for functional food, cosmetics and tissue engineering because of their favorable biological features, such as excellent biodegradability, biocompatibility and weak antigenicity [5,6]. At present, some consumers have paid close attention to the safety of mammalian collagens because of the outbreaks of bovine spongiform encephalopathy, foot mouth disease and other prions disease. In addition, use of mammalian collagen is a hurdle in the development of kosher and halal products due to some religious factors [3,7]. Therefore, the enormous demand for collagen from alternative resources such as aquatic byproducts (skin, bone, swim bladder, scale and fins) has increased for many years due to no dietary restriction and risk of disease transmission [3,8]. Furthermore, effective use of aquatic byproducts to produce high value-added products is an important way to increase the income to the fish processor and protect the environment [9].

An imbalance in pro-oxidant/antioxidant can cause oxidative stress, which further trigger the accumulated reactive oxygen species (ROS) production and result in cell damage and many health disorders, such as skin damage, diabetes mellitus, cancer and inflammatory diseases [10,11]. Therefore, researchers have continued to show an interest in screening naturally-derived antioxidants including collagens and their peptides. Acid-soluble collagen (ASC) and pepsin-soluble collagen (PSC) from swim bladders of miiuy croaker could scavenge 1,1-diphenyl-2-picrylhydrazyl (DPPH) radical, hydroxyl radical, superoxide anion radical and 2,2′-azino-bis-3-ethylbenzothiazoline-6-sulfonic acid (ABTS) radical in a dose-dependent manner and the radical scavenging activity of PSC was higher than that of ASC at all concentrations [12]. Zhuang et al. reported that jellyfish collagen (JC) and jellyfish collagen hydrolysate (JCH) alleviated UV-induced abnormal changes of antioxidant defense systems such as superoxide dismutase (SOD) and glutathione peroxidase (GSH-Px). In addition, JCH with lower molecular weight as compared to JC provides a much stronger protection against UV-induced photoaging [13]. Therefore, antioxidant collagens and collagen peptides derived from marine fish have gained enormous interest in nutraceutical, pharmaceutical and cosmeceutical industries.

Fish scales are composed of protein and collagen of connective tissue (41 to 81%) and calcium-deficient hydroxyapatite. For now, approximately 49,000 tons of fish scales are generated in the de-scaling process of aquatic products. However, large quantities of scales are discarded as waste during processing and filleting due to lower economic value, which give rise to some additional ecological environmental problems especially in developing countries. Effective use of those resources not only solves the problem of environmental pollution but also increases economic returns for the fishery industry. Therefore, collagens have been isolated from scales of some kinds of fish [14–20] and those results indicated that fish scale collagens are more appropriate as the alternative of pig skin collagen than fish skin collagen [21,22]. Miiuy croaker (*Miichthys miiuy*) is an important and highly consumed aquaculture species in China and Japan and it has been widely cultured since late 1990s because of its fast growth, various feeding habit and high medicinal and economic values [23]. Therefore, making full use of miiuy croaker scales to produce medical products with higher value will further accelerate the development of the miiuy croaker aquaculture industry. However, there was little information available about the extraction of collagen from the scales of miiuy croaker. In addition, there are some differences in structure and amino acid composition of collagens from different fish scales due to the living environment and species, which further influence the physicochemical and bioactive properties of collagens. Therefore, acid-soluble collagen (ASC-MC) and pepsin-soluble collagen (PSC-MC) from the scales of miiuy croaker (*M. miiuy*) were prepared and their physicochemical and antioxidant properties were characterized for their potential applications in the cosmetic and biomedical industries.

2. Results and Discussion

2.1. Proximate and Yield Analysis

Chemical compositions of scale from miiuy croaker, as well as the ASC-MC and PSC-MC derived from them are presented in Table 1. The main components of the scales were ash (47.31 g/100 g), moisture (26.37 g/100 g), protein (19.42 g/100 g) and fat (6.97 g/100 g). The high ash content (47.31 g/100 g) detected in the scales was mainly because of the calcium-deficient hydroxyappatite in the upper osseous layer and lower fibrillar plate of scales. The ash content of miiuy croaker scale was higher than those of the scales from redspot goatfish (42.31%) [23], croceine croaker (46.73%) [4] and deep-sea redfish (39.4%) [24] but lower than that of the scales from redlip croaker (48.49%) [4]. The protein content of the scales from miiuy croaker was higher than that of the scales from redlip croaker (18.47%) [4] but lower than those of the scales from redspot goatfish (34.46%) [23], croceine croaker (20.33%) [4], silver carp (37.91%) and carp (43.43%) [25]. The data indicated that the vast majority (>95%) of inorganic substances were removed from the scales of miiuy croaker by demineralization process. As shown in Table 1, ASC-MC and PSC-MC presented the similar chemical compositions, which had high content of protein (93.19 ± 1.80 and 94.87 ± 1.89 g/100 g for ASC-MC and PSC-MC, respectively) and low contents of moisture (5.18 ± 0.43 and 4.37 ± 0.32 g/100 g for ASC-MC and PSC-MC, respectively), ash (1.15 ± 0.54 and 0.92 ± 0.39 g/100 g for ASC-MC and PSC-MC, respectively) and fat (0.50 ± 0.15 and 0.34 ± 0.08 g/100 g for ASC-MC and PSC-MC, respectively). Those data indicated that the impurities in scales were effectively removed through the extraction process of collagens.

Table 1. Chemical compositions of miiuy croaker scales, acid-soluble collagen (ASC-MC) and pepsin-soluble collagen (PSC-MC) from the scales of miiuy croaker (*M. miiuy*).

Sample	Proximate Compositions (g/100 g Dry Weight)				Yield (%)
	Moisture	Fat	Ash	Protein	Dry Weight Basis
Scales	26.37 ± 0.18 [a]	6.94 ± 0.43 [a]	47.31 ± 3.07 [a]	19.42 ± 0.86 [a]	
ASC-MC	5.18 ± 0.43 [b]	0.50 ± 0.15 [b]	1.15 ± 0.54 [b]	93.19 ± 1.80 [b]	0.64 ± 0.07 [a]
PSC-MC	4.37 ± 0.32 [b]	0.34 ± 0.08 [b]	0.92 ± 0.39 [b]	94.87 ± 1.89 [b]	3.87 ± 0.15 [b]

All values are mean ± SD (n = 3); [a–b] Values with different letters in the same column indicate significant difference ($p < 0.05$).

ASC-MC and PSC-MC were isolated from the scales of miiuy croaker (*M. miiuy*) with yields of 0.64 ± 0.07% and 3.87 ± 0.15% of dry weight basis, respectively. The yield of PSC-MC was 6.05-fold higher than that of ASC and it could be supposed that there were many interchain cross-links at the telopeptide region, leading to the low solubility of collagen in acid [4,8]. With further limited pepsin digestion, the cross-linked molecules at the telopeptide region were cleaved and resulted in further extraction. So, pepsin has been used to isolate collagen from the scales of redlip croakers [4], croceine croaker [15], grass carp [17], seabass [19], spotted golden goatfish [20] and snakehead [25]. Thus, pepsin could be used as an aid for increasing the extraction yield of collagen from the byproducts of miiuy croaker and other aquatic products.

2.2. Amino Acid Analysis

The amino acid compositions of type I collagen from calf skin (CSC), ASC-MC and PSC-MC from the scales of miiuy croaker were expressed as amino acid residues per 1000 total amino acid residues and presented in Table 2. The results indicated that ASC-MC and PSC-MC had similar amino acid compositions, with glycine (Gly) as the most abundant amino acid, followed by alanine (Ala), proline (Pro) and hydroxyproline (Hyp). Low contents of cysteine (Cys), tyrosine (Tyr), hydroxylysine (Hyl) and histidine (His) were also observed. In general, Gly represents about one-third of the total residues and is normally spaced at the beginning of typical tripeptide repetitions (Gly-X-Y, X is mostly Pro and Y is Hyp) present in areas of collagens that do not include the first 10 or so amino acids at the C-terminus and the last 14 or so amino acids at the N-terminus [3]. Moreover, Gly, as the smallest amino acid with only a hydrogen atom side chain, allows the three helical chains to form the final superhelix. In addition, Gly content of ASC-MC (341.8 residues/1000 residues) was higher than those (328–341 residues/1000 residues) of ASC from scales of Japanese seabass [26], deep-sea redfish [24], redspot goatfish [23] and common carp [27] but lower than those of scales ASC from *Labeo rohita* (361 residues/1000 residues), *Catla catla* (353 residues/1000 residues) [28], redlip croaker (351.4 residues/1000 residues) and crocine croaker (347.1 residues/1000 residues) [4]. The Gly content of PSC-MC (344.5 residues/1000 residues) was higher than those (276–350 residues/1000 residues) of PSC from scales of Japanese seabass (337 residues/1000 residues) [26], Nile tilapia (276 residues/1000 residues) [29], redspot goatfish (340 residues/1000 residues) [23] and snakehead fish (327.1 residues/1000 residues) [25] but lower than those of scales black drum 345 residues/1000 residues), sheepshead (347 residues/1000 residues) [30], *L. rohita* (361 residues/1000 residues), *C. catla* (353 residues/1000 residues) [28], bighead carp (350 residues/1000 residues) [31] and crocine croaker (347.1 residues/1000 residues) [4].

Table 2. Amino acid composition of type I collagen from calf skin (CSC), acid-soluble collagen (ASC-MC) and pepsin-soluble collagen (PSC-MC) from the scales of miiuy croaker (*M. miiuy*) (residues/1000 residues).

Amino Acid	ASC-MC	PSC-MC	CSC
Hydroxyproline (Hyp)	85.6 ± 3.3	84.8 ± 2.5	95.1 ± 2.4
Aspartic acid/asparagine (Asp)	39.6 ± 1.5	41.2 ± 1.7	45.7 ± 2.1
Threonine (Thr)	25.7 ± 1.1	27.1 ± 1.0	18.4 ± 0.8
Serine (Ser)	31.4 ± 1.3	25.5 ± 1.1	33.2 ± 0.9
Glutamine/glutamic acid (Glu)	61.9 ± 2.2	63.3 ± 3.5	75.9 ± 3.3
Proline (Pro)	112.0 ± 1.9	110.4 ± 2.9	121.5 ± 3.4
Glycine (Gly)	341.8 ± 4.2	344.5 ± 3.2	330.6 ± 4.6
Alanine (Ala)	122.3 ± 3.7	120.1 ± 3.5	119.7 ± 2.7
Cysteine (Cys)	2.3 ± 0.1	3.1 ± 0.1	0.0
Valine (Val)	22.4 ± 0.5	23.6 ± 0.7	21.5 ± 0.7
Methionine (Met)	14.3 ± 0.4	13.9 ± 0.6	6.1 ± 0.3
Isoleucine (Ile)	12.7 ± 0.5	11.5 ± 0.6	11.4 ± 0.5
Leucine (Leu)	22.7 ± 0.8	24.6 ± 0.9	23.4 ± 0.4
Tyrosine (Tyr)	5.9 ± 0.3	4.6 ± 0.3	3.7 ± 0.5
Phenylalanine (Phe)	14.4 ± 0.9	15.3 ± 1.1	3.3 ± 0.6
Hydroxylysine (Hyl)	6.2 ± 0.3	6.6 ± 0.4	7.7 ± 0.4
Lysine (Lys)	25.5 ± 1.0	24.8 ± 0.8	26.5 ± 1.1
Histidine (His)	7.6 ± 0.3	8.5 ± 0.5	5.3 ± 0.3
Arginine (Arg)	45.7 ± 1.5	46.6 ± 1.3	51.0 ± 1.4
Total	1000.0	1000.0	1000.0
Imino acid (Pro + Hyp)	197.6	195.2	216.6

All data are presented as the mean ± SD of triplicate results.

As shown in Table 2, the imino acid (Pro + Hyp) content of ASC-MC was 197.6 residues/1000 residues, which was analogous to those (192–204 residues/1000 residues) of ASC from scales of common carp [27], Japanese sardine [26], redspot goatfish [23] and *C. catla* [28] but significantly higher than that (160 residues/1000 residues) of ASC from deep-sea redfish scales [24]. The imino acid content of PSC-MC was 195.2 residues/1000 residues, which were similar to those (189–198.1 residues/1000 residues) of scale PSC from seabream [30], snakehead [25], redspot goatfish [23] and black drum [30] but significantly higher than that (156 residues/1000 residues) of scale PSC from bighead carp [31].

Pyrrolidine rings of imino acid enforced constraints on the conformation of the polypeptide chain and helped to strengthen the thermal stability of triple helix. It has been verified that Hyp has played an important role in stabilizing the triple-stranded helix of collagen by hydrogen bonds [6,25]. Therefore, the content of imino acid is very important for the structural integrity of collagen. So, the helices of ASC-MC and PSC-MC might be more unstable than that of CSC (216.6 residues/1000 residues) because of their low contents of imino acid.

2.3. SDS-PAGE and Peptide Hydrolysis Patterns of ASC-MC and PSC-MC

2.3.1. SDS-PAGE Pattern of ASC-MC and PSC-MC

SDS-PAGE pattern is commonly applied to determine the type and composition of collagen on the subunit composition, electrophoretic mobility and intensity of the band. Similar protein patterns of ASC-MC, PSC-MC and type I collagen from calf skin (CSC) were observed in Figure 1. ASC-MC and PSC-MC were composed of two different α chains (α1 and α2) with molecular weight (MW) of about 121.3 and 114.9 kDa, respectively. High molecular weight component of β (dimers) chains were also observed. Moreover, the α1-chain:α2-chain band intensity ratio of ASC-MC and PSC-MC was approximate 2:1. The result of Figure 1 including α chains (α1 and α2) and type I collagen of calf skin (Lane 4) suggested that ASC-MC and PSC-MC from the scales of miiuy croaker were mainly composed of type I collagen ($[\alpha1]_2\alpha2$). This finding was agreement with the scale collagens from tilapia [18], snakehead fish [25], Japanese sardine [26], *L. rohita* and *C. catla* [28].

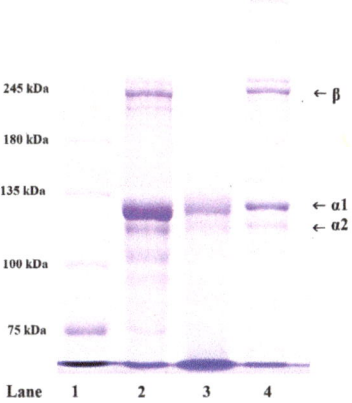

Figure 1. SDS-PAGE patterns of acid-soluble collagen (ASC-MC) and pepsin-soluble collagen (PSC-MC) from the scales of miiuy croaker (*M. miiuy*). Lane 1. marker protein; lane 2. ASC-MC; lane 3. PSC-MC; lane 4. type I collagen of calf skin.

2.3.2. Peptide Hydrolysis Patterns of ASC-MC and PSC-MC

Peptide hydrolysis patterns of ASC-MC and PSC-MC from the scales of miiuy croaker (*M. miiuy*) are presented in Figure 2. After digested by trypsin at pH of 2.5, 37 °C for 3 h, the high MW components including α-chains (α1 and α2) and β-chains almost entirely disappeared with a concomitant generation of lower MW peptide fragments ranging broadly from 20.0 to 100.0 kDa. Compared peptide hydrolysis patterns of ASC-MC and PSC-MC with that of CSC, it could be found that CSC was more tolerant to digestion by trypsin at the same conditions because the peptide fragments with high molecular weights were more than that of ASC-MC and PSC-MC, which was agreement with the analysis that the helices of ASC-MC and PSC-MC might be more unstable than that of CSC because of the lower content of imino acid. In addition, PSC-MC was easier to digestion by trypsin than ASC-MC as indicated by a greater band intensity of lower MW peptide fragments ranging from 20.0 to 43.0 kDa. Therefore, ASC-MC, PSC-MC and CSC might have some different in their primary structures and sequence amino acids, which will be our future work.

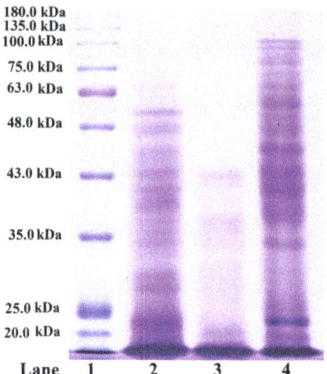

Figure 2. Peptide hydrolysis patterns of acid-soluble collagen (ASC-MC) and pepsin-soluble collagen (PSC-MC) from the scales of miiuy croaker (*M. miiuy*). Lane 1. marker protein; lane 2. ASC-MC; lane 3. PSC-MC; lane 4. type I collagen of pig skin (CSC).

2.4. Ultraviolet (UV) Spectra

It is well known that the maximum absorption wavelength of protein in the near ultraviolet region is 280 nm because of the absorbance (280 nm) of aromatic amino acids such as Phe, Trp and Tyr [8]. Previous reports indicated that the protein might be collagen if there was a maximum absorption near 210–240 nm [4,22]. The UV absorption data of ASC-MC and PSC-MC were shown in Figure 3. The maximum absorption peaks of CSC, ASC-MC and PSC-MC were at 220 nm, which was related to the groups C=O, –COOH and $CONH_2$ in polypeptides chains of collagens [22]. Very weak absorbance measurements were obtained at 280 nm due to low concentrations of aromatic amino acids in ASC (20.3 residues/1000 residues) and PSC (19.9 residues/1000 residues) (Table 1). Similar findings were reported in collagens from skin of loach (218 nm) [32], body wall of sea cucumber (220 nm) [33] and channel catfish (232 nm) [34].

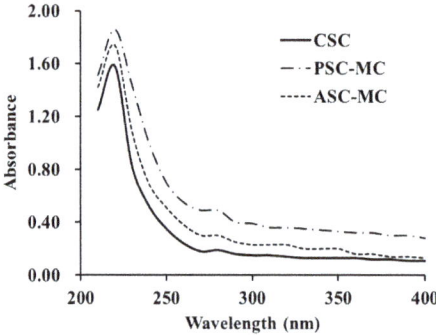

Figure 3. UV spectra of type I collagen from calf skin (CSC) and acid-soluble collagen (ASC-MC) and pepsin-soluble collagen (PSC-MC) from the scales of miiuy croaker (*M. miiuy*).

2.5. Fourier-Transform Infrared Spectroscopy (FTIR)

FTIR spectrum is a powerful technique to research the structure and of collagens and configuration of polypeptide chain and the frequencies relate to the nature of the molecular bonds and their structure and chemical environment [35]. Collagen structure is distinguished by the formation of a right-handed triple superhelical rod consisting of three almost identical polypeptide chains. Each polypeptide chain forms a left-handed helix and consists of repeating triplets (Gly-Xaa-Yaa) [12,36]. In that collagen structure, three polypeptide strands were held together in a helical conformation by a single interstrand N-H(Gly)···O=C(Xaa) hydrogen bond per triplet [35,37]. Therefore, the characteristic peaks of amide A, B, I, II and III band contain a lot of valuable information on the right-handed triple helical conformation of collagen [4,12]. The FTIR spectra of ASC-MC, PSC-MC and CSC were shown in Figure 4 and similar FTIR spectra of ASC-MC, PSC-MC and CSC were observed. The major peaks, including amide A, amide B, amide I, amide II and amide III, could be found in amide band region and assigned in Table 3, which arise from the vibration of the peptide groups and provide information about the secondary structure of ASC-MC, PSC-MC and CSC.

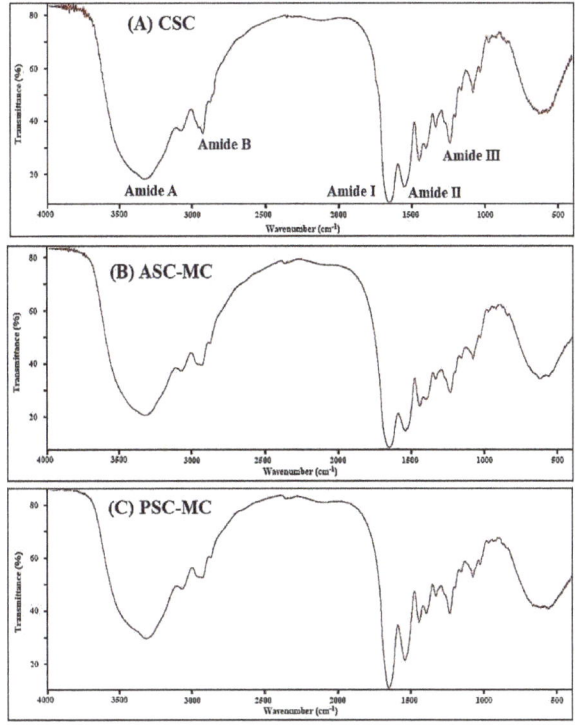

Figure 4. FTIR spectra of type I collagen from calf skin (CSC) (**A**) and acid-soluble collagen (ASC-MC) (**B**) and pepsin-soluble collagen (PSC-MC) (**C**) from the scales of miiuy croaker (*M. miiuy*).

The band of amide A is bound up with the N-H stretching frequency. The wavenumber of a free N-H stretching vibration is located next to the range 3400–3440 cm^{-1} and the wavenumber would move to lower frequency if the N-H group participated in the formation of a hydrogen-bond [8,38]. Figure 4 showed that the amide A wavenumbers of ASC-MC and PSC-MC were in 3415 and 3424 cm^{-1}. The data illustrated that some N-H groups in ASC-MC and PSC-MC contributed to the formation of hydrogen bonding and the hydrogen-bonding numbers of ASC-MC were more than that of PSC-MC. However, the amide A wavenumbers of ASC-MC and PSC-MC were lower than that of CSC (3426 cm^{-1}), which indicated that the structure stability of ASC-MC and PSC-MC was weaker than that of CSC. The amide B band is related to asymmetric stretch vibrations of $-NH_3^+$ and =C–H and the shift of amide B to higher wavenumber is associated with an increase in free $NH-NH_3^+$ groups from lysine residues of N-terminal [8,12]. The wavenumbers of amide B band of CSC, ASC-MC and PSC-MC were found at positions of 2940, 2937 and 2936 cm^{-1}, respectively. The result indicated that the free $-NH_3^+$ groups of PSC-MC was fewer than those of ASC-MC and CSC.

Table 3. FTIR spectra peak locations of CSC (type I collagen from calf skin), acid-soluble collagen (ASC-MC) and pepsin-soluble collagen (PSC-MC) from the scales of miiuy croaker (*M. miiuy*).

Properties	Peak Wavenumber (cm^{-1})			Assignment
	ASC-MC	PSC-MC	CSC	
Amide A	3415	3424	3426	NH stretch coupled with hydrogen bond
Amide B	2937	2936	2940	CH$_2$ asymmetrical stretch
Amide I	1658	1655	1660	C=O stretch/hydrogen bond coupled with COO–
Amide II	1543	1547	1541	NH bend coupled with CN stretch
Amide III	1239	1237	1241	NH bend coupled with CN stretch

Amide I, amide II and amide III bands are bound up with the triple helical structure of collagen, resulting from C=O stretching, N–H bending and C–H stretching, respectively [9,26]. The amide I band with strong absorbance in the range of 1600–1700 cm^{-1} is primarily associated with the C=O stretching vibration along the polypeptide backbone or a hydrogen bond coupled with COO– and the decrease of molecular order will make the peak shift to lower wavenumber [19]. Amide I band of ASC-MC was found at 1658 cm^{-1} and slight lower wavenumber (1655 cm^{-1}) was found for PSC-MC. The result indicated that partial telopeptides were degraded by pepsin during the preparation process of PSC-MC, which caused the missing of active amino acids (Lys, Hyl and His) at telopeptide region of PSC-MC molecular [8].

The amide II band representing the N–H bending vibration coupled with C–N stretching vibration generally occurs in the range of 1550–1600 cm^{-1}, which specifies the number of NH groups involved in hydrogen bonding with the adjacent α-chain; therefore, the lower wavenumber of the amide II band is related to the increased of hydrogen bonds by NH groups, which is attributed to collagen's higher structure order [12]. The wavenumbers of CSC, ASC-MC and PSC-MC were found to be 1541, 1543 and 1547 cm^{-1}, respectively, which indicated that the hydrogen bonding in CSC and ASC-MC was more than that of PSC-MC and the finding is consistent with the result of peptide hydrolysis patterns.

Amide III band absorption was arisen from wagging vibrations of CH$_2$ groups from the Gly backbone and Pro side-chains, which is weak and associated with the triple helix structure of collagen [12]. Figure 4 showed the amide III bands of CSC, ASC-MC and PSC-MC were located at wavenumbers of 1241, 1239 and 1237 cm^{-1}, respectively. The result indicated that hydrogen bonds were involved in CSC, ASC-MC and PSC-MC. In addition, the intensity ratio between Amide III band and 1450 cm^{-1} band has been used to elucidate the triplehelical structure of collagen and the absorption ratio between amide III (CSC 1241 cm^{-1}, ASC-MC 1239 cm^{-1} and PSC-MC 1237 cm^{-1}) and 1452 cm^{-1} (CSC), 1451 cm^{-1} (ASC-MC) or 1448 cm^{-1} (PSC-MC) bands was approximately equal to 1.0, which confirmed that ASC-MC and PSC-MC have maintained a high extent of intact triple helix structures. In addition, the amide I and amide A bands on ASC-MC and PSC-MC suggested that the structure of ASC-MC was more stable than that of PSC-MC due to more hydrogen-bonding and partial telopeptides in ASC-MC molecular but the structures of ASC-MC and PSC-MC were more unstable than that of CSC on the information of their FTIR spectra.

2.6. Viscosity and Denaturation Temperature (T_d)

Collagen consists of amino acids wound together to form triple-helices to form of elongated fibrils and the triple helix structure could be depolymerized and transformed to the unordered coil configuration if the intramolecular hydrogen bond was broken by high temperature, which is along with the changes of physical characteristics, such as solubility decrease, precipitation and viscosity reducing. Therefore, viscosity measurement is often applied to research the thermos stability of collagen [4,8].

As shown in Figure 5, the relative viscosities of ASC-MC and PSC-MC solutions showed a similar rapid decline trend at the concentration of 0.6% when temperature increased from 4 to 44 °C. Denaturation temperature (T_d) is the temperature at which the triple-helix structure of collagen deforms to a random coil structure. The T_d values of ASC-MC and PSC-MC were 32.2 and 29.0 °C, which were similar to those of some warm and tropical fish species, such as skipjack tuna (29.7 °C), paper nautilus (27 °C), ocellate puffer (28 °C), eel (29.3 °C), Japanese seabass (26.5 °C) and ayu (29.7 °C) [39] and higher than those of cold-water fish species, such as Alaska pollack (16.8 °C), Baltic cod (15.0 °C) and Argentine hake (10.0 °C) [40]. However, the T_d values of ASC-MC and PSC-MC were lower than those of CSC (35.9 °C). The finding further confirmed that the helix structures of ASC-MC and PSC-MC were more unstable than those of collagens from mammals. A low T_d value is an undesirable property in the manufacturing process and for biomaterials because denaturation drastically changes the biological, mechanical and physicochemical properties of collagen [41]. At present, chemical crosslinking using glutaraldehyde, carbodiimide or physical treatments including ultraviolet irradiation and dehydrothermal treatment usually was used to improve the thermal stability of collagen from aquatic animals [41]. The T_d and viscosity of PSC-MC were slightly lower than this of ASC-MC, which might be caused by MW reduction in the telopeptide region induced by pepsin hydrolysis.

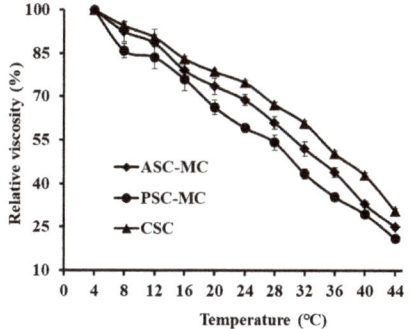

Figure 5. Relative viscosity changes of acid-soluble collagen (ASC-MC) and pepsin-soluble collagen (PSC-MC) from the scales of miiuy croaker (*M. miiuy*) in deionized water. All data are presented as the mean ± SD of triplicate results.

2.7. Solubility

Solubility of collagen is the most important factor and excellent index for their functionality. Knowledge of collagen solubility can give useful information on the potential utilization of proteins and their functionality, especially in foams, emulsions and gels [42]. In addition, solubility is the main characteristic of collagens selected for use in liquid foods and beverages. Except influenced by amino acid composition and sequence, molecular weight and conformation, solubility of collagen is affected by environmental factors, such as pH, ionic strength, type of solvent, temperature and processing conditions [43]. Therefore, the influence of pH and ionic strength (NaCl concentration) on solubility of ASC-MC and PSC-MC was measured and the results were shown in Figure 6.

2.7.1. Effect of pH

Collagen to be soluble should be able to interact as much as possible with the solvent. Collagen-water interactions increase at pH values higher or lower than the isoelectric point (p*I*) because Collagen carries a positive or negative charge [43]. However, collagens have a net zero charge at the p*I*, attractive forces predominate and molecules tend to associate, resulting in insolubility. Figure 6A depicted that ASC-MC, PSC-MC and CSC were more easily dissolved in acid solution (pH 1–5) and the solubility significantly decreased at pH 5–7. The maximum solubility of ASC-MC was achieved at pH 1 and the solubility of PSC-MC reached maxima at pH 1–3. Similar result was reported for scale collagens from redspot goatfish [23], snakehead [25], *C. catla* [28], croceine and redlip croakers [4]. The minimum solubility of ASC-MC and PSC-MC was at pH 7. However, the solubility of

ASC-MC and PSC-MC showed a slight upward trend when pH value was higher than 7. The present data indicated that the pIs of ASC-MC and PSC-MC were about pH 7 and the data were in agreement with previous reports that the collagen pIs were usually at pH 6–9 [23]. At the same pH value, PSC-MC had higher solubility than ASC-MC, which was in line with that of PSC from scales of redspot goatfish [23], croceine and redlip croakers [4]. The finding could be due to the predominance of weaker bonds and lower cross-linking degree of PSC.

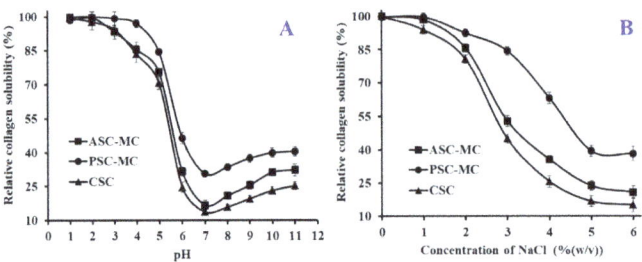

Figure 6. Solubilities of acid-soluble collagen (ASC-MC) and pepsin-soluble collagen (PSC-MC) from the scales of miiuy croaker (*M. miiuy*) in 0.5 M acetic acid at different pH (**A**) and NaCl concentrations (**B**). All data are presented as the mean ± SD of triplicate results.

2.7.2. Effect of NaCl Concentration

The functionality of collagens can be studied more effectively if a systematic study is first made of the protein solubility under various ionic conditions [43]. The mechanism of the ionic strength effect on protein solubility probably involves solvation, electrostatic and salting in and salting out phenomena [8]. Low concentrations of neutral salts may increase the solubility of proteins. Chloride ions increase solubility by electrostatic repulsion after binding to the positively charged protein groups. As presented in Figure 6B, the solubility of ASC-MC, PSC-MC and CSC showed similar pattern with slightly difference when NaCl concentrations ranged from 0 to 6%. The solubility of ASC-MC, PSC-MC and CSC remained high level (more than 90%) when the NaCl concentration was lower than 1% and rapidly reduced if NaCl concentration was between 1 and 5%, after which the solubility of ASC-MC, PSC-MC and CSC was slowly reduced when the NaCl concentration was ranged from 5 to 6%. The result was like the solubility of scale collagens from redspot goatfish [23], snakehead [25], bighead carp [27], croceine and redlip croakers [4]. The solubility changes of ASC-MC, PSC-MC and CSC might be due to the 'salting out' effect resulted from the relatively high NaCl concentration. An ionic strength increase could enhance the hydrophobic-hydrophobic interactions of protein chains and increase the competition for water with the ionic salts, which led to protein precipitation [4]. These solubility behaviors of ASC-MC, PSC-MC and CSC with pH and NaCl concentration changes might play an important role in their preparation process.

2.8. Zeta Potential

Zeta potential, also known as electrokinetic potential, is the potential difference across phase boundaries between solids and liquids and often used to describe double-layer properties of a colloidal dispersion [12]. Therefore, the zeta potential is a key indicator of the stability of colloidal dispersions and macromolecules with a high zeta potential have low propensity to form aggregates [44]. The zeta potentials of the ASC-MC, PSC-MC and CSC at various pH values were presented in Figure 7 and showed the similar tendency. ASC-MC and PSC-MC were positively charged at pH 2–6 and negatively charged at pH 7–11. The Zeta potential data revealed when the zeta net charges of ASC-MC and PSC-MC were zero, their potential values and pI values were 6.66 and 6.81, respectively, which consistent with the result obtained in effect of pH on solubility that the pIs of ASC-MC and PSC-MC were about pH 7. The difference in pI values between ASC-MC and PSC-MC might be due to the removal of PSC telopeptides by pepsin. Collagen from various fish skins had different p*I* values, such as ASC from scales and skin of tilapia (6.82 and 6.42 respectively) [29], ASC and PSC from skin of loach (6.42 and 6.51 respectively) [32] and PSC from skin of bamboo shark (6.12) [45]. The differences in collagen p*I* values might due to amino acid sequences and distribution of amino acid residues.

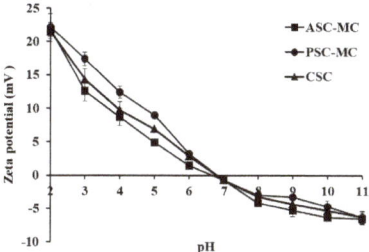

Figure 7. Zeta potentials of acid-soluble collagen (ASC-MC) and pepsin-soluble collagen (PSC-MC) from the scales of miiuy croaker (*M. miiuy*) at different pH levels. All values were mean ± SD.

2.9. Collagen Ultrastructure

Ultrastructure and surface area of collagen are important to evaluate its potential applications in biomedicine and biomedicine engineering [23,30]. Scanning electron microscopy (SEM) ultrastructure of ASC-MC and PSC-MC from the scales of miiuy croaker were observed in Figure 8. ASC-MC presented irregular dense sheet-like film linked by random-coiled filaments under SEM (Figure 8A) and the surface was partially wrinkled, possibly because of dehydration during lyophilizing. The fibrillar structure of PSC-MC was also found in Figure 8B. SEM ultrastructure of ASC-MC and PSC-MC was similar to those of collagens from skin and bone of Spanish mackerel [15], gutted silver carp [30], swim bladder of carp [23] and skin of Amur sturgeon [46]. In addition, the sheet-like film structure of ASC-MC and the fibrillar structure of PSC-MC at the same concentration (5% (w/v)) suggested that there were some differences in the primary structures between ASC-MC and PSC-MC. Previous reports suggested that collagens with interconnectivity, fibrillary and sheet-like film structures have the potentiality to be used in new tissue formation, cell seeding, growth, wound healing and mass transport and migration [30]. In general, the microscopic structure of ASC-MC and PSC-MC indicated that they may be the suitable biomaterial for different medical applications.

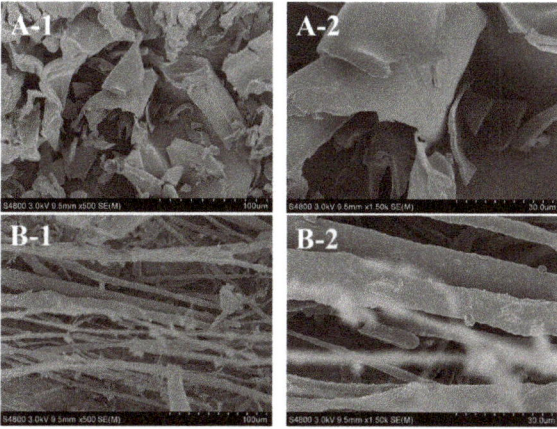

Figure 8. SEM images of acid-soluble collagen (ASC-MC) and pepsin-soluble collagen (PSC-MC) from the scales of miiuy croaker (*M. miiuy*). (**A**): ASC-MC; (**B**): PSC-MC. 1: (×500); 2: (×1500).

2.10. Antioxidant Activity

Oxidative stress is associated with the pathogenesis of many chronic diseases and excessive free radicals generated in metabolism are a potential reason for the oxidative stress of human body [11,47]. Reactive oxygen species (ROS), such as superoxide and hydroxyl radical, are observed to possess the strong capacity to attack biological macromolecules, which further cause cell injury and play an important role in developing process of chronic diseases [3,48]. In addition, the radical scavenging activity is an important property for skin photoaging and ultraviolet damage of cosmeceutical products [49,50]. Therefore, the radical scavenging activity of the fish collagen is an important characteristic for evaluating its potential application.

The antioxidant properties of ASC-MC and PSC-MC were evaluated using DPPH radical, hydroxyl radical, superoxide anion radical and ABTS radical scavenging assays and shown in Figure 9. The present results indicated that the antioxidant capacities (DPPH radical, hydroxyl radical, superoxide anion radical and ABTS radical scavenging activities) of ASC-MC and PSC-MC were positively correlated with their tested concentration ranged from 0 to 5 mg/mL. The DPPH radical scavenging activity of PSC-MC was significantly higher than those of ASC-MC and CSC at the same concentrations except the concentrations of 1.5 and 2.5 mg/mL ($p < 0.05$) and the hydroxyl radical scavenging activity of PSC-MC showed the same trend and was significantly higher than those of ASC-MC and CSC at the same concentrations except the concentrations of 0.5 mg/mL ($p < 0.05$). Furthermore, PSC-MC showed significantly higher superoxide anion radical and ABTS radical scavenging activity than PSC-MC did at the same concentrations ($p < 0.05$). However, there were no significant difference between ASC-MC and CSC on hydroxyl radical, superoxide anion radical and ABTS radical scavenging activities at most tested concentrations ($p > 0.05$). In addition, the radical scavenging activities of ASC-MC, PSC-MC and CSC were significantly lower than those of the positive control of ascorbic acid and glutathione (GSH), which was agreed with the previous reports that small molecular including oligopeptides (2–9 amino acid residues) showed high radical scavenging activities than macromolecules because they were easily accessible to active radicals to provide potential effects in reaction mixture [51,52].

Moreover, the scavenging capability of PSC-MC on hydroxyl radical (Figure 9B) and superoxide anion radical (Figure 9C) was higher than those of DPPH radical and ABTS radical. In the human body, superoxide anion radical is the most common free radical generated in vivo. It can produce hydrogen peroxide and hydroxyl radical through dismutation and other types of reactions in vivo. Both superoxide anion radical and its derivatives including hydroxyl radical are cell damaging, which can cause damage to DNA and membrane of cell [15]. Therefore, the damage caused by the highly reactive free radicals is widely accepted as the primary reason for skin damage, inflammation and skin aging [11]. In biological systems, SODs can catalyze superoxide radicals into hydrogen peroxide and oxygen with a reaction rate 10,000-fold higher than that of spontaneous dismutation. Therefore, ASC-MC and PSC-MC might have a high antioxidant activity similar to that of SOD and could be served as hydroxyl radical and superoxide radical scavenger in cosmeceutical products for reducing the radical damage in skin aging.

The skin aging process can be divided into intrinsic aging and photoaging. Skin photoaging is a premature skin-aging damage after repeated exposure to ultraviolet (UV) radiation, mainly characterized by oxidative stress and inflammatory disequilibrium, which makes skin show the typical symptoms of photoaging such as coarse wrinkling, dryness, irregular pigmentation and laxity [53]. ROS are thought to be involved in cancer, aging and various inflammatory disorders. Therefore, more and more attention has been paid to utilize fish-derived collagen, gelatin and peptides for protecting skin from photoaging due to their excellent antioxidant activity and skin-repairing ability [12]. Chen et al. reported that gelatin hydrolysate (CH) with average molecular weight of 1200 Da from pacific cod skin can improved pathological changes of collagen fibers and significantly inhibited collagen content reduction in photoaging skin. Moreover, CH can effectively protect against UV irradiation-induced skin photoaging by inhibiting the expression and the activity of matrix metalloproteinases [54,55]. Wang et al.

reported that the collagen polypeptides from *Apostichopus japonicus* showed protective effects against ultraviolet radiation-induced skin photoaging [56]. Hou et al. reported collagen polypeptide fractions of CP1 (2 kDa < MW < 6 kDa) and CP2 (MW < 2 kDa) from cod skin could protect skin structures against UV-induced wrinkle formation and destruction and they also provided good moisture absorption and retention properties [57]. Sun et al. reported that tilapia gelatin peptides (TGP) could protect skin lipid and collagen from the UV radiation damages through alleviating the UV-induced abnormal changes of antioxidant indicators and repairing the endogenous collagen synthesis [1]. Therefore, the present finding suggested that ASC-SC and PSC-SC from the scales of miiuy croaker might be served as hydroxyl radical and superoxide anion radical scavenger in cosmeceutical products for protecting skins from photoaging and ultraviolet damage.

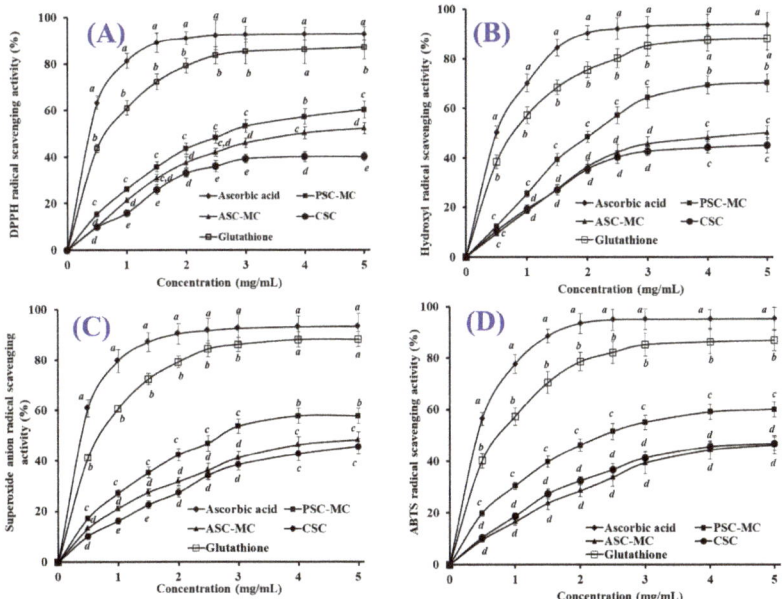

Figure 9. DPPH radical (**A**), hydroxyl radical (**B**), superoxide anion radical (**C**) and ABTS radical (**D**) scavenging activities of CSC and acid-soluble collagen (ASC-MC) and pepsin-soluble collagen (PSC-MC) from the scales of miiuy croaker (*M. miiuy*). Ascorbic acid and glutathione were designed as positive controls to compare with the sample groups. All the values were mean ± SD. $^{a-e}$ Values with same letters indicated no significant difference of different sample at same concentrations ($p > 0.05$).

3. Experimental Section

3.1. Chemicals and Reagents

The scales of miiuy croaker (*M. miiuy*) were obtained from Zhejiang Hailisheng Group Co. Ltd., in Zhoushan City, Zhejiang Province of China. High molecular weight markers and type I collagen from calf skin (CSC) were used as the standards and bought from Sigma-Aldrich (St. Louis, MO, USA). All other reagents used were of analytical grade.

3.2. Extraction of Scale Collagens

3.2.1. Pretreatment of Scales

The extraction procedure of scale collagens of miiuy croaker was according to the method described by Matmaroh et al. [20]. The scales were added to 0.1 M NaOH solution with a material/liquid ratio of

1:10 (w/v) and stirred for 6 h and NaOH solution was replaced each 3 h. Afterwards, the scales were rinsed using cold tap water until the pH value of washing water got to 7.0–7.5 and demineralized using EDTA-2Na (0.5 M, pH 7.4) with a material/liquid ratio of 1:10 (w/v) and stirred for 48 h and EDTA-2Na solution was renewed every 12 h. The pretreated scales were cleaned with a scale/cold tap water ratio of 1:20 (w/v) for three times.

3.2.2. Extraction of Acid-Soluble Collagen (ASC-MC)

The pretreated scales were soaked in 0.5 M acetic acid solution with a material/liquid ratio of 1:15 (w/v) for 48 h. The extracting solution was filtered using a cheesecloth and the collagen was precipitated from the filtrate using 2.5 M NaCl solution. The precipitates were collected by centrifugation at 20,000× g for 30 min at 4 °C, re-dissolved in a minimum volume of 0.5 M acetic acid solution and dialyzed against 25 volumes of 0.1 M acetic acid solution for 12 h. Thereafter, the dialyzed solution was dialyzed against 25 volumes of distilled water for 48 h and distilled water was changed each 12 h. The final dialysate was lyophilized.

3.2.3. Extraction of Pepsin-Soluble Collagen (PSC-MC)

The scale residues from ASC-MC preparation were soaked in 0.5 M acetic acid solution containing 1% porcine pepsin (w/w) at a solvent/scale ratio of 15:1 (v/w) for 48 h at 4 °C. Thereafter, other processes were carried with the identical manner as the ASC-MC preparation.

3.3. Proximate Analysis

Moisture, ash and fat contents of scale and collagens were determined using the methods of Association of Official Agricultural Chemists (AOAC) method (2003) with the method numbers of 950.46B, 920.153 and 960.39 (a), respectively. Protein content was measured using the Kjeldahl method and an auto protein analyzer (Kjeltec 2400 auto-analyzer, Hillerød, Denmark). The converting factor of 6.25 was used for calculation of protein content [7].

3.4. Amino Acid Analysis

Tested samples were hydrolyzed in 6 M HCl at 110 °C for 24 h and the hydrolysates were vaporized and the residues were dissolved in 25 mL citric acid buffer solution. An aliquot of 0.05 mL was applied to an automated amino acid analyzer (HITACHI 835-50 Amino Acid Analyzer, Tokyo,, Japan). Then the degrees of Pro and Lys hydroxylation (%) were calculated as follows:

Degrees of Pro hydroxylation (%) = Hyp content/(Hyp content + Pro content) × 100%.
Degrees of Lys hydroxylation (%) = Hyl content/(Hyl content + Lys content) × 100%.

3.5. Electrophoretic Pattern

Electrophoretic patterns of ASC-MC and PSC-MC were determined using the previous method [9], using 7.5% resolving gel and 4% stacking gel. Collagen samples were suspended in 5% (w/v) SDS prior to incubation at 85 °C for 1 h. The mixture was centrifuged at 5,000× g for 10 min for removing undissolved debris. The samples (about 20 µL) were mixed with the sample loading buffer (60 mM Tris-HCl, pH 8.0, containing 25% glycerol, 2% SDS, 0.1% bromophenol blue) at the ratio of 4:1 (v/v) in the presence of β-ME, then applied to sample wells and electrophoresed in an electrophoresis instrument (AE-6200, ATTO Corporation, Tokyo, Japan). The electrophoresis was carried out for about 4 h at a constant voltage of 100 V. After electrophoresis, gel was stained with 0.1% (w/v) Coomassie blue R-250 in 45% (v/v) methanol and 10% (v/v) acetic acid.

3.6. Peptide Hydrolysis Patterns

Peptide hydrolysis patterns of ASC-MC and PSC-MC were measured on the method described by Wu et al. [4]. Collagen solutions (3.5 M) dissolved in acetic acid solution (0.5 M) were hydrolyzed for

3.0 h at 37 °C after adding trypsin with a substrate/enzyme ratio of 20:1 (w/w) and the hydrolysis was terminated in boiled water for 5 min after the addition of SDS-PAGE sample buffer. SDS-PAGE with 12.0% separating gels was used to measure the molecular weight of peptides.

3.7. UV Measurements

The UV adsorption spectra of ASC-MC and PSC-MC were recorded using the method of Yu et al. [22], using a spectrophotometer (UV-1800, Mapada Instruments Co., Ltd., Shanghai, China) from 200 to 400 nm. The sample was prepared by dissolving the collagen in 0.5 M acetic acid solution with a sample/solution ratio of 1:1 000 (w/v).

3.8. FTIR Spectral Analysis

The IR spectra of ASC-MC and PSC-MC were recorded in KBr disks with a FTIR spectrophotometer (Nicolet 6700, Thermo Fisher Scientific Inc., Waltham, MA, USA). The mixture at a sample to potassium bromide (KBr) ratio of 1:100 (w/w) was pressed into a disk for spectrum recording. The IR spectra in the range of 4000–400 cm^{-1} with automatic signal gain were collected in 32 scans at a resolution of 4 cm^{-1} and were ratioed against a background spectrum recorded from the clean empty cell.

3.9. Viscosity

Viscosity of ASC-MC and PSC-MC was measured using the previous method [9]. All the samples were dissolved in deionized water with the vibration of THZ-100 shaker (Shanghai Yiheng Technical Co., Ltd., Shanghai, China), to obtain a concentration of 0.6% (w/v) and 500 mL solutions were subjected to viscosity measurement using a NDJ-8S viscometer (Jingtian Instruments Co., Ltd., Shanghai, China) with appropriate spindles (from No.4 to No.1) and an appropriate speed. All the sample solutions were heated from 4 to 44 °C with a heating rate of 4 °C/min and the solution was held for 30 min prior to viscosity determination at the designated temperature. The relative viscosity was calculated in comparison with that obtained at 4 °C and T_d was defined as the temperature at which relative viscosity was 0.5.

3.10. Solubility

Effects of pH and NaCl concentration on the collagen solubility were measured using the previous method [9]. Collagen solutions (3.5 M) were prepared using 0.5 M acetic acid solution and stirred for 24 h at 4 °C. The solutions were centrifuged at 10,000× g for 15 min at 4 °C and the resulting supernatants were used for measuring solubility of collagen.

3.10.1. Effect of pH on Solubility

Sample solution (8 mL) was transferred to a 50 mL centrifuge tube and the pH was adjusted with either 6 M NaOH or 6 M HCl to obtain the final pH ranging from 1 to 11. The volume of solution was made up to 10 ml by deionized water previously adjusted to the same pH as the sample solution. The solution was centrifuged at 15,000× g for 60 min at 4 °C. For all the samples, protein content in the supernatant was measured. Then the relative solubility was calculated in the comparison with that of be obtained at the pH giving the highest solubility.

3.10.2. Effect of NaCl on Solubility

Sample solution (5 mL) was mixed with 5 mL of NaCl in 0.5 M acetic acid at various concentrations to give the final concentrations of 0%, 1%, 2%, 3%, 4%, 5% and 6%. The mixture was stirred continuously at 4 °C for 30 min, followed by centrifuging at 15,000× g for 60 min at 4 °C.

3.11. Zeta Potential

Zeta potentials of ASC-MC and PSC-MC were measured on the previous method [29]. ASC-MC and PSC-MC were dissolved in 0.05 M acetic acid to a final con-centration of 0.2 mg/mL and incubated at 4 °C for 48 h. The zeta potentials of ASC-MC and PSC-MC were determined using a NanoBrook Omni zeta potential analyzer (Brookhaven Instruments Corporation, Holtsville, NY, USA) as reported by Chen et al. [29]. The pH of the samples (20 mL) was adjusted across a pH range (3–11) with 1 M KOH and 1 M HCl. The p*I*s of ASC-MC and PSC-MC were determined from the pH value that resulted in a zero zeta potential.

3.12. Collagen Ultrastructure

The morphological characteristics of ASC-MC and PSC-MC were studied by SEM using Hitachi TM-1000 (Tokyo, Japan). Collagen was re-dissolved in 0.5 M acetic acid at a concentration of 5% (w/v), followed by dialyzing against distilled water. The collagen was lyophilized in a freeze dryer (EYELA FD-1000, Tokyo Rikakikai Co., LTD, Tokyo, Japan) and the sample was sputter coated for 90 s with gold using a JEOL JFC-1200 (Tokyo Rikakikai Co., Ltd., Tokyo, Japan) fine coater. The morphologies of the electro spun fibers and membrane were observed using Hitachi TM-1000 (Hitachi High-Technologies Co., Ltd., Tokyo, Japan).

3.13. Antioxidant Activity

The radical (DPPH radical, hydroxyl radical, superoxide anion radical and ABTS radical) scavenging activity and lipid peroxidation inhibition assays were performed according to previously reported methods [58,59].

3.14. Statistical Analysis

All experiments were carried out in triplicate. An ANOVA test using the software of SPSS 19.0 (Statistical Program for Social Sciences, SPSS Corporation, Chicago, IL, USA) as applied to compare the average values of each treatment. Duncan's multiple range test ($p < 0.05$) was used to measure the significant differences between the parameters means.

4. Conclusions

In the experiment, acid-soluble collagen (ASC-MC) and pepsin-soluble collagen (PSC-MC) from the scales of miiuy croaker (*M. miiuy*) were isolated and characterized. Amino acid composition, SDS-PAGE pattern, UV spectra and FTIR confirmed that ASC-MC and PSC-MC were mainly composed of type I collagen. The antioxidant capacities of ASC-MC and PSC-MC were positively correlated with their tested concentration ranged from 0 to 5.0 mg/mL and the radical scavenging activity of PSC-MC was significantly higher than that of ASC-MC at most tested concentrations ($p < 0.05$). The present result suggested that ASC-SC and PSC-SC from the scales of miiuy croaker could be served as substitutes of skin collagens from mammalian and aquatic products in cosmeceutical products for protecting skins from photoaging and ultraviolet damage by scavenging reactive oxide species. Therefore, this study provides scientific basis for the medical application of scale collagens of miiuy croaker (*M. miiuy*).

Author Contributions: B.W. and C.-F.C. conceived and designed the experiments. L.-Y.L. and Y.H. performed the experiments. L.-Y.L. and Y.-Q.Z. analyzed the data. C.-F.C. and B.W. contributed the reagents, materials and analytical tools and wrote the paper.

Funding: This work was funded by the National Natural Science Foundation of China (NSFC) (No.81673349), the International S&T Cooperation Program of China (2012DFA30600), Natural Science Foundation of Zhejiang Province, China (LY15C190010) and Science and Technology Program of Zhoushan (2016C41016).

Acknowledgments: The authors thank Prof. Sheng-Long Zhao of Zhejiang Ocean University for his valuable help in identifying the experiment material.

Conflicts of Interest: The authors declare no conflicts of interest.

References

1. Sun, L.; Li, B.; Song, W.; Si, L.; Hou, H. Characterization of Pacific cod (*Gadus macrocephalus*) skin collagen and fabrication of collagen sponge as a good biocompatible biomedical material. *Process Biochem.* **2017**, *63*, 229–235. [CrossRef]
2. Bua, Y.; Elangoa, J.; Zhang, J.; Bao, B.; Guo, R.; Palaniyandi, K.; Robinson, J.S.; Geevaretnam, J.; Regenstein, J.M.; Wu, W. Immunological effects of collagen and collagen peptide from blue shark cartilage on 6T-CEM cells. *Process Biochem.* **2017**, *57*, 219–227. [CrossRef]
3. Pal, G.K.; Suresh, P.V. Sustainable valorisation of seafood by-products: Recovery of collagen and development of collagen-based novel functional food ingredients. *Innov. Food Sci. Emerg.* **2016**, *37*, 201–215. [CrossRef]
4. Wu, Q.Q.; Li, T.; Wang, B.; Ding, G.F. Preparation and characterization of acid and pepsin-soluble collagens from scales of croceine and redlip croakers. *Food Sci. Biotechnol.* **2015**, *24*, 2003–2010. [CrossRef]
5. Liu, X.; Dan, N.; Dan, W. Preparation and characterization of an advanced collagen aggregatefrom porcine acellular dermal matrix. *Int. J. Biol. Macromol.* **2016**, *88*, 179–188. [CrossRef] [PubMed]
6. Tziveleka, L.; Ioannou, E.; Tsiourvas, D.; Berillis, P.; Foufa, E.; Roussis, V. Collagen from the marine sponges *Axinella cannabina* and *Suberites carnosus*: isolation and morphological, biochemical, and biophysical characterization. *Mar. Drugs* **2017**, *15*, 152. [CrossRef] [PubMed]
7. Chi, C.F.; Wang, B.; Li, Z.R.; Luo, H.Y.; Ding, G.F. Characterization of acid-soluble collagens from the cartilages of scalloped hammerhead (*Sphyrna lewini*), red stingray (*Dasyatis akajei*), and skate (*Raja porosa*). *Food Sci. Biotechnol.* **2013**, *22*, 909–916. [CrossRef]
8. Li, Z.R.; Wang, B.; Chi, C.F.; Zhang, Q.H.; Gong, Y.D.; Tang, J.J.; Luo, H.Y.; Ding, G.F. Isolation and characterization of acid soluble collagens and pepsin soluble collagens from the skin and bone of spanish mackerel (*Scomberomorous niphonius*). *Food Hydrocolloid.* **2013**, *31*, 103–113. [CrossRef]
9. Chi, C.F.; Wang, B.; Li, Z.R.; Luo, H.Y.; Ding, G.F.; Wu, C.W. Characterization of acid-soluble collagen from the skin of hammerhead shark (*Sphyrna lewini*). *J. Food Biochem.* **2014**, *38*, 236–247. [CrossRef]
10. Zheng, Z.; Si, D.; Ahmad, B.; Li, Z.; Zhang, R. A novel antioxidative peptide derived from chicken blood corpuscle hydrolysate. *Food Res. Int.* **2018**, *106*, 410–419. [CrossRef] [PubMed]
11. Zhao, W.H.; Luo, Q.B.; Pan, X.; Chi, C.F.; Sun, K.L.; Wang, B. Preparation, identification, and activity evaluation of ten antioxidant peptides from protein hydrolysate of swim bladders of miiuy croaker (*Miichthys miiuy*). *J. Funct. Foods* **2018**, *47*, 503–511. [CrossRef]
12. Zhao, W.H.; Chi, C.F.; Zhao, Y.Q.; Wang, B. Preparation, physicochemical and antioxidant properties of acid- and pepsin-soluble collagens from the swim bladders of miiuy croaker (*Miichthys miiuy*). *Mar. Drugs* **2018**, *16*, 161. [CrossRef] [PubMed]
13. Zhuang, Y.; Hou, H.; Zhao, X.; Zhang, Z.; Li, B. Effects of collagen and collagen hydrolysate from jellyfish (*Rhopilema esculentum*) on mice skin photoaging induced by UV irradiation. *J. Food Sci.* **2009**, *74*, H183–H188. [CrossRef] [PubMed]
14. Bhagwat, P.K.; Dandge, P.B. Isolation, characterization and valorizable applications of fish scale collagen in food and agriculture industries. *Biocatal. Agric. Biotechnol.* **2016**, *7*, 234–240. [CrossRef]
15. Wang, B.; Wang, Y.; Chi, C.; Hu, F.; Deng, S.; Ma, J. Isolation and characterization of collagen and antioxidant collagen peptides from scales of croceine croaker (*Pseudosciaena crocea*). *Mar. Drugs* **2013**, *11*, 4641–4661. [CrossRef] [PubMed]
16. Sankar, S.; Sekar, S.; Mohan, R.; Rani, S.; Sundaraseelan, J.; Sastry, T.P. Preparation and partial characterization of collagen sheet from fish (*Lates calcarifer*) scales. *Int. J. Biol. Macromol.* **2008**, *42*, 6–9. [CrossRef] [PubMed]
17. Liu, Y.; Ma, D.; Wang, Y.; Qin, W. A comparative study of the properties and self-aggregation behavior of collagens from the scales and skin of grass carp (*Ctenopharyngodon idella*). *Int. J. Biol. Macromol.* **2018**, *106*, 516–522. [CrossRef] [PubMed]
18. Huang, C.Y.; Kuo, J.M.; Wu, S.J.; Tsai, H.T. Isolation and characterization of fish scale collagen from tilapia (*Oreochromis sp.*) by a novel extrusion–hydro-extraction process. *Food Chem.* **2016**, *190*, 997–1006. [CrossRef] [PubMed]
19. Chuaychan, S.; Benjakul, S.; Kishimura, H. Characteristics of acid- and pepsin-soluble collagens from scale of seabass (*Lates calcarifer*). *LWT-Food Sci. Technol.* **2015**, *63*, 71–76. [CrossRef]

20. Matmaroh, K.; Benjakul, S.; Prodpran, T.; Encarnacion, A.B.; Kishimura, H. Characteristics of acid soluble collagen and pepsin soluble collagen from scale of spotted golden goatfish (*Parupeneus heptacanthus*). *Food Chem.* **2011**, *129*, 1179–1186. [CrossRef] [PubMed]
21. Wang, J.K.; Yeo, K.P.; Chun, Y.Y.; Tan, T.T.Y.; Choong, C. Fish scale-derived collagen patch promotes growth of blood and lymphatic vessels in vivo. *Acta Biomater.* **2017**, *63*, 246–260. [CrossRef] [PubMed]
22. Yu, D.; Chi, C.F.; Wang, B.; Ding, G.F.; Li, Z. Characterization of acid and pepsin soluble collagens from spine and skull of skipjack tuna (*Katsuwonus pelamis*). *Chin. J. Nat. Med.* **2014**, *12*, 712–720. [CrossRef]
23. Che, R.; Sun, Y.; Sun, D.; Xu, T. Characterization of the miiuy croaker (*Miichthys miiuy*) transcriptome and development of immune-relevant genes and molecular markers. *PLoS ONE* **2014**, *9*, e94046. [CrossRef] [PubMed]
24. Wang, L.; An, X.; Yang, F.; Xin, Z.; Zhao, L.; Hu, Q. Isolation and characterization of collagens from the skin, scale and bone of deep-sea redfish (*Sebastes mentella*). *Food Chem.* **2008**, *108*, 616–623. [CrossRef] [PubMed]
25. Liu, W.; Li, G.; Miao, Y.; Wu, X. Preparation and characterization of pepsin solubilized type I collagen from the scales of snakehead (*Ophiocephalus Argus*). *J. Food Biochem.* **2009**, *33*, 20–37. [CrossRef]
26. Nagai, T.; Izumi, M.; Ishii, M. Fish scale collagen. Preparation and partial characterization. *Int. J. Food Sci. Technol.* **2004**, *39*, 239–244. [CrossRef]
27. Duan, R.; Zhang, J.; Du, X.; Yao, X.; Konno, K. Properties of collagen from skin, scale and bone of carp (*Cyprinus carpio*). *Food Chem.* **2009**, *112*, 702–706. [CrossRef]
28. Pati, F.; Adhikari, B.; Dhara, S. Isolation and characterization of fish scale collagen of higher thermal stability. *Bioresour. Technol.* **2010**, *101*, 3737–3742. [CrossRef] [PubMed]
29. Chen, J.; Li, L.; Yi, R.; Xu, N.; Gao, R.; Hong, B. Extraction and characterization of acid-soluble collagen from scales and skin of tilapia (*Oreochromis niloticus*). *LWT-Food Sci. Technol.* **2016**, *66*, 453–459. [CrossRef]
30. Ogawa, M.; Portier, R.J.; Moody, M.W.; Bell, J.; Schexnayder, M.A.; Losso, J.N. Biochemical properties of bone and scale collagens isolated from the subtropical fish black drum (*Pogonia cromis*) and sheepshead seabream (*Archosargus probatocephalus*). *Food Chem.* **2004**, *88*, 495–501. [CrossRef]
31. Shoulders, M.D.; Raines, R.T. Collagen structure and stability. *Annu. Rev. Biochem.* **2009**, *78*, 929–958. [CrossRef] [PubMed]
32. Wang, J.; Pei, X.; Liu, H.; Zhou, D. Extraction and characterization of acid-soluble and pepsin-soluble collagen from skin of loach (*Misgurnus anguillicaudatus*). *Int. J. Biol. Macromol.* **2018**, *106*, 544–550. [CrossRef] [PubMed]
33. Cui, F.X.; Xue, C.H.; Li, Z.J.; Zhang, Y.Q.; Dong, P.; Fu, X.Y.; Gao, X. Characterization and subunit composition of collagen from the body wall of sea cucumber *Stichopus japonicus*. *Food Chem.* **2007**, *100*, 1120–1125. [CrossRef]
34. Liu, H.Y.; Li, D.; Guo, S.D. Studies on collagen from the skin of channel catfish (*Ictalurus punctaus*). *Food Chem.* **2007**, *101*, 621–625. [CrossRef]
35. Noreen, R.; Moenner, M.; Hwu, Y.; Petibois, C. FTIR spectro-imaging of collagens for characterization and grading of gliomas. *Biotechnol. Adv.* **2012**, *30*, 1432–1446. [CrossRef] [PubMed]
36. Luo, Q.B.; Chi, C.F.; Yang, F.; Zhao, Y.Q.; Wang, B. Physicochemical properties of acid- and pepsin-soluble collagens from the cartilage of Siberian sturgeon. *Environ. Sci. Pollut. Res. Int.* **2018**, *25*, 31427–31438. [CrossRef] [PubMed]
37. Cheheltani, R.; McGoverin, C.M.; Rao, J.; Vorp, D.A.; Kiani, M.F.; Pleshko, N. Fourier transform infrared spectroscopy to quantify collagen and elastin in an in vitro model of extracellular matrix degradation in aorta. *Analyst* **2014**, *139*, 3039–3047. [CrossRef] [PubMed]
38. Doyle, B.B.; Bendit, E.G.; Blout, E.R. Infrared spectroscopy of collagen and collagen-like polypeptides. *Biopolymers* **1975**, *14*, 937–957. [CrossRef] [PubMed]
39. Jongjareonrak, A.; Benjakul, S.; Visessanguan, W.; Nagai, T.; Tanaka, M. Isolation and characterisation of acid and pepsin-solubilised collagens from the skin of Brownstripe red snapper (*Lutjanus vitta*). *Food Chem.* **2005**, *93*, 475–484. [CrossRef]
40. Zhang, Y.; Liu, W.T.; Li, G.Y.; Shi, B.; Miao, Y.Q.; Wu, X.H. Isolation and partial characterization of pepsin-soluble collagen from the skin of grass carp (*Ctenopharyngodon idella*). *Food Chem.* **2007**, *103*, 906–912. [CrossRef]
41. El-Rashidy, A.A.; Gad, A.; Abu-Hussein, A.-H.; Habib, S.I.; Badr, N.A.; Hashem, A.A. Chemical and biological evaluation of Egyptian Nile Tilapia (*Oreochromis niloticas*) fish scale collagen. *Int. J. Biol. Macromol.* **2015**, *79*, 618–826. [CrossRef] [PubMed]

42. Latorre, M.E.; Lifschitz, A.L.; Purslow, P.P. New recommendations for measuring collagen solubility. *Meat Sci.* **2016**, *118*, 78–81. [CrossRef] [PubMed]
43. Zayas, J.F. Solubility of proteins. In *Functionality of Proteins in Food*; Zayas, J.F., Ed.; Springer: Berlin, Germany, 1997; pp. 6–75.
44. Ferraro, V.; Gaillard-Martinie, B.; Sayd, T.; Chambon, C.; Anton, M.; Santé-Lhoutellier, V. Collagen type I from bovine bone. Effect of animal age, bone anatomy and drying methodology on extraction yield, self-assembly, thermal behaviour and electrokinetic potential. *Int. J. Biol. Macromol.* **2017**, *97*, 55–66. [CrossRef] [PubMed]
45. Kittiphattanabawon, P.; Benjakul, S.; Visessanguan, W.; Kishimura, H.; Shahidi, F. Isolation and characterisation of collagen from the skin of brownbanded bamboo shark (*Chiloscyllium punctatum*). *Food Chem.* **2010**, *119*, 1519–1526. [CrossRef]
46. Wang, L.; Liang, Q.; Chen, T.; Wang, Z.; Xu, J.; Ma, H. Characterization of collagen from the skin of Amur sturgeon (*Acipenser schrenckii*). *Food Hydrocolloid.* **2014**, *38*, 104–109. [CrossRef]
47. Pan, X.; Zhao, Y.Q.; Hu, F.Y.; Wang, B. Preparation and identification of antioxidant peptides from protein hydrolysate of skate (*Raja porosa*) cartilage. *J. Funct. Foods* **2016**, *25*, 220–230. [CrossRef]
48. Tao, J.; Zhao, Y.Q.; Chi, C.F.; Wang, B. Bioactive peptides from cartilage protein hydrolysate of spotless smoothhound and their antioxidant activity in vitro. *Mar. Drugs* **2018**, *16*, 100. [CrossRef] [PubMed]
49. Gómez-Guillén, M.C.; Giménez, B.; López-Caballero, M.E.; Montero, M.P. Functional and bioactive properties of collagen and gelatin from alternative sources: A review. *Food Hydrocolloid.* **2011**, *25*, 1813–1827. [CrossRef]
50. Hu, F.Y.; Chi, C.F.; Wang, B.; Deng, S.G. Two novel antioxidant nonapeptides from protein hydrolysate of skate (*Raja porosa*) muscle. *Mar. Drugs* **2015**, *13*, 1993–2009. [CrossRef] [PubMed]
51. Sila, A.; Bougatef, A. Antioxidant peptides from marine by-products: Isolation, identification and application in food systems. A review. *J. Funct. Foods* **2016**, *21*, 10–26. [CrossRef]
52. Chi, C.F.; Hu, F.Y.; Wang, B.; Li, T.; Ding, G.F. Antioxidant and anticancer peptides from protein hydrolysate of blood clam (*Tegillarca granosa*) muscle. *J. Funct. Foods* **2015**, *15*, 301–313. [CrossRef]
53. Kong, S.Z.; Li, D.D.; Luo, H.; Li, W.J.; Huang, Y.M.; Li, J.C.; Hu, Z.; Huang, N.; Guo, M.H.; Chen, Y.; et al. Anti-photoaging effects of chitosan oligosaccharide in ultraviolet-irradiated hairless mouse skin. *Exp. Gerontol.* **2018**, *103*, 27–34. [CrossRef] [PubMed]
54. Chen, T.; Hou, H.; Fan, Y.; Wang, S.; Chen, Q.; Si, L.; Li, B. Protective effect of gelatin peptides from pacific cod skin against photoaging by inhibiting the expression of MMPs via MAPK signaling pathway. *J. Photochem. Photobiol. B Biol.* **2016**, *165*, 34–41. [CrossRef] [PubMed]
55. Chen, T.; Hou, H. Protective effect of gelatin polypeptides from Pacific cod (*Gadus macrocephalus*) against UV irradiation-induced damages by inhibiting inflammation and improving transforming growth Factor-β/Smad signaling pathway. *J. Photochem. Photobiol. B Biol.* **2016**, *162*, 633–640. [CrossRef] [PubMed]
56. Wang, Y.; Wang, J.F.; Gao, S.; Zhao, Q.; Liu, Z.D.; Liang, Y.F. Protective effect of collagen polypeptides from Apostichopus japonicus on the skin of photoaging-model mice induced by ultraviolet irradiation. *J. China Pharm. Univ.* **2008**, *39*, 64–67.
57. Hou, H.; Li, B.; Zhang, Z.; Xue, C.; Yu, G.; Wang, J.; Bao, Y.; Bu, L.; Sun, J.; Peng, Z. Moisture absorption and retention properties, and activity in alleviating skin photodamage of collagen polypeptide from marine fish skin. *Food Chem.* **2012**, *135*, 1432–1439. [CrossRef] [PubMed]
58. Li, Z.; Wang, B.; Chi, C.; Luo, H.; Gong, Y.; Ding, G. Influence of average molecular weight on antioxidant and functional properties of collagen hydrolysates from *Sphyrna lewini*, *Dasyatis akjei* and *Raja porosa*. *Food Res. Int.* **2013**, *51*, 283–293. [CrossRef]
59. Li, X.R.; Chi, C.F.; Li, L.; Wang, B. Purification and identification of antioxidant peptides from protein hydrolysate of scalloped hammerhead (*Sphyrna lewini*) cartilage. *Mar. Drugs* **2017**, *15*, 61. [CrossRef] [PubMed]

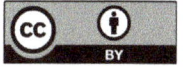

© 2018 by the authors. Licensee MDPI, Basel, Switzerland. This article is an open access article distributed under the terms and conditions of the Creative Commons Attribution (CC BY) license (http://creativecommons.org/licenses/by/4.0/).

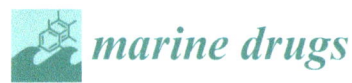

Article

Anti-Photoaging Effects of Low Molecular-Weight Fucoidan on Ultraviolet B-Irradiated Mice

Young-In Kim [1,2,†], Won-Seok Oh [1,†], Phil Hyun Song [3,†], Sungho Yun [4], Young-Sam Kwon [4], Young Joon Lee [5], Sae-Kwang Ku [6], Chang-Hyun Song [6,*] and Tae-Ho Oh [1,*]

1. Department of Veterinary Internal Medicine, College of Veterinary Medicine, Kyungpook National University, Daegu 41566, Korea; kimyoungin@kpclab.co.kr (Y.-I.K.); owsvcs@hanmail.net (W.-S.O.)
2. KPC Corporation, Gwangju 12773, Korea
3. Department of Urology, College of Medicine, Yeungnam University, Daegu 42415, Korea; sph04@yu.ac.kr
4. Department of Veterinary Surgery, College of Veterinary Medicine, Kyungpook National University, Daegu 41566, Korea; shyun@knu.ac.kr (S.Y.); kwon@knu.ac.kr (Y.-S.K.)
5. Department of Preventive Medicine, College of Korean Medicine, Daegu Haany University, Gyeongsan 38610, Korea; gksxntk@dhu.ac.kr
6. Department of Anatomy and Histology, College of Korean Medicine, Daegu Haany University, Gyeongsan 38610, Korea; gucci200@hanmail.net
* Correspondence: dvmsong@dhu.ac.kr (C.-H.S.); thoh@knu.ac.kr (T.-H.O.); Tel.: +82-53-819-1822 (C.-H.S.); +82-53-950-5959 (T.-H.O.); Fax: +82-53-819-1822 (C.-H.S.); +82-53-950-7488 (T.-H.O.)
† These authors contributed equally to this paper.

Received: 20 July 2018; Accepted: 17 August 2018; Published: 18 August 2018

Abstract: Ultraviolet (UV) B exposure induces DNA damage and production of reactive oxygen species (ROS), which causes skin photoaging through signaling pathways of inflammation and modulation of extracellular matrix remodeling proteins, collagens, and matrix metalloproteinase (MMP). As low molecular-weight fucoidan (LMF) has potential antioxidant and anti-inflammatory properties, we examined the protective effects of LMF against UVB-induced photoaging. A UVB-irradiated mouse model was topically treated with myricetin or LMF at 2.0, 1.0 and 0.2 mg/cm^2 (LMF2.0, LMF1.0 and LMF0.2, respectively) once a day for 15 weeks. Wrinkle formation, inflammation, oxidative stress, MMP expression, and apoptosis in the treated regions were compared with those in a distilled water-treated photoaging model (UVB control). LMF treatments, particularly LMF2.0 and LMF1.0, significantly inhibited the wrinkle formation, skin edema, and neutrophil recruitment into the photo-damaged lesions, compared with those in the UVB control. While LMF decreased interleukin (IL)-1β release, it increased IL-10. The LMF treatment inhibited the oxidative stresses (malondialdehyde and superoxide anion) and enhanced endogenous antioxidants (glutathione). Additionally, LMF reduced the mRNA expression of MMP-1, 9, and 13. The histopathological analyses revealed the anti-photoaging effects of LMF exerted via its antioxidant, anti-apoptotic, and MMP-9-inhibiting effects. These suggest that LMF can be used as a skin-protective remedy for photoaging.

Keywords: skin-aging; UVB; low molecular-weight; fucoidan; antioxidant; anti-inflammation; MMP

1. Introduction

Along with the increasing aging population and their demands for maintaining youthful skin, a development of skin anti-aging agents has attracted attention in the pharmaceutical and cosmetic science fields. Skin aging is divided into intrinsic chronological aging and extrinsic aging caused by various external stimuli, mainly ultraviolet (UV) radiation, called photoaging. In particular, UVB comprising 5–10% of all UV wavelengths is considered as the main cause of skin photoaging characterized by wrinkles, thickness, laxity, roughness, and pigmentation [1]. The mechanism involves a direct DNA damage and formation of photoproducts including cyclobutane pyrimidine dimers and pyrimidine (1,2) pyrimidine photoproducts. The photoproducts trigger apoptosis, cytokine release, immunosuppression, and signal transduction, severely followed by carcinogenesis [2]. In addition, repetitive exposure to UVB increases intracellular reactive oxygen species (ROS), leading to oxidative DNA damage, and activation of inflammation and extracellular matrix (ECM) remodeling proteins including matrix metalloproteinases (MMPs) [3]. Currently, UVB-induced photoaging has recently increased because of progressive depletion of the ozone layer, and thus optimal anti-photoaging remedies are required to increase treatment options.

Basic photoaging prevention is simply blocking sunlight through protective clothing or filters. However, because UVB exposure has positive effects on vitamin (Vt.) D3 synthesis, particularly in chronic kidney disease patients, the strict photoprotection may need additional vitamin (Vt.) D supplementation [4]. Additionally, the method is not effective for treating skin that is already photo-damaged. Thus, many topical treatments have been evaluated to reduce photoaging; retinoids, known as Vt. A (i.e., tretinoin, tazarotene, adapalene, retinol and retinaldehyde, alitretinoin), are drugs shown to reverse skin aging. However, only two topical retinoids, tretinoin and tazarotene, have received U.S. Food and Drug Administration approval for treating photoaging [5]. The other anti-photoaging reagents available include numerous natural antioxidants such as ascorbic acid (Vt. C) and tocopherol (Vt. E), as well as medicinal plant extracts including polyphenolic compounds, particularly flavonoids [4,5]. For example, myricetin, a flavonoid found in several foods (i.e., onions, berries, grapes, and red wines), has shown anti-photoaging effects through its antioxidant and anti-inflammatory properties [6,7]. The beneficial effects have encouraged researchers to develop photo-protective products from natural sources [8–11].

Fucoidan, found mainly in marine brown algae, is a complex sulfated polysaccharide, which has various pharmacological properties including antioxidant, anti-inflammatory, anticoagulant, antiviral, and anticancer effects [12,13]. Furthermore, unlike native fucoidan with a high molecular-weight of approximately 20,000 kDa, low molecular-weight fucoidan (LMF)—less than 10 kDa—has shown more biological activities because of its high absorption and bioavailability [13]. However, a few studies have examined the anti-photoaging effect of fucoidans, which include three in vitro studies demonstrating the down-regulating effects on MMP-1 [14–16] and one in vivo study showing inhibitory effects on inflammation and MMP-1 expression following oral administration [17]. We previously showed that topical application of LMF has dermal wound healing effects with anti-inflammatory and antioxidant activities and modulates ECM rebuilding factors, such as transforming growth factor (TGF)-β1, fibroblast growth factor (FGF)-2, and MMPs [18]. It suggests that LMF also exerts biological effects involved in anti-photoaging.

To produce LMF, enzymatic hydrolysis methods are more advantageous than acid-hydrolysis or other conventional techniques; the method is non-toxic because enzymes are converted into water-soluble materials, and high bioactive compound yield and enhanced antioxidant activities are achieved [19]. Previously, fucoidan from Gamte, *Ecklonia cava* distributed along Korean coasts, has shown high antioxidant effects in a DPPH (1,1-diphenyl-2-picrylhydrazyl) free radical scavenging assay [19]. Therefore, we examined the anti-photoaging effects of LMF isolated from *E. cava*, using an enzymatic hydrolysis technique in UVB-irradiated mice, and the underlying mechanisms of these effects.

2. Results

2.1. Body Weight Changes

Body weights were normal in the UVB-irradiated mice (UVB control) compared with those of non-irradiated normal mice (Intact). The body weight changes did not differ among any groups regardless of the treatments (Figure 1).

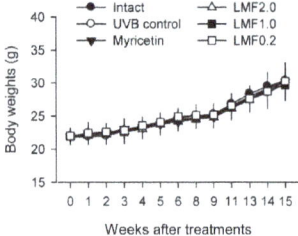

Figure 1. Non-irradiated normal mice and one group of UV (ultraviolet) B-irradiated mice were topically treated with distilled water (Intact and UVB control, respectively). The other four groups of UVB-irradiated mice were treated with myricetin (Myricetin) or low molecular-weight fucoidan (LMF) at 2.0, 1.0, and 0.2 mg/cm^2 (LMF2.0, LMF1.0, and LMF0.2, respectively). The body weights were measured every week after treatment, and expressed as means ± SD of eight mice per group.

2.2. Wrinkle Formation and Edema in UVB-Irradiated Skin

To examine the protective effects of LMF on photo-damages, skin wrinkle formation and tissue weights of the cutaneous edema were assessed. The UVB-irradiated dorsal back skin and its replicas showed evident wrinkle formation, but no skin cancer lesions were found. The wrinkle formation was observed to be severe in the UVB control group, whereas it was mild in the Myricetin and LMF groups (Figure 2A). Indeed, wrinkle length and depth in the skin replicas were significantly increased in the UVB control group compared with those in the intact, however, these values were decreased in the Myricetin and LMF groups compared with those in the UVB control (Figure 2B,C) ($p < 0.05$). In particular, the wrinkling degree did not differ between the LMF2.0 or LMF1.0 and the intact group. Wrinkle lengths were decreased by 37.4%, 46.1%, 39.5%, and 24.7% in the Myricetin, LMF2.0, LMF1.0, and LMF0.2 groups, respectively, and wrinkle depths were decreased by 32.5%, 52.3%, 41.3%, and 33.8%, respectively, compared with the corresponding values in the UVB control. Similarly, skin weight was significantly increased in the UVB control compared with that in the intact, but decreased in the Myricetin and LMF groups, especially in the LMF2.0 and LMF1.0 (Figure 2D) ($p < 0.05$). Decreases of 41.4%, 60.9%, 51.0%, and 42.1% in the Myricetin, LMF2.0, LMF1.0, and LMF0.2, respectively, were found compared with those in the UVB control group.

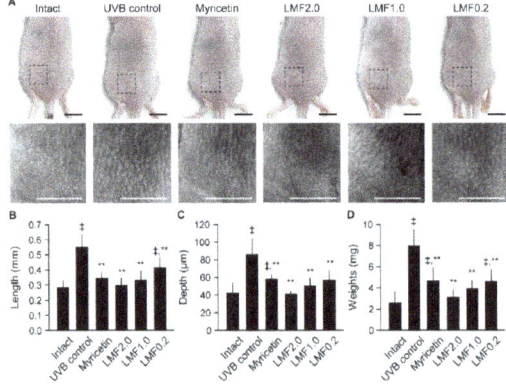

Figure 2. After treatments for 15 weeks, the left dorsal back skin (upper) and its replicas (lower) were observed (**A**). Scale bars indicate 10 mm. Wrinkle length (**B**) and depth (**C**) were assessed from the skin replicas. The dermal tissues were sampled and weighed (**D**). Values were expressed as means ± SD of 8 mice per group. ‡ $p < 0.01$ vs. intact and ** $p < 0.01$ vs. UVB control.

2.3. UVB-Irradiated Skin Inflammation

UVB irradiation leads to leukocyte infiltration by dilating dermal blood vessels and increasing vascular hypermeability [8]. Thus, the skin myeloperoxidase (MPO) was assessed as a proinflammatory enzyme in the granulocytes. Consistently, the skin MPO activities were significantly increased in the UVB control compared with those in the intact ($p < 0.05$) (Figure 3A), indicating enhanced neutrophil recruitment to UVB-irradiated skin lesions. However, MPO activities were decreased in the Myricetin and LMF groups ($p < 0.05$). In addition, the dermal levels of IL-1β, a cytokine stimulating neutrophil, were increased in the UVB control compared with those in the intact, but decreased in the Myricetin and LMF groups compared with those in the UVB control (Figure 3B) ($p < 0.05$). In contrast, the level of IL-10, an anti-inflammatory cytokine, was significantly increased in the Myricetin and LMF groups compared with that in the UVB control (Figure 3C) ($p < 0.05$).

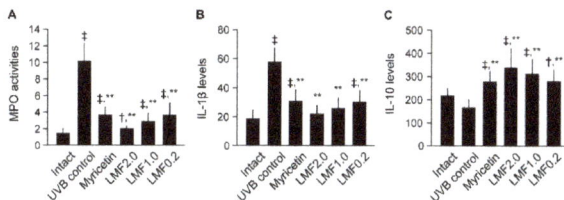

Figure 3. After treatments for 15 weeks, myeloperoxidase (MPO) activity (neutrophils × 10^5 per mg of tissue protein, **A**) and skin levels of IL-1β and IL-10 (pg per 100 mg of protein, **B** and **C**, respectively) were assessed in UVB-irradiated skins. Values were expressed as means ± SD of 8 mice per group. ‡ $p < 0.01$, † $p < 0.05$ vs. intact, and ** $p < 0.01$ vs. UVB control.

2.4. Antioxidant Activities in UVB-Irradiated Skin

The skin contents of glutathione (GSH) as an endogenous antioxidant were measured, and level of malondialdehyde (MDA) for lipid peroxidation and superoxide anion were assessed for the oxidative stress (Table 1). The GSH content was significantly decreased in the UVB control compared with that in the intact, but increased in the Myricetin and LMF groups ($p < 0.05$). In contrast, the levels of MDA and superoxide anion were significantly increased in the UVB control compared with those in the intact, but decreased in the Myricetin and LMF groups, particularly in the LMF2.0 ($p < 0.05$). The higher GSH and the lower levels of MDA and superoxide suggest antioxidant effects of LMF on the UVB-damaged skins. The antioxidant activities were further examined by measuring the mRNA expression levels of GSH reductase, an enzyme that regenerates GSH from the oxidized disulfide form, and Nox2, a nicotinamide adenine dinucleotide phosphate (NADPH) oxidase related to ROS formation (Table 2). The mRNA expression of GSH reductase was significantly lower in the UVB control than in the intact, but higher in the Myricetin and LMF groups than in the UVB control ($p < 0.05$). In contrast, Nox2 expression was higher in the UVB control than in the intact, but lower in the Myricetin and LMF groups than in the UVB control ($p < 0.05$).

2.5. mRNA Expression of MMPs Related to Skin Photoaging

As UV radiation stimulates MMPs to promote the breakdown of collagen [20], the skin remodeling process was examined by detecting the mRNA expression of MMP-1, MMP-9, and MMP-13 (Table 2). These expressions were significantly up-regulated in the UVB control compared with that in the intact ($p < 0.05$). However, they were significantly down-regulated in the Myricetin and LMF groups compared with that in the UVB control ($p < 0.05$).

Table 1. Antioxidant activities in ultraviolet (UV) B-irradiated skins.

	GSH (µM/mg)	MDA (nM/mg)	Superoxide Anion (NBT Reduction)
Intact	1.47 ± 0.62	0.34 ± 0.11	0.36 ± 0.08
UVB control	0.41 ± 0.09 ‡	1.68 ± 0.41 ‡	1.03 ± 0.18 ‡
Myricetin	0.95 ± 0.15 †,**	0.69 ± 0.20 ‡,**	0.56 ± 0.16 ‡,**
LMF2.0	1.44 ± 0.14 **	0.40 ± 0.10 **	0.36 ± 0.08 **
LMF1.0	1.36 ± 0.20 **	0.51 ± 0.13 †,**	0.49 ± 0.08 †,**
LMF0.2	0.94 ± 0.18 †,**	0.67 ± 0.13 ‡,**	0.56 ± 0.15 ‡,**

Non-irradiated normal group and one group of UVB-irradiated mice were topically treated with distilled water (intact and UVB control, respectively). The other four groups of UVB-irradiated mice were treated with myricetin at 0.32 ng/cm^2 (Myricetin) or low molecular-weight fucoidan (LMF) at 2.0, 1.0, and 0.2 mg/cm^2 (LMF2.0, LMF1.0, and LMF0.2, respectively). After treatment for 15 weeks, the glutathione (GSH), malondialdehyde (MDA) and superoxide anions were assessed in the skin tissues and they were normalized to the tissue proteins. Values are expressed as means ± SD of eight mice. NBT = nitroblue tetrazolium. ‡: $p < 0.01$ and †: $p < 0.05$ vs. intact, and **: $p < 0.01$ vs. UVB control.

Table 2. Tissue mRNA expressions in UVB-irradiated skins.

	MMP-1	MMP-9	MMP-13	GSH Reductase	Nox2
Intact	1.04 ± 0.09	1.07 ± 0.10	1.06 ± 0.07	1.01 ± 0.09	1.01 ± 0.08
UVB control	2.02 ± 0.20 ‡	1.93 ± 0.23 ‡	2.29 ± 0.25 ‡	0.79 ± 0.15 ‡	1.71 ± 0.22 ‡
Myricetin	1.34 ± 0.18 ‡,**	1.31 ± 0.14 ‡,**	1.47 ± 0.21 ‡,**	1.28 ± 0.16 ‡,**	1.22 ± 0.14 ‡,**
LMF2.0	1.06 ± 0.09 **	1.12 ± 0.08 **	1.15 ± 0.07 †,**	1.93 ± 0.19 ‡,**	1.06 ± 0.08 **
LMF1.0	1.20 ± 0.09 †,**	1.16 ± 0.09 †,**	1.26 ± 0.05 ‡,**	1.58 ± 0.36 ‡,**	1.12 ± 0.08 †,**
LMF0.2	1.33 ± 0.14 ‡,**	1.28 ± 0.09 ‡,**	1.47 ± 0.17 ‡,**	1.30 ± 0.12 ‡,**	1.22 ± 0.05 ‡,**

After treatment for 15 weeks, expressions of mRNA for matrix metalloprotease (MMP)-1, -9, and -13, GSH reductase and nicotinamide adenine dinucleotide phosphate (NADPH) oxidase 2 (Nox2) were assessed. Values are expressed as means ± SD of eight mice for relative mRNA expressions per β-actin. ‡: $p < 0.01$, †: $p < 0.05$ vs. intact, and **: $p < 0.01$ vs. UVB control.

2.6. Histopathological Changes

The UVB control exhibited increased epithelial thickness and microfold formation with hyperplasia and hypertrophy of the epidermal keratinocytes in hematoxylin-eosin stains (Figure 4). In addition, the UVB control showed increases in altered collagen deposition in the Masson's trichrome (MT) stains. However, the histopathological changes appeared to be reversed in the Myricetin and LMF groups. Histomorphometric analyses revealed significant increases in epithelial thickness, microfolds, infiltrated inflammatory cells, and regions occupying collagen fibers in the UVB control compared with those in the intact ($p < 0.05$) (Table 3). However, the changes were significantly inhibited in the Myricetin and LMF groups compared with those in the UVB control ($p < 0.05$).

Table 3. Histopathological changes on UVB-irradiated skins.

	Microfolds (Folds/mm)	Epi. Thickness (µm)	IF Cells (Cells/mm^2)	Collagen Fiber (%/mm^2)
Intact	10.50 ± 3.63	20.54 ± 2.52	9.50 ± 2.98	45.31 ± 5.75
UVB control	74.75 ± 10.94 ‡	48.28 ± 5.04 ‡	269.50 ± 50.65 ‡	82.54 ± 8.20 ‡
Myricetin	39.50 ± 13.73 ‡,**	30.26 ± 5.08 ‡,**	204.50 ± 51.29 ‡,*	59.32 ± 6.17 ‡,**
LMF2.0	19.63 ± 4.17 ‡,**	26.75 ± 4.04 ‡,**	31.00 ± 7.19 ‡,**	48.44 ± 2.97 **
LMF1.0	38.63 ± 5.10 ‡,**	30.63 ± 2.04 ‡,**	61.25 ± 14.57 ‡,**	55.72 ± 7.89 ‡,**
LMF0.2	56.88 ± 5.99 ‡,**	32.89 ± 3.83 ‡,**	140.00 ± 38.37 ‡,**	59.77 ± 8.94 ‡,**

After treatments for 15 weeks, microfolds, epithelial (Epi.) thickness, and inflammatory (IF) cells were assessed in hematoxylin-eosin stains in Figure 4, and relative regions of collagen fiber was assessed in Masson's trichrome stains. Values are expressed as means ± SD of eight mice. ‡: $p < 0.01$ vs. intact, **: $p < 0.01$, and *: $p < 0.05$ vs. UVB control.

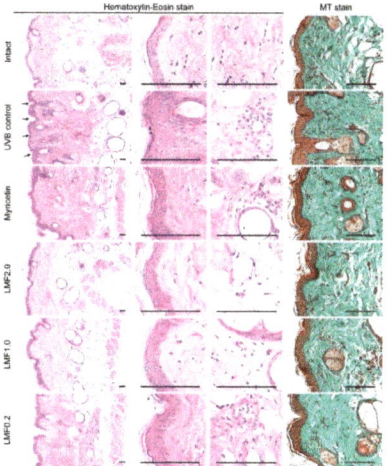

Figure 4. Skin tissue sections were stained with hematoxylin and eosin or Masson's trichrome (MT). Arrows indicate epithelial microfolds formed. Scale bars indicate 100 μm.

2.7. Immunohistochemistry

Immunostaining for nitrotyrosine and 4-hydroxynonenal (4-HNE), as markers of oxidative stress, and caspase-3 and cleaved poly (adenosine diphosphate-ribose) polymerase (PARP), as markers of apoptosis, showed more intense signals in the UVB control than in the intact. The MMP-9 was also detected more in the UVB control than the intact (Figure 5). However, the tendencies were decreased in the Myricetin and LMF groups. Histomorphometric analyses revealed significant increases in immunoreactive cells for nitrotyrosine, 4-HNE, caspase-3, PARP, and MMP-9 in the UVB control compared with those in the intact ($p < 0.05$) (Table 4). However, the immunoreactive cells were significantly reduced in the Myricetin and LMF groups ($p < 0.05$).

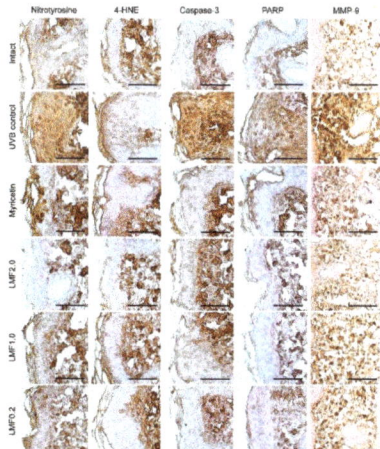

Figure 5. Skin tissue sections were immunostained for nitrotyrosine and 4-hydroxynonenal (4-HNE), as markers of oxidative stress; caspase-3 and poly (adenosine diphosphate-ribose) polymerase (PARP) as markers of apoptosis; and matrix metalloproteinase (MMP)-9. Next, the sections were counterstained with hematoxylin. Scale bars indicate 50 μm.

Table 4. Immunohistochemistry in UVB-irradiated skins.

	Nitrotyrosine	4-HNE	Caspase-3	PARP	MMP-9
Intact	12.00 ± 4.21	12.50 ± 3.07	17.38 ± 3.25	15.13 ± 3.04	31.25 ± 8.58
UVB control	86.88 ± 10.11 ‡	78.00 ± 10.72 ‡	83.50 ± 10.17 ‡	79.13 ± 11.00 ‡	81.75 ± 11.62 ‡
Myricetin	50.00 ± 6.70 ‡,**	43.13 ± 12.17 ‡,**	32.00 ± 6.55 ‡,**	38.88 ± 8.01 ‡,**	51.88 ± 8.04 ‡,**
LMF2.0	21.38 ± 4.44 ‡,**	19.50 ± 2.56 ‡,**	21.13 ± 2.90 †,**	21.13 ± 2.53 ‡,**	43.00 ± 5.13 ‡,**
LMF1.0	36.25 ± 5.65 ‡,**	33.00 ± 3.70 ‡,**	26.13 ± 4.22 ‡,**	23.88 ± 3.14 ‡,**	48.63 ± 5.01 ‡,**
LMF0.2	50.25 ± 6.11 ‡,**	39.75 ± 4.53 ‡,**	30.25 ± 3.20 ‡,**	36.75 ± 5.01 ‡,**	53.00 ± 8.02 ‡,**

After treatments for 15 weeks, immunostains in Figure 5 were examined; immunostains for nitrotyrosine, 4-hydroxynonenal (4-HNE), and caspase-3 and cleaved poly (adenosine diphosphate-ribose) polymerase (PARP) were assessed as epidermal immunoreactive cells per 100 epithelial cells, and matrix metalloprotease (MMP)-9 was assessed as relative immunoreactive regions per regions of interests (%). Values are expressed as means ± SD of eight mice. ‡: $p < 0.01$, †: $p < 0.05$ vs. intact, and **: $p < 0.01$ vs. UVB control.

3. Discussion

Similar to the clinical symptoms of chronic UV exposure, our UVB-irradiated model exhibited increased winkle formation and dermal thickness, and decreased skin elasticity [1]. However, LMF treatment inhibited photoaging by enhancing antioxidant, anti-inflammatory, and anti-apoptotic activities and inhibiting ECM degradation through down-regulating UV-responsive genes encoding MMP-1, MMP-9, and MMP-13. Because the LMF treatment was mostly absorbed before the irradiation, the results seemed to be involved in photo-protective effects rather than UV filtering effects. Although only one in vivo study has demonstrated the anti-photoaging effects of native fucoidan via oral administration [17], this is the first study to show that LMF ameliorates UBV-induced photoaging via topical application.

UVB irradiation induces ROS production and deteriorates the antioxidant defense system, leading to a state of oxidative stress [21]. Here, UVB irradiation up-regulated the mRNA expression of Nox2 as an ROS producer and increased the dermal contents of superoxide anion and MDA, while it reduced dermal GSH contents by down-regulating GSH reductase. However, LMF treatment inhibited the progression to oxidative stress and enhanced innate antioxidant activities. Immunostaining for nitrotyrosine or 4-HNE also revealed that LMF exert a strong antioxidant activity against photo-damage. To date, fucoidans from various algae, including *Porphyra haitanesis*, *Ulva pertusa*, *F. vesiculosus*, *Laminaria japonica*, and *Ecklonia kurome* have been shown to possess antioxidant properties [13]. The beneficial effects are thought to be conferred by the chemical compositions of fucoidans such as sulfate, monosaccharide, sugar residue [18,22]. It suggests that LMF has substantial fucose and sulfate content as a natural antioxidants involved in modulating a number of oxidative stress-mediated diseases including photoaging.

With the antioxidant activities, LMF treatment showed anti-inflammatory effects on UVB-irradiated skins, which was supported by inhibiting edema and neutrophil recruitment to photo-damaged lesions. The anti-inflammatory activities of LMF may contribute to decreasing IL-1β and increasing IL-10 levels. The imbalance between ROS production and the antioxidant defense system is known to cause skin inflammation through complex pathways [23]. ROS activate mitogen-activated protein kinase (MAPK) signaling transduction pathways. MAPK pathways activate nuclear factor (NF)-κB and activator protein-1 (AP-1), which enhances the release of inflammatory cytokines such as tumor necrosis factor-α, IL-1β, IL-6, and IL-8 [21,24]. In particular, Nox2 and superoxide anion contribute to stimulating neutrophil infiltration. In this context, the antioxidant effects of LMF may result in inhibition of the inflammatory progress. However, the anti-photoaging effects of LMF likely occur through interactive mechanisms between antioxidant and anti-inflammatory effects. For example, because fucoidan directly inhibits neutrophil infiltration by blocking selectin [25], the reduced neutrophils may be linked to inhibition of the release of free oxygen radicals by reducing MPO activities. In addition, because IL-1β activates Nox complexes as producers of ROS and IL-10 inhibits the NF-κB pathways, the decreased IL-1β and increased IL-10 may be linked to inhibited production of ROS and further release of inflammatory cytokine [26]. Thus, the antioxidant and anti-inflammatory effects of LMF have therapeutic potentials for treating skin photoaging.

Wrinkle formation is closely related to the degradation of ECM proteins via collagen fragmentation and MMP secretion [20]. MMPs are activated by excessive oxidative stress or inflammatory responses: oxidative stresses up-regulate MMPs including MMP-1, MMP-3, MMP-9, and MMP-13 through binding of AP-1 to MMPs, and pro-inflammatory cytokines also up-regulate MMPs and degrade dermal collagen elastin fibers [27]. Thus, the development of MMP inhibitors is considered a promising strategy for anti-photoaging. Some flavonoid compounds, such as naringenim, apigenin, wogonin, kaempferol, and quercetin, have been reported to inhibit the expression of MMP-1 and type I procollagen [28]. Here, LMF treatment down-regulated the gene expression of MMP-1, MMP-9 and MMP-13. Previous studies have shown that native fucoidans modulate MMP-1 expression in human fibroblasts [14–16]. Furthermore, L-fucose and fucose-rich polysaccharides have a direct relationship with increased synthesis of elastin and collagen by down-regulating MMPs, particularly MMP-2 and MMP-9 [29–31]. These results demonstrate that LMF attenuates connective tissue damage by inhibiting MMP activities and enhancing collagen synthesis.

In photoaging, a failure in the repair mechanisms of DNA damage leads to apoptosis through the AP-1 signaling pathway [32]. Various molecules, such as T4N5, photolyase, and thymidine dinucleotide, have been proven to be valuable for photoaging protection by enhancing the repair of DNA photo-damage [5]. Fucoidans isolated from various brown algae also have been reported to inhibit oxidative DNA damage in tumor cells [33,34] and diabetic cardiomyocytes [35]. The beneficial effects are involved in the interactions between fucoidans and growth factors including basic FGF [36] and TGF-β [37], suggesting their therapeutic potentials for tissue repair. Indeed, LMF decreased immunoreactive cells for caspase-3 and PARP in UVB-irradiated skin lesions, likely by inhibiting the MAPK pathways related to NF-κB and AP-1.

Overall, these results demonstrate the anti-photoaging effects of LMF on UVB-irradiated skin damage by cooperative interactions of antioxidant, anti-inflammatory, and MMP-inhibiting effects. Furthermore, fucoidan has been reported to inhibit melanin formation, which may be useful for developing treatments for hyperpigmentation [38]. Taken together, these finding suggest that LMF can serve as a potential agent for treating UV-related skin disease.

4. Materials and Methods

4.1. Reagents

LMF was kindly provided by Glucan Corp. Ltd. (Busan, Korea). To produce LMF, a commercial high molecular-weight fucoidan from Gamte, *E. cava* (Aqua Green Technology Co., Ltd., Jeju, Korea) was reduced by reacting fucoidan with fucoidanase isolated from *Pseudoalteromonas* sp. (strain 1493) for 2 h at 50 °C and pH 8 [9,39]. The resulting solution was filtered through 10 and 5 kDa ceramic membranes, and then lyophilized. The molecular weight was nearly 8 kDa according to gel permeation chromatography based on high-performance liquid chromatography analysis. Myricetin was purchased from Sigma-Aldrich (St. Louis, MO, USA). LMF and myricetin were dissolved in distilled water and acetone, respectively.

4.2. Animals

All animal experiments were performed according to the national regulations of the usage and welfare of laboratory animals and approved by the Institutional Animal Care and Use Committee in Daegu Haany University (Gyeongsan, Korea) (DHU2012-058, 20 October 2012). Six-week female HR-1 hairless mice (SLC, Shizuoka, Japan) were housed in a polycarbonate cage and maintained in a temperature (20–25 °C) and humidity (50–55%) controlled room with a 12-h light/dark cycle. Food and water were supplied ad libitum.

4.3. Skin Photoaging Model and Treatment

After eight day acclimatization, the mice were divided into six groups ($n = 8$/group) with similar body weights. In five groups, skin photoaging was induced by 0.18 J/cm^2 UVB irradiation three times a week using a UV crosslinker system emitting wavelengths of 254 nm, 312 nm, and 365 nm, with a peak emission at 312 nm (Hoefer Scientific Instruments, San Francisco, CA, USA), as described previously [40]. The remaining group was not irradiated with the off-system. Treatment was applied topically to the left dorsal back skin in a 1 × 1 cm area near the gluteal region in a volume of 200 µL as follows: the UVB non-irradiated group and one irradiated group were treated with distilled water (intact and UVB control, respectively), and other UVB-irradiated groups were treated with myricetin at 5 nM (0.32 ng/cm^2) (Myricetin) or LMF at 10 (2.0 mg/cm^2), 5 (1.0 mg/cm^2), and 1 mg/mL (0.2 mg/cm^2) (LMF2.0, LMF1.0, and LMF0.2, respectively). The application was performed once a day for 15 weeks. The body weight of mice was measured every week.

4.4. Macroscopic Analysis of UVB-Irradiated Skin

UVB-irradiated skin wrinkles were assessed in replicas of the mouse dorsal skins including the treated region using the Repliflo Cartridge Kit (CuDerm Corp., Dallas, TX, USA), as described previously [40]. Wrinkle shadows of the impression replicas were generated using an optical light with an angle of 40°. The black and white images were analyzed by Skin-Visiometer VL650 software (Courage & Khazaka, Cologne, Germany). Next, the dorsal skin was sampled using a punch with a 6-mm diameter, and the sample was weighed for skin edema. The skin samples, including other treated regions, were homogenized for biochemical analyses or fixed for histopathological analyses.

4.5. Measurement of Leukocyte Migration to UVB-Irradiated Skin

Leukocyte migration to UVB-irradiated skin damage was analyzed by the MPO assay [24]. The skin sample was homogenized in 50 mM K_2HPO_4 buffer (pH 6.0) containing 0.5% hexadecyltrimethylammonium bromide for 15 s on ice. After centrifuging at 1000× g for 2 min at 4 °C, the supernatants were mixed with the K_2HPO_4 buffer (pH 6.0) containing 0.167 mg/mL o-dianisidine dihydrochloride and 0.05% hydrogen peroxide, and the absorbance was assessed at 450 nm (OPTIZEN POP, Mecasys, Daejeon, Korea). The tissue protein was measured using the Lowry method. In comparison with a standard curve of neutrophils, MPO activity was expressed as the number of neutrophils/mg of protein.

4.6. Measurement of IL-1β and IL-10 in UVB-Irradiated Skin

The skin samples were homogenized as described previously [40]. IL-1β and IL-10 was assessed using an enzyme-linked immunosorbent assay kit (Abcam, Cambridge, UK) according to the manufacturer's instructions. The absorbance was measured at 490 nm using a microplate spectrophotometer reader (Tecan, Männedorf, Switzerland).

4.7. Antioxidant Activities in UVB-Irradiated Skin

To determine glutathione (GSH) contents, skin sample was homogenized in 100 mM NaH_2PO_4 buffer solution (pH 8.0) containing 5 mM ethylenediaminetetraacetic acid (1:3, w/w dilution). The homogenates were added with 30% trichloroacetic acid, and centrifuged twice at 1940× g for 6 min and then at 485× g for 10 min. The supernatant was added to 1 mg/mL o-phthalaldehyde (Sigma-Aldrich), and measured in a fluorescence spectrophotometer (RF-5301PC; Shimadzu Corp., Tokyo, Japan) (kexc = 350 nm; kem = 420 nm). Values were expressed as µM of GSH/mg of protein compared with a standard curve using diluted solutions of GSH (75 µM). Another tissue sample was homogenized at 10 mg/mL in 1.15% KCl, as described previously [40]. For MDA, the homogenates were added to 10% trichloroacetic acid, and centrifuged at 1000× g for 3 min. The supernatant was incubated with 0.67% thiobarbituric acid for 15 min at 100 °C, and then assessed at 535 and 572 nm using a spectrophotometer reader (Tecan). For superoxide anion, the homogenates were incubated with 1 mg/mL nitroblue tetrazolium (NBT, Sigma-Aldrich) for 1 h at 37 °C. The supernatant was removed and the formazan precipitates were solubilized with a mixture of 2 M potassium hydroxide and dimethyl sulfoxide. The reduction of NBT to formazan by superoxide anion was measured at 600 nm using a spectrophotometer reader (Tecan).

4.8. Quantitative Reverse Transcription Polymerase Chain Reaction (qRT-PCR) Analysis

Total skin tissue RNA was extracted using TRIzol reagent (Invitrogen, Carlsbad, CA, USA), as described previously [24,40]. RNA concentration and quality were analyzed using a CFX96™ Real-Time System (Bio-Rad, Hercules, CA, USA). The sample was treated with recombinant DNase I (DNA-free; Ambion, Austin, TX, USA) to remove contaminating DNA, and RNA was reverse-transcribed using a reagent High-Capacity cDNA Reverse Transcription Kit (Applied Biosystems, Foster City, CA, USA) according to the manufacturer's instructions. A total of 50 PCR cycles were performed as follows: 95 °C for 15 s, 60 °C for 20 s, and 72 °C for 30 s for denaturation, annealing, and extension, respectively. The primers used are listed in Table S1.

4.9. Histopathology

Skin samples were fixed in 10% neutral buffered formalin. The samples were paraffin-embedded and sectioned at a thickness of 3 μm. The sections were stained with hematoxylin and eosin (H&E) or Masson's trichrome (MT). In H&E, histomorphometric analyses were performed for epithelial microfolds (folds/mm of epithelium), epithelial thicknesses (μm), and inflammatory cells infiltrated in the dermis (cells/mm^2 of dermis), using a computer-assisted image analysis program (iSolution FL ver 9.1, IMT i-solution Inc., Vancouver, BC, Canada). In the MT stain, the area occupying collagen fiber (%/mm^2 of dermis) was assessed. The histopathologist was blinded to the treatment groups.

4.10. Immunohistochemistry

The other serial sections were deparaffinized and rehydrated, followed by antigen retrieval pretreatment in 10 mM citrate buffer for 20 min at 95–100 °C (Shi et al., 1993). The sections were immunostained using a Vectastain Elite ABC Kit (Vector Lab., Inc., Burlingame, CA, USA), as described previously [18,40]. Briefly, endogenous peroxidase was inactivated by 0.3% H_2O_2 for 30 min, and non-specific binding of proteins was blocked with normal horse serum for 1 h. The sections were incubated with primary rabbit polyclonal antibodies for cleaved caspase-3 (# 9661, Cell Signaling Technology Inc., Danvers, MA, USA, 1:400), cleaved PARP (# 9545, Cell Signaling Technology, 1:100), 4-HNE (# Ab 46545, Abcam, 1:100), nitrotyrosine (# 06-284, Millipore, Billerica, MA, USA, 1:200), or MMP-9 (# Ab 38898, Abcam, 1:100), overnight at 4 °C. The following day, the sections were incubated with biotinylated secondary antibody and then ABC reagents for 1 h each. Immunoreactivity was visualized using a peroxidase substrate kit (Vector Lab.) for 3 min, and counterstained with hematoxylin. All incubation procedures were carried out in a humidity chamber, and the sections were rinsed with 10 mM phosphate-buffered saline three times between each step. Cells or fibers occupying more than 30% of the immunoreactivity were regarded as positive, and analyzed using the iSolution program. The histopathologist was blinded to the groupings.

4.11. Statistical Analyses

Values are expressed as means ± standard deviation (SD) of eight sample sizes. Variance homogeneity was examined by using the Levene test. If no significance was detected, the data were analyzed by one way analysis of variance (ANOVA) followed by a least-significant differences multi-comparison (LSD) post hoc test. In a case of significances, a non-parametric Kruskal–Wallis H test was conducted, followed by the Mann–Whitney U (MW) post hoc test. The analyses focused mainly on the differences among treatment groups compared with the UVB control. A p-value < 0.05 indicated significance.

Supplementary Materials: The following are available online at http://www.mdpi.com/1660-3397/16/8/286/s1, Table S1: Primers used for quantitative RT-PCR.

Author Contributions: Y.-I.K., W.-S.O., P.H.S., and T.-H.O. conceived and designed the experiments; Y.-I.K., P.H.S., and S.-K.K. carried out the experiments and analyzed the data; S.Y., Y.-S.K., and Y.J.L. performed partially experiments and statistical analyses; Y.-I.K., W.-S.O., and P.H.S. drafted the paper; and C.-H.S. and T.-H.O. supervised and reviewed the manuscript. All authors read and approved the final manuscript.

Funding: This study was supported by the National Research Foundation of Korea grant funded by the Korean government (grant no. 2012R1A5A2A42671316), and by the 2016 Yeungnam University Research Grant.

Conflicts of Interest: The authors declare no conflict of interest.

References

1. Fisher, G.J.; Wang, Z.Q.; Datta, S.C.; Varani, J.; Kang, S.; Voorhees, J.J. Pathophysiology of premature skin aging induced by ultraviolet light. *N. Engl. J. Med.* **1997**, *337*, 1419–1428. [CrossRef] [PubMed]
2. Svobodova, A.; Walterova, D.; Vostalova, J. Ultraviolet light induced alteration to the skin. *Biomed. Pap. Med. Fac. Univ. Palacky Olomouc Czech Repub.* **2006**, *150*, 25–38. [CrossRef] [PubMed]
3. Finkel, T.; Holbrook, N.J. Oxidants, oxidative stress and the biology of ageing. *Nature* **2000**, *408*, 239–247. [CrossRef] [PubMed]
4. Krause, R. Vitamin D and UV exposure in chronic kidney disease. *Dermatoendocrinol* **2013**, *5*, 109–116. [CrossRef] [PubMed]
5. Antoniou, C.; Kosmadaki, M.G.; Stratigos, A.J.; Katsambas, A.D. Photoaging: Prevention and topical treatments. *Am. J. Clin. Dermatol.* **2010**, *11*, 95–102. [CrossRef] [PubMed]
6. Jung, S.K.; Lee, K.W.; Kim, H.Y.; Oh, M.H.; Byun, S.; Lim, S.H.; Heo, Y.S.; Kang, N.J.; Bode, A.M.; Dong, Z.; et al. Myricetin suppresses UVB-induced wrinkle formation and MMP-9 expression by inhibiting Raf. *Biochem. Pharmacol.* **2010**, *79*, 1455–1461. [CrossRef] [PubMed]
7. Sim, G.S.; Lee, B.C.; Cho, H.S.; Lee, J.W.; Kim, J.H.; Lee, D.H.; Kim, J.H.; Pyo, H.B.; Moon, D.C.; Oh, K.W.; et al. Structure activity relationship of antioxidative property of flavonoids and inhibitory effect on matrix metalloproteinase activity in UVA-irradiated human dermal fibroblast. *Arch. Pharm. Res.* **2007**, *30*, 290–298. [CrossRef] [PubMed]
8. Divya, S.P.; Wang, X.; Pratheeshkumar, P.; Son, Y.O.; Roy, R.V.; Kim, D.; Dai, J.; Hitron, J.A.; Wang, L.; Asha, P.; et al. Blackberry extract inhibits UVB-induced oxidative damage and inflammation through MAP kinases and NF-kappaB signaling pathways in SKH-1 mice skin. *Toxicol. Appl. Pharmacol.* **2015**, *284*, 92–99. [CrossRef] [PubMed]
9. Lim, J.Y.; Kim, O.K.; Lee, J.; Lee, M.J.; Kang, N.; Hwang, J.K. Protective effect of the standardized green tea seed extract on UVB-induced skin photoaging in hairless mice. *Nutr. Res. Pract.* **2014**, *8*, 398–403. [CrossRef] [PubMed]
10. Patwardhan, J.; Bhatt, P. Ultraviolet-B Protective Effect of Flavonoids from Eugenia caryophylata on Human Dermal Fibroblast Cells. *Pharmacogn. Mag.* **2015**, *11* (Suppl. 3), S397–S406. [PubMed]
11. Cavinato, M.; Waltenberger, B.; Baraldo, G.; Grade, C.V.C.; Stuppner, H.; Jansen-Durr, P. Plant extracts and natural compounds used against UVB-induced photoaging. *Biogerontology* **2017**, *18*, 499–516. [CrossRef] [PubMed]
12. Berteau, O.; Mulloy, B. Sulfated fucans, fresh perspectives: Structures, functions, and biological properties of sulfated fucans and an overview of enzymes active toward this class of polysaccharide. *Glycobiology* **2003**, *13*, 29R–40R. [CrossRef] [PubMed]
13. Senthilkumar, K.; Manivasagan, P.; Venkatesan, J.; Kim, S.K. Brown seaweed fucoidan: Biological activity and apoptosis, growth signaling mechanism in cancer. *Int. J. Biol. Macromol.* **2013**, *60*, 366–374. [CrossRef] [PubMed]
14. Moon, H.J.; Lee, S.H.; Ku, M.J.; Yu, B.C.; Jeon, M.J.; Jeong, S.H.; Stonik, V.A.; Zvyagintseva, T.N.; Ermakova, S.P.; Lee, Y.H. Fucoidan inhibits UVB-induced MMP-1 promoter expression and down regulation of type I procollagen synthesis in human skin fibroblasts. *Eur. J. Dermatol.* **2009**, *19*, 129–134. [PubMed]
15. Moon, H.J.; Lee, S.R.; Shim, S.N.; Jeong, S.H.; Stonik, V.A.; Rasskazov, V.A.; Zvyagintseva, T.; Lee, Y.H. Fucoidan inhibits UVB-induced MMP-1 expression in human skin fibroblasts. *Biol. Pharm. Bull.* **2008**, *31*, 284–289. [CrossRef] [PubMed]

16. Moon, H.J.; Park, K.S.; Ku, M.J.; Lee, M.S.; Jeong, S.H.; Imbs, T.I.; Zvyagintseva, T.N.; Ermakova, S.P.; Lee, Y.H. Effect of Costaria costata fucoidan on expression of matrix metalloproteinase-1 promoter, mRNA, and protein. *J. Nat. Prod.* **2009**, *72*, 1731–1734. [CrossRef] [PubMed]
17. Maruyama, H.; Tamauchi, H.; Kawakami, F.; Yoshinaga, K.; Nakano, T. Suppressive Effect of Dietary Fucoidan on Proinflammatory Immune Response and MMP-1 Expression in UVB-Irradiated Mouse Skin. *Planta Med.* **2015**, *81*, 1370–1374. [PubMed]
18. Park, J.H.; Choi, S.H.; Park, S.J.; Lee, Y.J.; Park, J.H.; Song, P.H.; Cho, C.M.; Ku, S.K.; Song, C.H. Promoting Wound Healing Using Low Molecular Weight Fucoidan in a Full-Thickness Dermal Excision Rat Model. *Mar. Drugs* **2017**, *15*, 112. [CrossRef] [PubMed]
19. Heo, S.J.; Park, E.J.; Lee, K.W.; Jeon, Y.J. Antioxidant activities of enzymatic extracts from brown seaweeds. *Bioresour. Technol.* **2005**, *96*, 1613–1623. [CrossRef] [PubMed]
20. Naylor, E.C.; Watson, R.E.; Sherratt, M.J. Molecular aspects of skin ageing. *Maturitas* **2011**, *69*, 249–256. [CrossRef] [PubMed]
21. Wang, X.F.; Huang, Y.F.; Wang, L.; Xu, L.Q.; Yu, X.T.; Liu, Y.H.; Li, C.L.; Zhan, J.Y.; Su, Z.R.; Chen, J.N.; et al. Photo-protective activity of pogostone against UV-induced skin premature aging in mice. *Exp. Gerontol.* **2016**, *77*, 76–86. [CrossRef] [PubMed]
22. Ale, M.T.; Mikkelsen, J.D.; Meyer, A.S. Important determinants for fucoidan bioactivity: A critical review of structure-function relations and extraction methods for fucose-containing sulfated polysaccharides from brown seaweeds. *Mar. Drugs* **2011**, *9*, 2106–2130. [CrossRef] [PubMed]
23. D'Orazio, J.; Jarrett, S.; Amaro-Ortiz, A.; Scott, T. UV radiation and the skin. *Int. J. Mol. Sci.* **2013**, *14*, 12222–12248. [CrossRef] [PubMed]
24. Campanini, M.Z.; Pinho-Ribeiro, F.A.; Ivan, A.L.; Ferreira, V.S.; Vilela, F.M.; Vicentini, F.T.; Martinez, R.M.; Zarpelon, A.C.; Fonseca, M.J.; Faria, T.J.; et al. Efficacy of topical formulations containing Pimenta pseudocaryophyllus extract against UVB-induced oxidative stress and inflammation in hairless mice. *J. Photochem. Photobiol. B* **2013**, *127*, 153–160. [CrossRef] [PubMed]
25. Tedder, T.F.; Steeber, D.A.; Chen, A.; Engel, P. The selectins: Vascular adhesion molecules. *FASEB J.* **1995**, *9*, 866–873. [CrossRef] [PubMed]
26. Weiss, E.; Mamelak, A.J.; La Morgia, S.; Wang, B.; Feliciani, C.; Tulli, A.; Sauder, D.N. The role of interleukin 10 in the pathogenesis and potential treatment of skin diseases. *J. Am. Acad. Dermatol.* **2004**, *50*, 657–675, quiz 676–678. [CrossRef] [PubMed]
27. Pittayapruek, P.; Meephansan, J.; Prapapan, O.; Komine, M.; Ohtsuki, M. Role of Matrix Metalloproteinases in Photoaging and Photocarcinogenesis. *Int. J. Mol. Sci.* **2016**, *17*, 868. [CrossRef] [PubMed]
28. Lim, H.; Kim, H.P. Inhibition of mammalian collagenase, matrix metalloproteinase-1, by naturally-occurring flavonoids. *Planta Med.* **2007**, *73*, 1267–1274. [CrossRef] [PubMed]
29. Isnard, N.; Peterszegi, G.; Robert, A.M.; Robert, L. Regulation of elastase-type endopeptidase activity, MMP-2 and MMP-9 expression and activation in human dermal fibroblasts by fucose and a fucose-rich polysaccharide. *Biomed. Pharmacother.* **2002**, *56*, 258–264. [CrossRef]
30. Robert, L.; Fodil-Bourahla, I.; Bizbiz, L.; Robert, A.M. Effect of L-fucose and fucose-rich polysaccharides on elastin biosynthesis, in vivo and in vitro. *Biomed. Pharmacother.* **2004**, *58*, 123–128. [CrossRef] [PubMed]
31. Fodil-Bourahla, I.; Bizbiz, L.; Schoevaert, D.; Robert, A.M.; Robert, L. Effect of L-fucose and fucose-rich oligo- and polysaccharides (FROP-s) on skin aging: Penetration, skin tissue production and fibrillogenesis. *Biomed. Pharmacother.* **2003**, *57*, 209–215. [CrossRef]
32. Kulms, D.; Schwarz, T. Molecular mechanisms involved in UV-induced apoptotic cell death. *Skin Pharmacol. Appl. Skin Physiol.* **2002**, *15*, 342–347. [CrossRef] [PubMed]
33. Hsu, H.Y.; Lin, T.Y.; Lu, M.K.; Leng, P.J.; Tsao, S.M.; Wu, Y.C. Fucoidan induces Toll-like receptor 4-regulated reactive oxygen species and promotes endoplasmic reticulum stress-mediated apoptosis in lung cancer. *Sci. Rep.* **2017**, *7*, 44990. [CrossRef] [PubMed]
34. Chen, L.M.; Liu, P.Y.; Chen, Y.A.; Tseng, H.Y.; Shen, P.C.; Hwang, P.A.; Hsu, H.L. Oligo-Fucoidan prevents IL-6 and CCL2 production and cooperates with p53 to suppress ATM signaling and tumor progression. *Sci. Rep.* **2017**, *7*, 11864. [CrossRef] [PubMed]
35. Yu, X.; Zhang, Q.; Cui, W.; Zeng, Z.; Yang, W.; Zhang, C.; Zhao, H.; Gao, W.; Wang, X.; Luo, D. Low molecular weight fucoidan alleviates cardiac dysfunction in diabetic Goto-Kakizaki rats by reducing oxidative stress and cardiomyocyte apoptosis. *J. Diabetes Res.* **2014**, *2014*, 420929. [CrossRef] [PubMed]

36. Matou, S.; Helley, D.; Chabut, D.; Bros, A.; Fischer, A.M. Effect of fucoidan on fibroblast growth factor-2-induced angiogenesis in vitro. *Thromb. Res.* **2002**, *106*, 213–221. [CrossRef]
37. McCaffrey, T.A.; Falcone, D.J.; Vicente, D.; Du, B.; Consigli, S.; Borth, W. Protection of transforming growth factor-beta 1 activity by heparin and fucoidan. *J. Cell. Physiol.* **1994**, *159*, 51–59. [CrossRef] [PubMed]
38. Wang, Z.J.; Xu, W.; Liang, J.W.; Wang, C.S.; Kang, Y. Effect of Fucoidan on B16 Murine Melanoma Cell Melanin Formation and Apoptosis. *Afr. J. Tradit. Complement. Altern. Med.* **2017**, *14*, 149–155. [CrossRef] [PubMed]
39. Bilan, M.I.; Kusaykin, M.I.; Grachev, A.A.; Tsvetkova, E.A.; Zvyagintseva, T.N.; Nifantiev, N.E.; Usov, A.I. Effect of enzyme preparation from the marine mollusk Littorina kurila on fucoidan from the brown alga Fucus distichus. *Biochemistry* **2005**, *70*, 1321–1326. [CrossRef] [PubMed]
40. Kang, S.J.; Choi, B.R.; Kim, S.H.; Yi, H.Y.; Park, H.R.; Song, C.H.; Ku, S.K.; Lee, Y.J. Beneficial effects of dried pomegranate juice concentrated powder on ultraviolet B-induced skin photoaging in hairless mice. *Exp. Ther. Med.* **2017**, *14*, 1023–1036. [CrossRef] [PubMed]

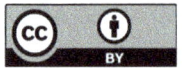

© 2018 by the authors. Licensee MDPI, Basel, Switzerland. This article is an open access article distributed under the terms and conditions of the Creative Commons Attribution (CC BY) license (http://creativecommons.org/licenses/by/4.0/).

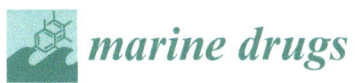

Article

Protective Effect of Sulfated Polysaccharides from Celluclast-Assisted Extract of *Hizikia fusiforme* Against Ultraviolet B-Induced Skin Damage by Regulating NF-κB, AP-1, and MAPKs Signaling Pathways In Vitro in Human Dermal Fibroblasts

Lei Wang [1], WonWoo Lee [2], Jae Young Oh [1], Yong Ri Cui [1], BoMi Ryu [1,*] and You-Jin Jeon [1,*]

[1] Department of Marine Life Sciences, Jeju National University, Jeju 63243, Korea; comeonleiwang@163.com (L.W.); ojy0724@naver.com (J.Y.O.); chyr6019@126.com (Y.R.C.)
[2] Freshwater Bioresources Utilization Division, Nakdonggang National Institute of Biological Resources, Sangju 37242, Korea; 21cow@naver.com
* Correspondence: bmryu@jejunu.ac.kr (B.R.); youjinj@jejunu.ac.kr (Y.-J.J.); Tel.: +82-64-754-3475 (B.R. & Y.-J.J.); Fax: +82-64-756-3493 (B.R. & Y.-J.J.)

Received: 12 June 2018; Accepted: 14 July 2018; Published: 17 July 2018

Abstract: Our previous study evaluated the antioxidant activities of sulfated polysaccharides from Celluclast-assisted extract of *Hizikia fusiforme* (HFPS) *in vitro* in Vero cells and *in vivo* in zebrafish. The results showed that HFPS possesses strong antioxidant activity and suggested the potential photo-protective activities of HFPS. Hence, in the present study, we investigated the protective effects of HFPS against ultraviolet (UV) B-induced skin damage *in vitro* in human dermal fibroblasts (HDF cells). The results indicate that HFPS significantly reduced intracellular reactive oxygen species (ROS) level and improved the viability of UVB-irradiated HDF cells in a dose-dependent manner. Furthermore, HFPS significantly inhibited intracellular collagenase and elastase activities, remarkably protected collagen synthesis, and reduced matrix metalloproteinases (MMPs) expression by regulating nuclear factor kappa B (NF-κB), activator protein 1 (AP-1), and mitogen-activated protein kinases (MAPKs) signaling pathways in UVB-irradiated HDF cells. These results suggest that HFPS possesses strong UV protective effect, and can be a potential ingredient in the pharmaceutical and cosmetic industries.

Keywords: *Hizikia fusiforme*; sulfated polysaccharides; ultraviolet-B; MMPs; NF-κB; AP-1; MAPKs

1. Introduction

In humans, skin is the largest organ of the integumentary system. It undergoes chronological aging similar to other organs. Skin is in direct exposure to the outside environment and therefore it undergoes aging as a consequence of environmental damage [1]. Ultraviolet (UV) irradiation from sunlight is the primary environmental factor that induces human skin aging and results in pigment accumulation and wrinkle formation. Human skin is frequently affected by oxidative stress caused by continuous exposure to UV irradiation from sunlight. Skin exposed to UV and environmental oxidizing pollutants is associated with diverse abnormal reactions including inflammatory responses, epidermal hyperplasia, the breakdown of collagen, and melanin accumulation [2,3].

UV can be classified into three subtypes of UVA, UVB, and UVC, based on the wavelength. UVB has a medium wavelength and is thought to bring more cellular stress to humans compared to the other two subtypes [4–6]. UVB is known to be associated with human health through stimulating reactive oxygen species (ROS) generation [7,8]. The excessive ROS subsequently activate cell signaling pathways including nuclear factor kappa B (NF-κB), activator protein 1 (AP-1), and mitogen-activated protein kinases (MAPKs), which stimulate matrix metalloproteinases (MMPs) expression [9]. MMPs are a class of structurally similar enzymes, and play a major role in physiological and pathological tissue remodeling. The imbalance of MMP expression could lead to cartilage, cardiac, and cancer-related diseases [10]. MMPs degrade the collagenous extra cellular matrix (ECM) in connective tissues, which is the main factor of wrinkling. Therefore, an ideal MMP inhibitor or an agent that reduces the expression of MMPs may be effective against wrinkle formation, and could be thought as a promising candidate to be used as an ingredient in the cosmetic industry.

Marine organisms are rich resources of several natural compounds such as polyphenol, polysaccharide, sterol, and peptide, which possess various bioactivities including antioxidant, anticancer, anti-inflammatory, anti-obesity, antihypertensive, anti-diabetes, and UV protective activities [11–20]. *Hizikia fusiforme* (*H. fusiforme*) is an edible brown seaweed, which is distributed in the areas of the northwest Pacific, including Korea, China, and Japan. *H. fusiforme* has been utilized as a traditional medicine and functional food. It contains various compounds, which possesses several of bioactivities, especially polysaccharides. Many studies have reported that polysaccharides from *H. fusiforme* possess various bioactivities such as antioxidant, anti-inflammatory, anti-angiogenic, anticancer, osteoprotective, and immunostimulatory activities [21–24]. Our previous research displayed that sulfated polysaccharides from Celluclast-assisted extract of *H. fusiforme* (HFPS) possess strong free radical scavenging activity and protective effects on H_2O_2-induced oxidative stress *in vitro* in Vero cells and *in vivo* in zebrafish [25]. These results suggest that HFPS may possess photo-protective activity. However, the protective effects of HFPS against UVB-induced skin damage have not yet been reported. Thus, the purpose of the present study was to investigate the protective effect of HFPS against UVB-induced skin damage *in vitro* in human dermal fibroblasts (HDF cells).

2. Results and Discussion

2.1. HFPS Inhibits Collagenase from Clostridium Histolyticum and Elastase from Porcine Pancreas

Both collagenase and elastase belong to proteases that break down proteins. Collagenase is the enzyme that breaks the peptide bonds in collagen, which is the key component of animal ECM. Elastase is the enzyme that breaks down elastin, which is an elastic fiber. Collagen and elastin together determine the mechanical properties of the connective tissue. In human skin, degradation of collagen leads to decreased skin thickness, and degradation of elastin results in losing skin elasticity. These are the major characteristics of wrinkle formation in aged skin. Thus, a collagenase or elastase inhibitor could be thought as an agent to reduce skin aging.

In this study, the inhibitory effects of HFPS against commercial collagenase and elastase were measured. As shown in Figure 1, HFPS inhibits collagenase and elastase in a dose-dependent manner. The collagenase inhibitory rates of HFPS were 13.46%, 22.58%, and 49.77% at the concentrations of 50, 100, and 200 μg/mL, respectively (Figure 1A); and the elastase inhibitory rates of HFPS were 18.78%, 38.14%, and 56.53% at the concentrations of 50, 100, and 200 μg/mL, respectively (Figure 1B). These results indicate that HFPS may possess the activity against skin aging through inhibition of collagenase and elastase.

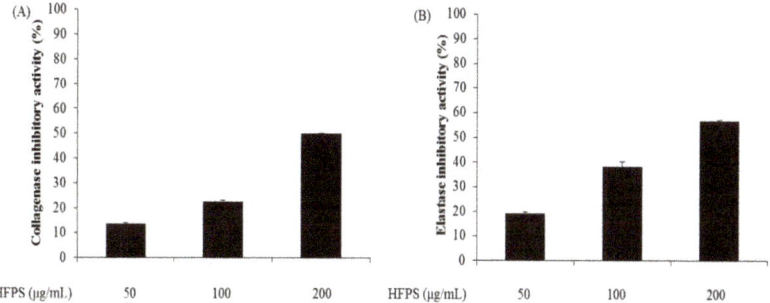

Figure 1. HFPS inhibits commercial collagenase and elastase: (**A**) collagenase inhibitory activity of HFPS; and (**B**) elastase inhibitory activity of HFPS. The experiments were conducted in triplicate, and the data are expressed as the means ± standard error (SE).

2.2. HFPS Promotes HDF Cell Proliferation and UVB Irradiation Damages HDF Cells

Skin is continuously exposed to UVB from sunlight, thus it is a major target of oxidative stress [26]. UVB-induced skin cell oxidative stress leads to cell damage, resulting in skin photoaging. Over the past decades, with industrial development, the oxidizing pollutants in the air and UV irradiated to the earth have increased. This is becoming a serious issue that threatens the skin health of humans. Therefore, finding nontoxic and effective agents that can protect dermic damage would be valuable for medical and cosmetic industries.

As the first step to evaluate protective effects and mechanisms of HFPS against UVB-induced skin damage in HDF cells, we employed various levels of UVB irradiation to induce cell damage in HDF cells, and determined the cytotoxicity of HFPS at different concentrations on HDF cells. As Figure 2 shows, UVB irradiation significantly decreased the viability of HDF cells in a dose-dependent manner (Figure 2A). Furthermore, the optimal UVB dose applied to HDF cells based on the 50% growth inhibitory dose was determined to be 50 mJ/cm^2. We then assessed the effect of HFPS alone on HDF cells. The cytotoxicity results (Figure 2B) suggest that HFPS is non-toxic on HDF cells and promotes HDF cells proliferation in a dose-dependent manner. This promotion of proliferation was comparable in cells treated with 100 µg/mL and 50 µg/mL samples. From these results, 50 mJ/cm^2 was determined as the optimal UVB dose applied to HDF cells and 100 µg/mL was selected as the maximum concentration of HFPS for further study.

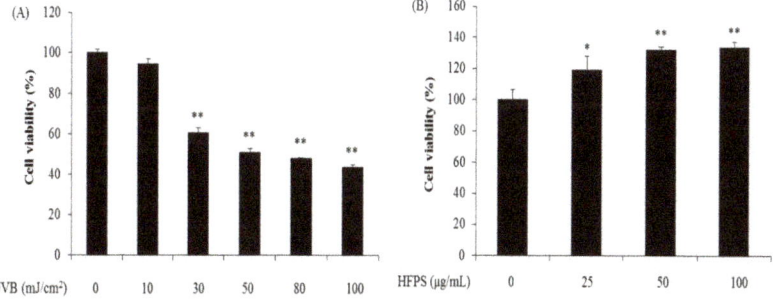

Figure 2. UVB irradiation damages HDF cells and HFPS promotes HDF cell proliferation: (**A**) cytotoxicity of UVB irradiation on HDF cells; and (**B**) proliferation effect of HFPS on HDF cells. Cell viability was measured by 3-(4-5-dimethyl-2yl)-2-5-diphenyltetrazolium bromide (MTT) assay. The data are expressed as the means ± SE ($n = 3$), * $p < 0.05$, ** $p < 0.01$ as compared to control group.

2.3. HFPS Improves Cell Viability and Scavenges Intracellular ROS Generated in UVB-Irradiated HDF Cells

UVB irradiation induces skin damage though stimulated intracellular ROS generation [27]. Recently, identification of ROS scavengers from natural resources has been given more attention. Our previous study isolated phlorotannins from marine algal, *Ecklonia cava*, and evaluated their UV protective effect. The results displayed that phlorotannins reduced intracellular ROS induced by UVB irradiation and improved cell viability in a dose-dependent manner [26]. Zeng et al. investigated the protective effect of polysaccharides from *Ganoderma lucidum* against UVB-induced photoaging. The results suggest that polysaccharides from *Ganoderma lucidum* significantly reduced ROS levels and improved the viability of UVB-irradiated cells [28].

In the present study, HDF cells were pretreated with HFPS and irradiated with UVB at a dose of 50 mJ/cm^2. Cell viability was subsequently measured by MTT assay and intracellular ROS level was analyzed by DCF-DA assay. As Figure 3 shows, cell viability was decreased while intracellular ROS level was increased after UVB irradiation. Treatment with increasing concentrations of HFPS (25, 50, and 100 µg/mL) improved cell viability by 11.78%, 14.97%, and 19.21% (Figure 3A) and intracellular ROS scavenging by 21.95%, 36.44%, and 48.14% (Figure 3B). These results indicate that HFPS possesses a protective effect against UVB-induced cellular damage via ROS clearance in HDF cells.

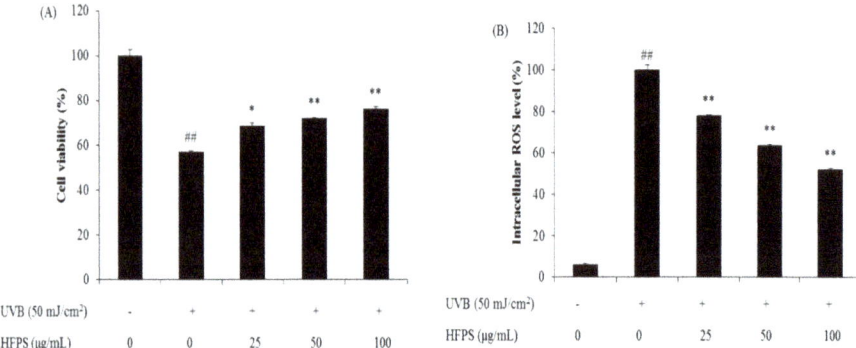

Figure 3. Protective effects of HFPS against UVB-induced HDF cell damage: (**A**) protective effects of HFPS against UVB-induced HDF cell damage; and (**B**) intracellular ROS scavenging effect of HFPS in UVB-irradiated HDF cells. Cell viability was measured by MTT assay and intracellular ROS level was measured by DCF-DA assay. The data are expressed as the means ± SE (n = 3). * p < 0.05, ** p < 0.01 as compared to UVB-exposed group and ## p < 0.01 as compared to control group.

2.4. HFPS Inhibits Intracellular Collagenase and Elastase Activities in UVB-Irradiated HDF Cells

Aged skin is thin and inelastic due to degradation of collagen and elastin in the ECM of connective tissue. Collagenase and elastase are key enzymes during collagen and elastin degradation. UVB stimulates the activities of fibroblast collagenase and elastase in the dermis consequently causing wrinkle formation [29,30]. As Figure 4 shows, the relative collagenase and elastase activities of UVB-irradiated HDF cells were significantly increased compared with non-irradiated cells. However, relative activities of both enzymes were decreased in the cells pretreated with HFPS in a dose-dependent manner. These results suggest that HFPS may act as an inhibitor of fibroblast collagenase and elastase and may prevent wrinkle formation induced by UVB irradiation.

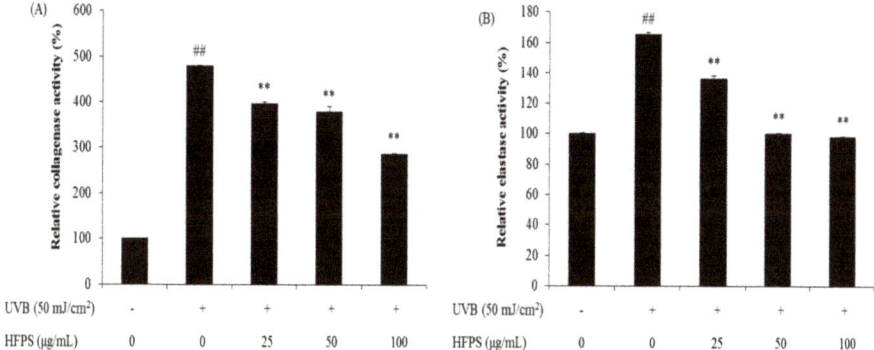

Figure 4. HFPS inhibits intracellular collagenase and elastase activities in UVB-irradiated HDF Cells: (**A**) relative collagenase activity; and (**B**) relative elastase activity. The data are expressed as the means ± SE (n = 3). * $p < 0.05$, ** $p < 0.01$ as compared to UVB-exposed group and ## $p < 0.01$ as compared to control group.

2.5. HFPS Protects Collagen Synthesis and Reduces MMPs Expression Levels in UVB-Irradiated HDF Cells

MMPs, particularly MMP-2 and MMP-9, have been identified as being central to degradation of ECM [31]. In addition, MMP-1 degrades two major structural proteins, type I and type III collagen [32]. Collagen is synthesized as a precursor molecule, procollagen, which contains additional peptide sequences. These sequences are cleaved off during collagen secretion, thus, a number of sequences can indirectly reflect collagen synthesis level. We determined procollagen type I carboxy-terminal peptide (PIP) to investigate collagen synthesis level.

As Figure 5 shows, UVB irradiation significantly decreased collagen synthesis in HDF cells, and HFPS dose-dependently protects collagen synthesis (Figure 5A). Furthermore, MMPs' expression levels were significantly increased in UVB-irradiated HDF cells but decreased in HFPS pretreated cells (Figure 5B–F). These results suggest that HFPS effectively protects collagen synthesis and reduces the expression of MMPs.

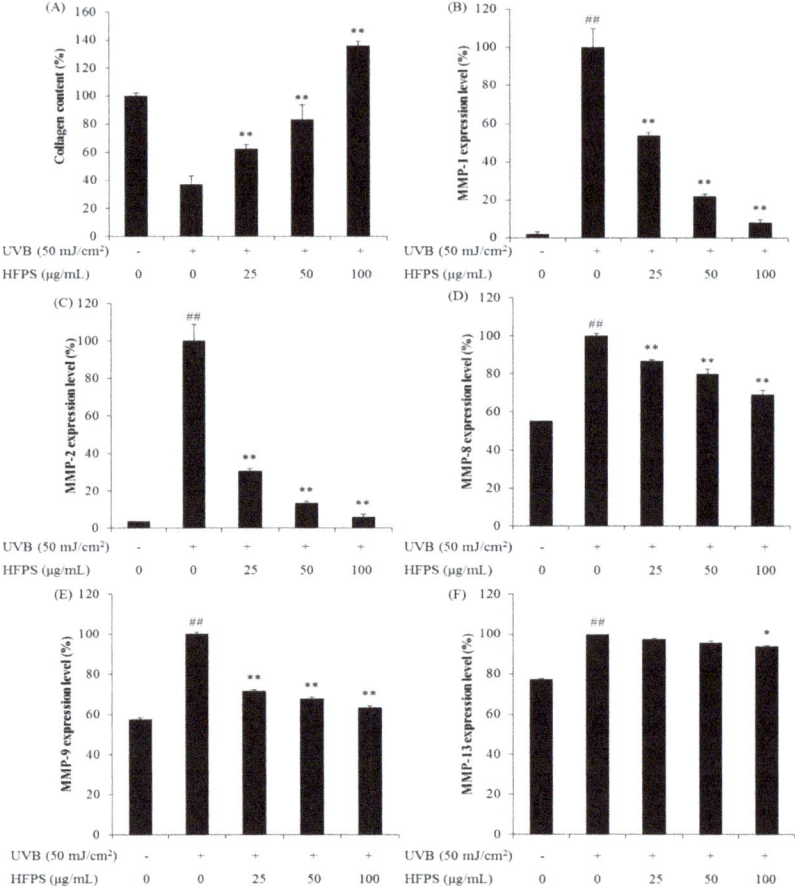

Figure 5. HFPS improve collagen synthesis and reduces MMPs expression in UVB-irradiated HDF cells: (**A**) collagen synthesis level in UVB-irradiated HDF cells; (**B**) MMP-1 expression level in UVB-irradiated HDF cells; (**C**) MMP-2 expression level in UVB-irradiated HDF cells; (**D**) MMP-8 expression level in UVB-irradiated HDF cells; (**E**) MMP-9 expression level in UVB-irradiated HDF cells; and (**F**) MMP-13 expression level in UVB-irradiated HDF cells. Collagen synthesis level was reflected by the amounts of PIP, and the amounts of PIP and MMPs were measured by the commercially ELISA kits, based on the manufacturer's instructions. The data are expressed as the means ± SE (n = 3). * $p < 0.05$, ** $p < 0.01$ as compared to UVB-exposed group and ## $p < 0.01$ as compared to control group.

2.6. HFPS Inhibits Nuclear Factor Kappa B (NF-κB) Activation, Reduces Activator Protein 1 (AP-1) Phosphorylation, and Suppresses Mitogen-Activated Protein Kinases (MAPKs) Activation in UVB-Induced HDF Cells

NF-κB is a protein complex that controls cytokine production, transcription of DNA, and cell survival. NF-κB plays an important role in immune responses, and dysregulation of NF-κB is associated with various diseases such as cancer, inflammation, and aging [33]. Many studies have reported that UVB irradiation can activate NF-κB, and the activation of NF-κB can induce MMPs expression [34–36]. As Figure 6 shows, UVB irradiation significantly increases nuclear levels of NF-κB (p65 and p50); however, HFPS treatment remarkably reduces nuclear NF-κB levels in UVB-irradiated HDF cells in a dose-dependent manner.

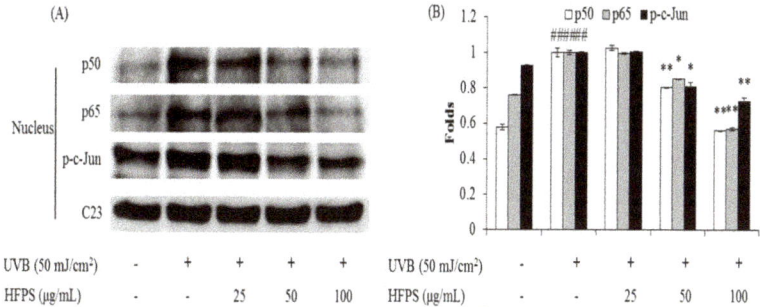

Figure 6. HFPS inhibits UVB-induced NF-κB activation and reduces AP-1 phosphorylation in UVB-irradiated HDF cells: (**A**) the inhibitory effects of HFPS on UVB-induced NF-κB related (p65 and p50) protein expression and AP-1 phosphorylation; and (**B**) relative amounts of NF-κB expressions and AP-1 phosphorylation levels. The relative amounts of NF-κB expressions and AP-1 phosphorylation were compared with C23. The data are expressed as the means ± SE ($n = 3$). * $p < 0.05$, ** $p < 0.01$ as compared to UVB-exposed group and ## $p < 0.01$ as compared to control group.

MAPKs are a type of protein kinases, which are involved in directing cellular responses to different stimuli, such as heat shock, mitogens, and pro-inflammatory cytokines. MAPKs regulate various cell functions including proliferation, differentiation, gene expression, cell survival and apoptosis [37,38]. The activation of MAPKs occurs through the phosphorylation of p38, Jun N-terminal kinase (JNK), and extracellular-regulated protein (ERK) signaling pathways. AP-1(c-Jun) is a nuclear transcription factor, which is phosphorylated after the activated MAPKs were translocated to the nucleus [39]. Subsequently, the expression of MMPs is up-regulated [33,40]. In the present study, the activated AP-1 and MAPKs levels were detected by Western blot analysis. The results indicate that UVB irradiation significantly phosphorylates AP-1 and HFPS remarkably reduces the phosphorylated AP-1 (p-c-Jun) levels in a dose-dependent manner (Figure 6). In addition, HFPS treatment effectively suppresses UVB-induced p38, JNK, and ERK phosphorylation in UVB-irradiated HDF cells (Figure 7). These results indicate that HFPS regulates NF-κB activation, AP-1 phosphorylation, and MAPKs activation in UVB-induced HDF cells.

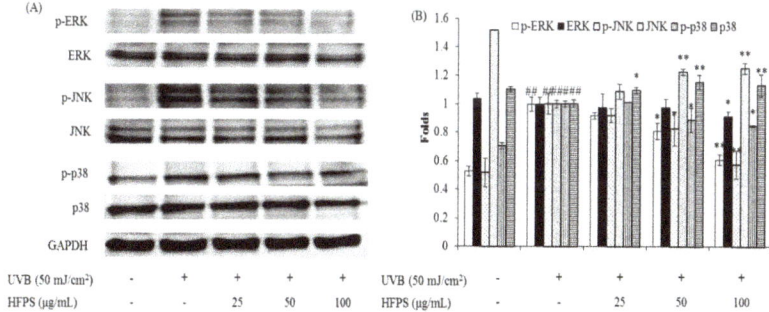

Figure 7. HFPS suppress MAPKs activation in UVB-irradiated HDF cells: (**A**) the inhibitory effects of HFPS on UVB-induced MAPKs activation; and (**B**) relative amounts of activated MAPKs levels. The relative amounts of activated MAPKs levels were compared with GAPDH. The data are expressed as the means ± S.E ($n = 3$). * $p < 0.05$, ** $p < 0.01$ as compared to UVB-exposed group and ## $p < 0.01$ as compared to control group.

3. Materials and Methods

3.1. Materials and Reagents

The fluorescent probe 2′, 7′-dichlorodihydroflurescin diacetate (DCFH-DA), dimethyl sulfoxide (DMSO), 3-(4-5-dimethyl-2yl)-2-5-diphynyltetrasolium bromide (MTT), 1 × phosphate buffered saline (PBS), collagenase from clostridium histolyticum, elastase from porcine pancreas, azo dye-impregnted collagen, and N-succinyl-Ala-Ala-Ala-p-nitroanilide were purchased from Sigma Co. (St. Louis, MO, USA). The Dulbecco's modified Eagle medium (DMEM), Ham's Nutrient Mixtures medium (F-12), penicillin/streptomycin, and fetal bovine serum (FBS) were purchased from Gibco BRL (Life Technologies, Burlington, ON, Canada). Antibodies against GAPDH, C23, p-c-Jun, NF-κB p65 and NF-κB p50, ERK and phospho-ERK, JNK and phospho-JNK, and p38 and phospho-p38 were purchased from Santa Cruz Biotechnology (Santa Cruz, CA, USA). Anti-rabbit IgG antibodies was purchased from Cell Signaling Technology (Beverly, MA, USA). PIP ELISA kit was purchased from TaKaRa Bio Inc. (Kusatsu, Japan) and Human MMP-1, 2, 8, 9, and 13 ELISA kits were purchased from GE Healthcare Life Sciences (Exeter, Devon, UK). All other chemicals used in this study were of analytical grade.

HFPS were prepared in our previous study. The separation and analysis procedures were described by Wang et al. [25]. In brief, the lyophilized *H. fusiforme* was hydrolyzed by Celluclast (Sigma, St. Louis, MO, USA, ≥700 units/g) at the optimal condition (pH 4.5, 50 °C) for 24 h and the polysaccharides (HFPS) were obtained by ethanol precipitation. HFPS contains 63.56% sulfated polysaccharides, which constitutes by glucose (5.95%), xylose (17.37%), galactose (23.15%), and fucose (53.53%).

3.2. Measurement of Enzyme Inhibitory Effects of HFPS

3.2.1. Measurement of Inhibitory Effect on Collagenase from Clostridium Histolyticum

To measure the collagenase inhibitory activity, a weight of 1 mg of azo dye-impregnated collagen was mixed with 800 µL of 0.1 M Tris-HCl (pH 7.0), 100 µL of 200 units/mL collagenase (stock solution), and 100 µL sample and incubated at 43 °C for 1 h under shaking condition. Subsequently, the reaction mixture was centrifuged at 3000 rpm for 10 min and the absorbance of the supernatant was detected at 550 nm in a microplate reader (BioTek Synergy HT, Woburn, MA, USA).

3.2.2. Measurement of Inhibitory Effect on Elastase from Porcine Pancreas

The elastase inhibitory activity was evaluated base on a method reported by Kraunsoe et al. (1996) [41]. In brief, the reaction mixture contained 650 µL of 1.015 mM N-succinyl-Ala-Ala-Ala-p-nitroanilide (dissolved in Tris-HCl, pH 8.0) and 50 µL of sample. The reaction mixture was vortexed and incubated for 10 min at 25 °C. After incubation, a volume of 50 µL of 0.0375 units/mL elastase enzyme solution was added to the reaction mixture and, following vortexing, the reaction mixture was incubated for 10 min at 25 °C in a water bath. The amount of released p-nitroaniline was assessed by measuring absorbance at 410 nm using a microplate reader.

3.3. Cell Culture and UVB Irradiation

HDF cells (ATCC® PCS20101™) were purchased from ATCC (American Type Culture Collection, Manassas, VA, USA). HDF cells were cultured in DMEM and F-12 mixed with a ratio of three to one supplemented with 10% heat-inactivated FBS, 100 unit/mL of penicillin and 100 µg/mL of streptomycin. Cells were sub-cultured every 5 days. Cells were incubated at 37 °C under humidified atmosphere containing 5% CO_2 in an incubator (Sanyo MCO-18AIC CO_2 Incubator, Moriguchi, Japan). UVB irradiation was carried out using a UVB meter (UV Lamp, VL-6LM, Vilber Lourmat, France), equipped with a fluorescent bulb emitting 280–320 nm wavelength with a peak at 313 nm. HDF cells were irradiated at a dose of 50 mJ/cm^2 of UVB in 1 × PBS. Cell medium was subsequently replaced with serum free medium and incubated until analysis.

3.4. Effect of HFPS on UVB-Irradiated HDF Cells

3.4.1. Cell Viability Assay

Cytotoxicity of HFPS on HDF cells was assessed by a colorimetric MTT assay. Briefly, cells were seeded at a concentration of 5.0×10^4 cells per well in 24-well plates. After 24 h, cells were treated with HFPS (25, 50, and 100 µg/mL) for 48 h, and their viabilities were determined by the method described previously [42,43].

3.4.2. Determination of Intracellular ROS Level and Cell Viability

For intracellular ROS level analysis, HDF cells were treated with HFPS and incubated for 30 min. Subsequently, cells were treated with DCFH-DA (stock, 500 µg/mL) and incubated for 30 min. After incubation, cells were exposed to UVB (50 mJ/cm^2) and incubated for 1 h at 37 °C. The fluorescence intensity of cells was determined according to the method described previously [44].

To analyze the protective effect of HFPS against UVB-induced cell damage, HDF cells were treated with HFPS and incubated for 2 h at 37 °C. Cells were then exposed to 50 mJ/cm^2 of UVB and incubated for 48 h. Cell viability was assessed by MTT assay using the protocol described previously [43,45].

3.4.3. Determination of Relative Intracellular Elastase and Collagenase Activities

HDF cells were seeded in 100 mm culture dishes at a density of 2.0×10^6 cells per dish and incubated for 24 h. Cells were pretreated with HFPS and incubated for 2 h. Following incubation, cells were irradiated with UVB. After 48 h incubation, cells were harvested and lysed with 0.1 M Tris-HCl (pH 7.6) buffer containing 1 mM PMSF and 0.1% Triton-X 100, followed by sonication for 5 min on ice. The lysates were centrifuged (4000 rpm, 20 min) at 4 °C. Supernatants were quantified for their protein content and were used as the fibroblastic enzyme solution. The relative elastase and collagenase activities were measured by the method described by Suganuma et al. [46].

3.4.4. Determination of Collagen Synthesis Level and MMPs Expression Levels by Enzyme-Linked Immunosorbent Assay (ELISA)

HDF cells were incubated with HFPS for 2 h, and exposed to UVB (50 mJ/cm^2). After 48 h incubation, the culture media were collected and used for assessment of MMPs expression levels and PIP level that reflect the level of collagen synthesis. The amounts of PIP and MMPs were measured by commercial ELISA kits, based on the manufacturer's instructions.

3.4.5. Western Blot Analysis

The effect of HFPS on the expressions of NF-κB, p-c-Jun, and MAPKs were assessed by Western blot analysis performed as described previously [43,47]. In brief, cells were pretreated with HFPS and irradiated with UVB. After 1 h (for MAPKs assay) or 6 h (for NF-κB and p-c-Jun assay) incubation, cells were harvested. Proteins were extracted with the PRO-PREP protein extraction kit (iNtRON Biotechnology, Sungnam, Korea). The protein level of each sample was measured by a BCA™ kit. Total proteins (50 µg) were separated on 10% sodium dodecyl sulfate (SDS)-polyacrylamide gels and transferred to pure nitrocellulose membranes. Membranes were blocked with 5% skim milk for 3 h at room temperature and incubated with primary antibodies overnight at 4 °C. After washing with TBS-T buffer, membranes were incubated with secondary antibodies for 3 h at room temperature. Finally, the protein bands were visualized using an ECL western blotting detection kit and exposed on X-ray films.

3.5. Statistical Analysis

The experiments were performed in triplicate. All data are expressed as the mean ± SE. Significant differences between the groups were determined using the unpaired Student's t-test (using Statistical

Product and Service Solutions 11.5 statistical software). Values of * $p < 0.05$, ** $p < 0.01$, and ## $p < 0.01$ were considered as significantly different.

4. Conclusions

In conclusion, in the present study, the protective effects of HFPS against UVB-induced skin damage *in vitro* in HDF cells were investigated. The results indicate that HFPS significantly protected collagen synthesis and reduced MMPs expression in UVB-irradiated HDF cells by regulating NF-κB, AP-1, and MAPKs signaling pathways. These results suggest that HFPS possess strong UV protective effect and has potential to be used as an ingredient in pharmaceutical and cosmetic industries.

Author Contributions: L.W., J.Y.O., and Y.-J.J. conceived and designed the experiments; L.W., B.R., W.L. and Y.R.C. performed experiments and analyzed data; L.W. and Y.-J.J. wrote the paper.

Funding: This research was supported by the 2017 scientific promotion program funded by Jeju National University.

Conflicts of Interest: The authors declare no conflicts of interest.

References

1. Fisher, G.J.; Kang, S.; Varani, J.; Bata-Csorgo, Z.; Wan, Y.; Datta, S.; Voorhees, J.J. Mechanisms of photoaging and chronological skin aging. *Arch. Dermatol.* **2002**, *138*, 1462–1470. [CrossRef] [PubMed]
2. Longstreth, J.; De Gruijl, F.; Kripke, M.; Abseck, S.; Arnold, F.; Slaper, H.; Velders, G.; Takizawa, Y.; Van der Leun, J. Health risks. *J. Photochem. Photobiol. B* **1998**, *46*, 20–39. [CrossRef]
3. Tanaka, K.; Hasegawa, J.; Asamitsu, K.; Okamoto, T. Magnolia ovovata extract and its active component magnolol prevent skin photoaging via inhibition of nuclear factor κB. *Eur. J. Pharmacol.* **2007**, *565*, 212–219. [CrossRef] [PubMed]
4. Ryu, B.; Ahn, B.-N.; Kang, K.-H.; Kim, Y.-S.; Li, Y.-X.; Kong, C.-S.; Kim, S.-K.; Kim, D.G. Dioxinodehydroeckol protects human keratinocyte cells from UVB-induced apoptosis modulated by related genes Bax/Bcl-2 and caspase pathway. *J. Photochem. Photobiol. B* **2015**, *153*, 352–357. [CrossRef] [PubMed]
5. Pathak, M.A.; Fanselow, D.L. Photobiology of melanin pigmentation: Dose/response of skin to sunlight and its contents. *J. Am. Acad. Dermatol.* **1983**, *9*, 724–733. [CrossRef]
6. Wang, L.; Ryu, B.; Kim, W.-S.; Kim, G.H.; Jeon, Y.-J. Protective effect of gallic acid derivatives from the freshwater green alga *Spirogyra* sp. against ultraviolet B-induced apoptosis through reactive oxygen species clearance in human keratinocytes and zebrafish. *Algae* **2017**, *32*, 379–388. [CrossRef]
7. Katiyar, S.K.; Bergamo, B.M.; Vyalil, P.K.; Elmets, C.A. Green tea polyphenols: DNA photodamage and photoimmunology. *J. Photochem. Photobiol. B* **2001**, *65*, 109–114. [CrossRef]
8. Pallela, R.; Na-Young, Y.; Kim, S.-K. Anti-photoaging and photoprotective compounds derived from marine organisms. *Mar. Drugs* **2010**, *8*, 1189–1202. [CrossRef] [PubMed]
9. Adil, M.D.; Kaiser, P.; Satti, N.K.; Zargar, A.M.; Vishwakarma, R.A.; Tasduq, S.A. Effect of *Emblica officinalis* (fruit) against UVB-induced photo-aging in human skin fibroblasts. *J. Ethnopharmacol.* **2010**, *132*, 109–114. [CrossRef] [PubMed]
10. Thomas, N.V.; Kim, S.-K. Metalloproteinase inhibitors: Status and scope from marine organisms. *Biochem. Res. Int.* **2010**, 845975. [CrossRef] [PubMed]
11. Ko, S.-C.; Jung, W.-K.; Lee, S.-H.; Lee, D.H.; Jeon, Y.-J. Antihypertensive effect of an enzymatic hydrolysate from Styela clava flesh tissue in type 2 diabetic patients with hypertension. *Nutr. Res. Pract.* **2017**, *11*, 396–401. [CrossRef] [PubMed]
12. Ko, J.-Y.; Kang, N.; Lee, J.-H.; Kim, J.-S.; Kim, W.-S.; Park, S.-J.; Kim, Y.-T.; Jeon, Y.-J. Angiotensin I-converting enzyme inhibitory peptides from an enzymatic hydrolysate of flounder fish (Paralichthys olivaceus) muscle as a potent anti-hypertensive agent. *Process Biochem.* **2016**, *51*, 535–541. [CrossRef]
13. Kang, M.-C.; Kang, N.; Ko, S.-C.; Kim, Y.-B.; Jeon, Y.-J. Anti-obesity effects of seaweeds of Jeju Island on the differentiation of 3T3-L1 preadipocytes and obese mice fed a high-fat diet. *Food Chem. Toxicol.* **2016**, *90* (Suppl. C), 36–44. [CrossRef] [PubMed]

14. Lee, W.; Kang, N.; Kim, E.-A.; Yang, H.-W.; Oh, J.-Y.; Fernando, I.P.S.; Kim, K.-N.; Ahn, G.; Jeon, Y.-J. Radioprotective effects of a polysaccharide purified from Lactobacillus plantarum-fermented Ishige okamurae against oxidative stress caused by gamma ray-irradiation in zebrafish *in vivo* model. *J. Funct. Foods* **2017**, *28* (Suppl. C), 83–89. [CrossRef]
15. Lee, S.-H.; Ko, S.-C.; Kang, M.-C.; Lee, D.H.; Jeon, Y.-J. Octaphlorethol A, a marine algae product, exhibits antidiabetic effects in type 2 diabetic mice by activating AMP-activated protein kinase and upregulating the expression of glucose transporter 4. *Food Chem. Toxicol.* **2016**, *91* (Suppl. C), 58–64. [CrossRef] [PubMed]
16. Lee, W.W.; Kim, W.S.; Ahn, G.; Kim, K.N.; Heo, S.J.; Cho, M.; Fernando, I.P.S.; Kang, N.; Jeon, Y.-J. Separation of glycine-rich proteins from sea hare eggs and their anti-cancer activity against U937 leukemia cell line. *Exeli J.* **2016**, *15*, 329–342.
17. Oh, J.-Y.; Fernando, I.S.; Jeon, Y.-J. Potential applications of radioprotective phytochemicals from marine algae. *Algae* **2016**, *31*, 403–414. [CrossRef]
18. Sanjeewa, K.K.A.; Fernando, I.P.S.; Samarakoon, K.W.; Lakmal, H.H.C.; Kim, E.-A.; Kwon, O.N.; Dilshara, M.G.; Lee, J.-B.; Jeon, Y.-J. Anti-inflammatory and anti-cancer activities of sterol rich fraction of cultured marine microalga Nannochloropsis oculata. *Algae* **2016**, *31*, 277–287. [CrossRef]
19. Kim, H.-H.; Kim, H.-S.; Ko, J.-Y.; Kim, C.-Y.; Lee, J.-H.; Jeon, Y.-J. A single-step isolation of useful antioxidant compounds from Ishige okamurae by using centrifugal partition chromatography. *Fish Aquat. Sci.* **2016**, *19*, 22. [CrossRef]
20. Kang, N.; Kim, S.-Y.; Rho, S.; Ko, J.-Y.; Jeon, Y.-J. Anti-fatigue activity of a mixture of seahorse (Hippocampus abdominalis) hydrolysate and red ginseng. *Fish. Aquatic. Sci.* **2017**, *20*, 3. [CrossRef]
21. Park, S.-Y.; Hwang, E.; Shin, Y.-K.; Lee, D.-G.; Yang, J.-E.; Park, J.-H.; Yi, T.-H. Immunostimulatory effect of enzyme-modified *Hizikia fusiforme* in a mouse model *in vitro* and ex vivo. *Mar. Biotechnol.* **2017**, *19*, 65–75. [CrossRef] [PubMed]
22. Baek, J.; Lim, S.-Y. Effect of *Hizikia fusiformis* extracts on reactive oxygen species mediated oxidative damage. *Int. J. Adv. Res. Biol. Sci.* **2017**, *4*, 120–126. [CrossRef]
23. Imbs, T.I.; Ermakova, S.P.; Malyarenko, O.S.; Isakov, V.V.; Zvyagintseva, T.N. Structural elucidation of polysaccharide fractions from the brown alga *Coccophora langsdorfii* and *in vitro* investigation of their anticancer activity. *Carbohyd. Polym.* **2016**, *135* (Suppl. C), 162–168. [CrossRef] [PubMed]
24. Oh, J.-H.; Kim, J.; Lee, Y. Anti-inflammatory and anti-diabetic effects of brown seaweeds in high-fat diet-induced obese mice. *Nutr. Res. Pract.* **2016**, *10*, 42–48. [CrossRef] [PubMed]
25. Wang, L.; Oh, J.Y.; Kim, H.S.; Lee, W.; Cui, Y.; Lee, H.G.; Kim, Y.-T.; Ko, J.Y.; Jeon, Y.-J. Protective effect of polysaccharides from Celluclast-assisted extract of *Hizikia fusiforme* against hydrogen peroxide-induced oxidative stress *in vitro* in Vero cells and *in vivo* in zebrafish. *Int. J. Biol. Macromol.* **2018**, *112*, 483–489. [CrossRef] [PubMed]
26. Heo, S.-J.; Ko, S.-C.; Cha, S.-H.; Kang, D.-H.; Park, H.-S.; Choi, Y.-U.; Kim, D.; Jung, W.-K.; Jeon, Y.-J. Effect of phlorotannins isolated from Ecklonia cava on melanogenesis and their protective effect against photo-oxidative stress induced by UV-B radiation. *Toxicol. In Vitro* **2009**, *23*, 1123–1130. [CrossRef] [PubMed]
27. Ko, S.-C.; Cha, S.-H.; Heo, S.-J.; Lee, S.-H.; Kang, S.-M.; Jeon, Y.-J. Protective effect of Ecklonia cava on UVB-induced oxidative stress: In vitro and *in vivo* zebrafish model. *J. Appl. Physiol.* **2011**, *23*, 697–708. [CrossRef]
28. Zeng, Q.; Zhou, F.; Lei, L.; Chen, J.; Lu, J.; Zhou, J.; Cao, K.; Gao, L.; Xia, F.; Ding, S. *Ganoderma lucidum* polysaccharides protect fibroblasts against UVB-induced photoaging. *Mol. Med. Rep.* **2017**, *15*, 111–116. [CrossRef] [PubMed]
29. Plastow, S.R.; Lovell, C.R.; Young, A.R. UVB-Induced collagen changes in the skin of the hairless albino mouse. *J. Invest. Dermatol.* **1987**, *88*, 145–148. [CrossRef] [PubMed]
30. Imokawa, G. Mechanism of UVB-Induced wrinkling of the skin: Paracrine cytokine linkage between keratinocytes and fibroblasts leading to the stimulation of elastase. *J. Invest. Dermatol. Symp. Proc.* **2009**, *14*, 36–43. [CrossRef] [PubMed]
31. Li, Y.H.; Wu, Y.; Wei, H.C.; Xu, Y.Y.; Jia, L.L.; Chen, J.; Yang, X.S.; Dong, G.H.; Gao, X.H.; Chen, H.D. Protective effects of green tea extracts on photoaging and photommunosuppression. *Skin Res. Technol.* **2009**, *15*, 338–345. [CrossRef] [PubMed]

32. Nikkari, S.T.; O'Brien, K.D.; Ferguson, M.; Hatsukami, T.; Welgus, H.G.; Alpers, C.E.; Clowes, A.W. Interstitial collagenase (MMP-1) expression in human carotid atherosclerosis. *Circulation* **1995**, *92*, 1393–1398. [CrossRef] [PubMed]
33. Zhang, M.; Hwang, E.; Lin, P.; Gao, W.; Ngo, H.T.; Yi, T.-H. Prunella vulgaris L. exerts a protective effect against extrinsic aging through NF-κB, MAPKs, AP-1, and TGF-β/Smad signaling pathways in UVB-Aged normal human dermal fibroblasts. *Rejuvenation Res.* **2018**. [CrossRef] [PubMed]
34. Hwang, B.-M.; Noh, E.-M.; Kim, J.-S.; Kim, J.-M.; Hwang, J.-K.; Kim, H.-K.; Kang, J.-S.; Kim, D.-S.; Chae, H.-J.; You, Y.-O. Decursin inhibits UVB-induced MMP expression in human dermal fibroblasts via regulation of nuclear factor-κB. *Int. J. Mol. Med.* **2013**, *31*, 477–483. [CrossRef] [PubMed]
35. Cooper, S.; Bowden, G. Ultraviolet B regulation of transcription factor families: Roles of nuclear factor-kappa B (NF-κB) and activator protein-1 (AP-1) in UVB-induced skin carcinogenesis. *Curr. Cancer Drug Targets* **2007**, *7*, 325–334. [CrossRef] [PubMed]
36. Bell, S.; Degitz, K.; Quirling, M.; Jilg, N.; Page, S.; Brand, K. Involvement of NF-κB signalling in skin physiology and disease. *Cell Signal.* **2003**, *15*, 1–7. [CrossRef]
37. Zhang, W.; Liu, H.T. MAPK signal pathways in the regulation of cell proliferation in mammalian cells. *Cell Res.* **2002**, *12*, 9. [CrossRef] [PubMed]
38. Rodríguez-Berriguete, G.; Fraile, B.; Martínez-Onsurbe, P.; Olmedilla, G.; Paniagua, R.; Royuela, M. MAP kinases and prostate cancer. *J. Signal. Ttransduct.* **2012**, *2012*, 169170. [CrossRef] [PubMed]
39. Cargnello, M.; Roux, P.P. Activation and function of the MAPKs and their substrates, the MAPK-activated protein kinases. *Microbiol. Mol. Biol. Rev.* **2011**, *75*, 50–83. [CrossRef] [PubMed]
40. Pittayapruek, P.; Meephansan, J.; Prapapan, O.; Komine, M.; Ohtsuki, M. Role of matrix metalloproteinases in photoaging and photocarcinogenesis. *Int. J. Mol. Sci.* **2016**, *17*, 868. [CrossRef] [PubMed]
41. Kraunsoe, J.A.; Claridge, T.D.; Lowe, G. Inhibition of human leukocyte and porcine pancreatic elastase by homologues of bovine pancreatic trypsin inhibitor. *Biochemistry* **1996**, *35*, 9090–9096. [CrossRef] [PubMed]
42. Kang, M.-C.; Kim, S.-Y.; Kim, E.-A.; Lee, J.-H.; Kim, Y.-S.; Yu, S.-K.; Chae, J.B.; Choe, I.-H.; Cho, J.H.; Jeon, Y.-J. Antioxidant activity of polysaccharide purified from *Acanthopanax koreanum* Nakai stems *in vitro* and *in vivo* zebrafish model. *Carbohyd. Polym.* **2015**, *127*, 38–46. [CrossRef] [PubMed]
43. Wang, L.; Fernando, I.S.; Kim, E.-A.; Jeon, Y.-J. Soft corals collected from Jeju Island; a potential source of anti-inflammatory phytochemicals. *J. Chitin Chitosan* **2016**, *21*, 247–254. [CrossRef]
44. Heo, S.-J.; Jeon, Y.-J. Protective effect of fucoxanthin isolated from Sargassum siliquastrum on UV-B induced cell damage. *J. Photochem. Photobiol. B* **2009**, *95*, 101–107. [CrossRef] [PubMed]
45. Wang, L.; Jo, M.-J.; Katagiri, R.; Harata, K.; Ohta, M.; Ogawa, A.; Kamegai, M.; Ishida, Y.; Tanoue, S.; Kimura, S.; et al. Antioxidant effects of citrus pomace extracts processed by super-heated steam. *LWT-Food Sci. Technol.* **2018**, *90*, 331–338. [CrossRef]
46. Suganuma, K.; Nakajima, H.; Ohtsuki, M.; Imokawa, G. Astaxanthin attenuates the UVA-induced up-regulation of matrix-metalloproteinase-1 and skin fibroblast elastase in human dermal fibroblasts. *J. Dermatol. Sci.* **2010**, *58*, 136–142. [CrossRef] [PubMed]
47. Lee, S.-H.; Han, J.-S.; Heo, S.-J.; Hwang, J.-Y.; Jeon, Y.-J. Protective effects of dieckol isolated from *Ecklonia cava* against high glucose-induced oxidative stress in human umbilical vein endothelial cells. *Toxicol. In Vitro* **2010**, *24*, 375–381. [CrossRef] [PubMed]

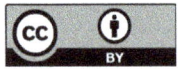

© 2018 by the authors. Licensee MDPI, Basel, Switzerland. This article is an open access article distributed under the terms and conditions of the Creative Commons Attribution (CC BY) license (http://creativecommons.org/licenses/by/4.0/).

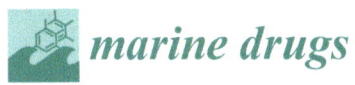

Article

The Suppressive Activity of Fucofuroeckol-A Derived from Brown Algal *Ecklonia stolonifera* Okamura on UVB-Induced Mast Cell Degranulation

Thanh Sang Vo [1], Se-Kwon Kim [2,*], BoMi Ryu [3], Dai Hung Ngo [4], Na-Young Yoon [5], Long Giang Bach [6], Nguyen Thi Nhat Hang [4,7] and Dai Nghiep Ngo [8,*]

1. NTT Institute of Hi-Technology, Nguyen Tat Thanh University, Ho Chi Minh City 700000, Vietnam; vtsang@ntt.edu.vn
2. Department of Marine Life Science, College of Ocean Science and Technology, Korea Maritime and Ocean University, Busan 606-791, Korea
3. School of Pharmacy, the University of Queensland, Brisbane QLD 4072, Australia; ryu.bomi@gmail.com
4. Faculty of Natural Sciences, Thu Dau Mot University, Thu Dau Mot City 820000, Binh Duong Province, Vietnam; hungdaingo83@yahoo.com (D.H.N.); hangntn@tdmu.edu.vn (N.T.N.H.)
5. Food and Safety Research Center, National Fisheries Research & Development, Busan 46083, Korea; dbssud@hanmail.net
6. Department of Science and Technology, Nguyen Tat Thanh University, Ho Chi Minh City 700000, Vietnam; blgiang@ntt.edu.vn
7. Faculty of Chemistry, University of Science-VNU-HCM City, 227 Nguyen Van Cu Street, Ho Chi Minh City 700000, Vietnam
8. Department of Biochemistry, Faculty of Biology and Biotechnology, University of Science, Vietnam National University, Ho Chi Minh City 700000, Vietnam
* Correspondence: sknkim@pknu.ac.kr (S.-K.K.); ndnghiep@hcmus.edu.vn (D.N.N.); Tel.: +82-51-629-6870 (S.-K.K.); +84-28-3830-0560 (D.N.N.)

Received: 14 October 2017; Accepted: 5 December 2017; Published: 4 January 2018

Abstract: UV light, especially UVB, is known as a trigger of allergic reaction, leading to mast cell degranulation and histamine release. In this study, phlorotannin Fucofuroeckol-A (F-A) derived from brown algal *Ecklonia stolonifera* Okamura was evaluated for its protective capability against UVB-induced allergic reaction in RBL-2H3 mast cells. It was revealed that F-A significantly suppress mast cell degranulation via decreasing histamine release as well as intracellular Ca^{2+} elevation at the concentration of 50 µM. Moreover, the inhibitory effect of F-A on IL-1β and TNF-α productions was also evidenced. Notably, the protective activity of F-A against mast cell degranulation was found due to scavenging ROS production. Accordingly, F-A from brown algal *E. stolonifera* was suggested to be promising candidate for its protective capability against UVB-induced allergic reaction.

Keywords: *Ecklonia stolonifera*; phlorotannin; Fucofuroeckol-A; anti-allergy; degranulation; mast cells

1. Introduction

Sunlight is a continuous spectrum of electromagnetic radiation that is divided into three major spectrums of wavelength such as ultraviolet, visible, and infrared [1]. The UV range is the most significant spectrum of sunlight with a wavelength from 10 nm to 400 nm, shorter than that of visible light but longer than X-rays. Ultraviolet (UV) radiation is divided into three distinct bands including UVA (320–400 nm), UVB (290–320 nm), and UVC (200–290 nm) in order of decreasing wavelength and increasing energy [2]. UVC light is absorbed by the atmosphere, while approximately 90–99% of UVA and 1–10% of UVB reaches the earth's surface [3]. Different wavelengths and energy associated with UV subdivision correspond to distinctly different effects on living tissue. UV light causes various biological reactions including acute inflammation and cancer, as in sunburn and eruptions of the skin [4,5]. Notably, it has been reported that mast cell activation including histamine release is involved in the UV-induced sunburn reaction [6]. At a low dose, UVB light inhibits histamine release from mast cells induced by compound 48/80 [7], A23187 [8], and substance P [9]. However, UVB light causes histamine release from rat peritoneal mast cells at doses higher than 7.8 kJ/m^2 [10]. Accordingly, UVB light can be applied as an allergic therapeutic at a low dose, whereas it is also a cause of allergic reaction from a high dose, such as exposure to outdoor sunlight. Thus, a protective agent that is able to block UVB from sunlight is necessary for humans when they go outside.

In recent years, seaweeds have served as an important source of bioactive natural substances that possess various pharmaceutical properties [11]. Among them, brown seaweed has been recognized as a rich source of phlorotannins, which are formed by the polymerization of phloroglucinol (1,3,5-tryhydroxybenzene) monomer units and biosynthesized through the acetate-malonate pathway [12]. Phlorotannins exhibit various beneficial bioactivities such as anti-oxidant, anti-cancer, anti-diabetic, anti-HIV, matrix metalloproteinase enzyme inhibition, and anti-hypertensive activities [13]. Notably, several phlorotannins from brown algae have been reported to be effective against allergic reaction in recent years. Dieckol, 6,6′-bieckol, and fucodiphloroethol G from *Ecklonia cava* were found to be strong inhibitors of histamine release from KU812 and RBL-2H3 cells with an IC$_{50}$ range of 27.8–55.1 µM [14,15]. Likewise, dioxinodehydroeckol and phlorofucofuroeckol A from *E. stolonifera* have been demonstrated to suppress intracellular calcium elevation and histamine release from CRA-1-stimulated KU812 cells [16]. Although the anti-allergic activities of phlorotannins have been well-evidenced, their protective effect against UVB-induced allergic reactions has been not reported. Meanwhile, phlorotannins (dieckol) from *E. cava* has been known to possess strong protective activity against UV-B radiation-induced DNA damage. Moreover, it can reduce the intracellular reactive oxygen species generated by gammaray radiation [17]. Therefore, phlorotannins from brown seaweeds are suggested as effective protective agents against UVB-induced damages. Accordingly, the present study was designed to evaluate the protective effects of phlorotannin Fucofuroeckol-A derived from brown algal *Ecklonia stolonifera* Okamura against UVB-induced mast cell activation.

2. Results and Discussion

2.1. Structure Elucidation of Phlorotannin

Fucofuroeckol-A (F-A) was isolated as a pale brown powder. The molecular formula was established as $C_{24}H_{14}O_{11}$. ^{1}H-NMR (400 MHz, DMSO-d_6) δ: 10.05 (1H, s, 14-OH), 9.88 (1H, s, 4-OH), 9.76 (1H, s, 10-OH), 9.44 (1H, s, 2-OH), 9.18 (2H, s, 3′, 5′-OH), 8.22 (1H, s, 8-OH), 6.71 (1H, s, H-13), 6.47 (1H, d, *J* = 1.1 Hz, H-11), 6.29 (1H, s, H-3), 6.25 (1H, d, *J* = 1.5 Hz, H-9), 5.83 (1H, s, H-4′), 5.76 (2H, d, *J* = 1.5 Hz, H-2′, 6′). Moreover, ^{13}C-NMR (100 MHz, DMSO-d_6) δ: 160.7 (C-1′), 158.8 (C-3′, 5′), 158.3 (C-11a), 157.6 (C-10), 150.5 (C-12a), 150.2 (C-8), 146.9 (C-2), 144.4 (C-14), 142.0 (C-4), 136.8 (C-15a), 133.6 (C-5a), 126.1 (C-14a), 122.6 (C-4a), 122.4 (C-1), 103.1 (C-6), 102.4 (C-7), 98.2 (C-3), 98.0 (C-9), 96.3 (C-4′), 94.6 (C-13), 93.7 (C-2′, 6′), 90.5 (C-11) (Figure 1).

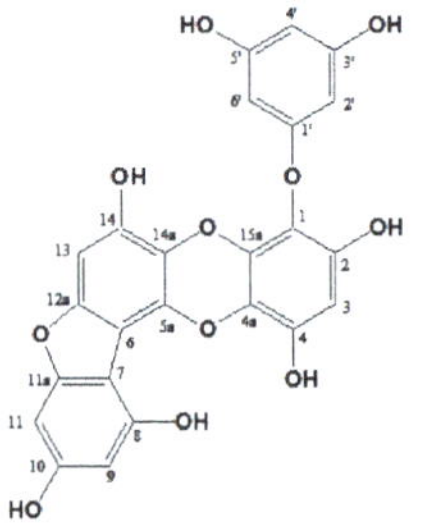

Figure 1. Chemical structures of Fucofuroeckol-A isolated from *E. stolonifera* Okamura.

2.2. Effect of F-A on Mast Cell Degranulation Induced by UVB

Although the reasons why allergies develop are not known, there are some substances that commonly cause an allergic reaction such as pet dander, bee stings, certain foods (nuts or shellfish), pollen, or molds [18]. Moreover, UV light, especially UVB, has also been reported to be able to trigger allergic reaction, leading to mast cell degranulation and histamine release [10]. Thus, compounds possessing protective activities against UVB light may influence its anti-allergic properties via the inhibition of mast cell degranulation and histamine release. Hence, the effect of F-A on mast cell degranulation was first evaluated by measuring histamine release induced by UVB. Figure 2 shows that F-A significantly decreases histamine release from the activated mast cells in a dose-dependent manner. The histamine release level upon pretreatment with 50 µM of F-A was 31%, as compared to the control group exposed to UVB alone (Figure 2A). On the other hand, its inhibitory effect on mast cell degranulation was also confirmed by testing cell morphological changes. In the normal condition, mast cells were generally branch-shaped with clear membranes, whereas the activated cells induced by UVB were round-shaped, and had reduced cell size, disrupted boundaries, and irregular surfaces. However, F-A-pretreated cells before being exposed to UVB exhibited a protective effect against the morphological changes (Figure 2B). This indicates that F-A is capable of protecting mast cells from UVB, thus blocking the mast cell degranulation and histamine release from the UVB-exposed mast cells.

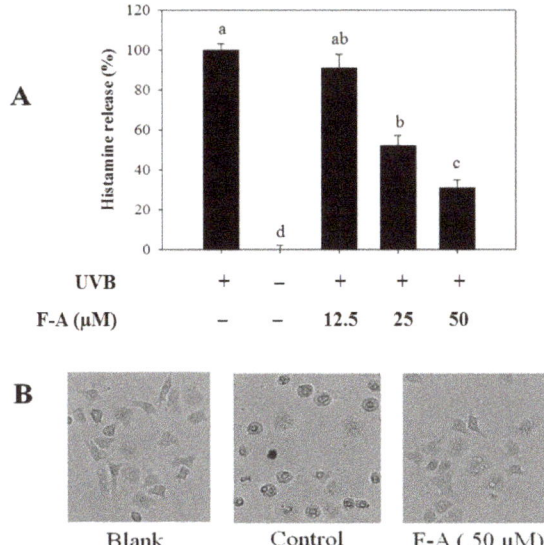

Figure 2. Effect of Fucofuroeckol-A (F-A) on mast cells degranulation in UVB-exposed RBL-2H3 cells. The cells were pretreated with F-A for 24 h before exposing to UVB for 60 min. (**A**) The levels of histamine release were measured via a spectrofluorometric assay. Each determination was made in three independent experiments, and the data are shown as means ± SD. Different letters a–d indicate significant difference among groups ($p < 0.05$) by Duncan's multiple-range test; (**B**) The representative images of the cells were assessed by using light microscopy (magnification, ×20).

2.3. Effect of F-A on Intracellular Ca^{2+} Elevation in UVB-Exposed RBL-2H3 Mast Cells

The process of mast-cell degranulation requires the elevation of intracellular Ca^{2+} levels. Intracellular Ca^{2+} elevation is important in the regulation of granule-plasma membrane fusion [19]. The increase in intracellular Ca^{2+} concentration is a necessary and sufficient stimulus for mast-cell degranulation. Thus, we also examined whether F-A alleviates the intracellular Ca^{2+} level in UVB-exposed RBL-2H3 mast cells. Figure 3 shows that UVB induced the elevation of intracellular Ca^{2+} level in mast cells. Meanwhile, the pretreatment of F-A caused significant inhibition of the intracellular Ca^{2+} elevation. Notably, the inhibitory effect of intracellular Ca^{2+} elevation was observed to be effective at a concentration of 50 µM of F-A pretreatment (Figure 3A). Similarly, the fluorescence intensity in photographs, shown in Figure 3B, also indicated that F-A remarkably decreased the intracellular Ca^{2+} density in RBL-2H3 mast cells exposed to UVB. As a result, the alleviative effects of F-A on intracellular Ca^{2+} elevation resulted in the inhibition of granule-plasma membrane fusion, thus reducing mast cell degranulation and histamine release from the activated mast cells. It is supported by previous reports that some anti-allergic drugs inhibit histamine release via the inhibition of intracellular Ca^{2+} elevation [20,21].

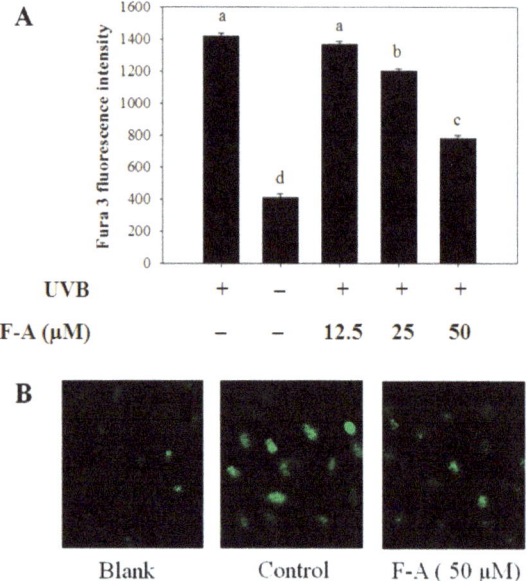

Figure 3. Effect of F-A on intracellular Ca^{2+} elevation in UVB-exposed RBL-2H3 mast cells. (**A**) The cells were pretreated with various doses of F-A for 24 h before incubating with Fura-3/AM for 60 min. The cells were then exposed to UVB for 10 min. The level of intracellular Ca^{2+} was monitored by a spectrofluorometric assay. Each determination was made in three independent experiments, and the data are shown as means ± SD. Different letters a–d indicate significant difference among groups ($p < 0.05$) by Duncan's multiple-range test; (**B**) The representative images of the cells were assessed by using light microscopy (magnification, ×20).

2.4. Effect of F-A on Cytokine Production in UVB-Exposed RBL-2H3 Mast Cells

Besides histamine release, mast cell degranulation also leads to the production of several cytokines, such as IL-1β and TNF-α. The excessive expression and production of these cytokines alter the local microenvironment and eventually lead to the recruitment of inflammatory cells such as neutrophils and eosinophils [22]. Therefore, the modulation of inflammatory cytokines from mast cells is a one of the key indicators of reduced allergic symptoms. Herein, the production levels of IL-1β (Figure 4A) and TNF-α (Figure 4B) were observed to increase in the culture supernatants of UVB-exposed RBL-2H3 mast cells. The amounts of IL-1β and TNF-α from the exposed cells were 121 ± 6 and 152 ± 11 pg/mL, respectively, whereas the correlative amounts of these cytokines in the non-exposed cells were 19 ± 4 and 31 ± 8 pg/mL, respectively. Conversely, these increases were considerably diminished in a concentration-dependent manner by F-A pretreatment. At the concentration of 50 μM, F-A reduced IL-1β and TNF-α levels to 58 ± 7 and 65 ± 12 pg/mL, respectively.

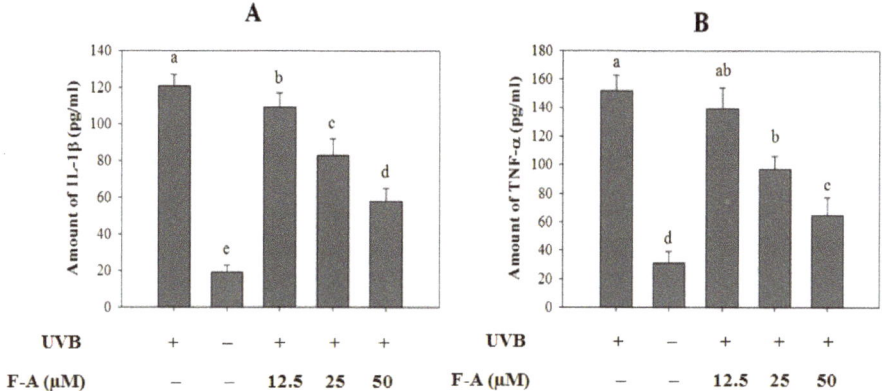

Figure 4. Effects of F-A on cytokine production in UVB-exposed RBL-2H3 mast cells. The cells were pretreated with various concentrations of F-A for 24 h before being exposed to UVB for 2 h. The production levels of IL-1β (**A**) and TNF-α (**B**) were quantified in culture media using commercial ELISA kits. Each determination was made in three independent experiments, and the data are shown as means ± SD. Different letters a–e indicate significant difference among groups ($p < 0.05$) by Duncan's multiple-range test.

2.5. Effect of F-A on ROS Production in UVB-Exposed RBL-2H3 Mast Cells

More importantly, the role of ROS as an inducer of Ca^{2+} elevation and degranulation in mast cells has been reported in numerous recent studies [23,24]. Meanwhile, the inhibition of ROS production by diphenyleneiodonium (DPI) or antioxidants such as (−)-epigallocatechin gallate resulted in the suppression of IgE-mediated histamine release [25]. Thus, ROS production is a potential target for the downregulation of mast cell degranulation. Accordingly, we attempted to determine whether F-A blocks ROS production in the activated mast cells using a dihydroethidium fluorescence indicator. A light microscope assay showed that the UVB-exposed cells significantly increased the fluorescence density of ROS in the control group (exposure to UVB only). However, the fluorescence density of ROS was markedly decreased by F-A pretreatments at a concentration of 50 μM, indicating the inhibitory effect of F-A on ROS production in UVB-exposed mast cells (Figure 5A). Many researchers have shown that phenolic compounds from marine algae have strong antioxidant activities on free radicals and possess radio-protective activity against UVB light [17,26,27]. These results suggested that the effective antioxidant activity and radio-protective activity of F-A significantly contributes to the depression of mast cell degranulation.

To exclude the possibility that the inhibitory activities of F-A were due to cytotoxicity, an MTT assay was performed in RBL-2H3 cells pretreated with various concentrations of F-A for 24 h before exposure to UVB (20 kJ/m^2) for 2 h. With the concentrations used in this study (12.5, 25, or 50 μM) and the exposure of UVB, none of the treatments affected cell viability (Figure 5B). Thus, the inhibitory activities of F-A on mast cell degranulation and ROS production were not due to any cytotoxic effect on RBL-2H3 cells.

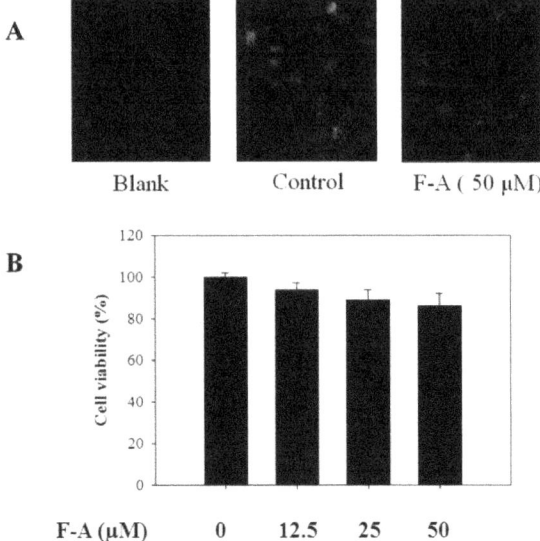

Figure 5. Effect of F-A on ROS production in UVB-exposed RBL-2H3 mast cells and cell viability. (**A**) The cells were pretreated with different doses of F-A for 24 h before being incubated with dihydroethidium for 60 min. The cells were then exposed to UVB for 60 min. The level of ROS production was monitored by a light microscope with 20× magnification; (**B**) The cells were pretreated with different concentrations of F-A for 24 h before being exposed to UVB for 2 h. Cell viability was demonstrated by the MTT method, and the results are expressed as a percentage of surviving cells over blank cells (no addition of F-A and UVB). Each determination was made in three independent experiments, and the data are shown as means ± SD.

3. Materials and Methods

3.1. Reagents and Materials

Fucofuroeckol-A (F-A) was kindly donated by Dr. Na-Young Yoon (Food and Safety Research Center, National Fisheries Research and Development, Busan, Korea). Enzyme immunoassay reagents for cytokine assays were purchased from R&D Systems (Minneapolis, MN, USA). Calcium-specific fluorescence probe (Fura-3/AM) was purchased from Santa Cruz Biotechnology Inc. (Santa Cruz, CA, USA). All other reagents were purchased from Sigma-Aldrich (St. Louis, MO, USA).

3.2. Cell Culture and Cell Viability Assay

RBL-2H3 mast cells were purchased from the Korean Cell Line Bank (Seoul, Korea). Cells were cultured in a humidified atmosphere containing 5% CO_2 at 37 °C using Dulbecco's Modified Eagle Medium (DMEM) supplemented with 10% heat-inactivated fetal bovine serum (FBS), 2 mM L-glutamine, 10 mM HEPES buffer, 100 U/mL of penicillin G, and 100 mg/mL of streptomycin.

The viability levels of RBL-2H3 cells was determined by MTT [3-(4,5-dimethyl-2-yl)-2,5-diphenyltetrazolium bromide] assay. The cells were grown in 96-well plates at a density of 2×10^5 cells/mL. Then, cells were washed with fresh medium and pretreated with different concentrations of F-A for 24 h before being exposed to UVB (20 kJ/m^2) for 2 h. Cells were rewashed and pretreated with MTT solution (1 mg/mL, final concentration) for 4 h. Finally, the supernatant was removed, and DMSO (100 µL) was added to solubilize the formed formazan salt. The amount of formazan salt was determined by measuring the absorbance at 540 nm using a microplate reader

(GENios® Tecan Austria GmbH, Grodig/Salzburg, Austria). Viability of cells was quantified as a percentage compared to blank.

3.3. Histamine Release Assay

RBL-2H3 cells were seeded into 24-well plates (2×10^5 cells/mL). Cells were pretreated with different concentrations of F-A (12.5, 25, or 50 µM) for 24 h before being exposed to UVB (20 kJ/m^2) for 60 min. Histamine release in the supernatants was determined as previously described [28]. Histamine release levels were calculated as a percentage compared to the control: Release ratio (%) = (T − B)/(C − B) × 100, where B is the group with neither stimulation nor the sample treatment, C is the stimulated group without treatment of the tested sample, and T is the stimulated group with the presence of the tested sample.

3.4. Measurement of the Intracellular Ca^{2+} Level

RBL-2H3 cells were seeded into black 96-well plates (2×10^5 cells/mL) and pretreated with F-A (12.5, 25, or 50 µM) for 24 h before being incubated with Fura-3/AM (2 µM, final concentration) for 60 min. The cells were then washed with Tyrode buffer and exposed to UVB (20 kJ/m^2) for 10 min. The Fura-3/AM fluorescence intensity was measured at an excitation wavelength of 360 nm and an emission wavelength of 528 nm using a microplate reader (GENios® Tecan Austria GmbH, Grodig/Salzburg, Austria). In addition, fluorescence images were visualized and photographed under a fluorescence microscope (CTR 6000, Leica, Wetzlar, Germany) after the addition of 2% paraformaldehyde.

3.5. Measurement of Cytokine Production

RBL-2H3 cells were seeded into 24-well plates (2×10^5 cells/mL) and pretreated with F-A (12.5, 25, or 50 µM) for 24 h before being exposed to UVB (20 kJ/m^2) for 2 h. The supernatants were collected, and the production of IL-1β and TNF-α were quantified by sandwich immunoassays following the protocol of R&D systems.

3.6. Measurement of ROS Production

RBL-2H3 cells were seeded into 12-well plates (1×10^4 cells/mL) and pretreated with F-A (12.5, 25, or 50 µM) for 24 h before being incubated with dihydroethidium (5 µM, final concentration) for 60 min at 37 °C. The cells were then washed with Tyrode buffer and exposed to UVB (20 kJ/m^2) for 60 min. The fluorescence intensity was visualized and photographed under a fluorescence microscope (CTR 6000, Leica, Wetzlar, Germany) after the addition of 2% paraformaldehyde.

3.7. Statistical Analysis

Data were analyzed using the analysis of variance (ANOVA) test of the statistical package for the social sciences (SPSS). The statistical differences among groups were assessed by using Duncan's multiple range tests. Differences were considered significant at $p < 0.05$.

4. Conclusions

In conclusion, this study determined that phlorotannin Fucofuroeckol-A derived from brown algal *Ecklonia stolonifera* Okamura possesses strong protective activity against UVB-induced allergic reaction. Its protective activity was revealed via scavenging ROS production, which might cause the inhibition of mast cell degranulation, histamine release, cytokine production, and intracellular Ca^{2+} elevation in UVB-exposed RBL-2H3 cells. Further study on the protective capability of Fucofuroeckol-A against UVB-induced allergic reaction on other mast cells as well as on an in vivo model will be performed to support its application as a novel cosmeceutical.

Acknowledgments: This research was funded by NTTU Foundation for Science and Technology Development under grant number: 2017.01.01. This research was also supported by a grant from Marine Bioprocess Research Center of the Marine Biotechnology Program funded by the Ministry of Oceans and Fisheries, Korea.

Author Contributions: Thanh Sang Vo was responsible for the experiment design, histamine release test, data processing, and manuscript preparation; Se-Kwon Kim was consulted for experiment design; BoMi Ryu was responsible for the cytokine production test; Dai Hung Ngo was responsible for the experiment design, intracellular Ca^{2+} elevation test, and manuscript preparation; Na-Young Yoon was responsible for the structure elucidation of phlorotannin; Long Giang Bach was responsible for English correction and structure elucidation of phlorotannin; Nguyen Thi Nhat Hang was responsible for English correction and statistical analysis; Dai Nghiep Ngo was responsible for the experiment design and ROS production test.

Conflicts of Interest: The authors declare no conflict of interest.

References

1. Soehnge, H.; Ouhtit, A.; Ananthaswamy, O.N. Mechanisms of induction of skin cancer by UV radiation. *Front. Biosci.* **1997**, *2*, D538–D551. [PubMed]
2. Tuchinda, C.; Srivannaboon, S.; Lim, W.H. Photoprotection by window glass, automobile glass and sunglasses. *J. Am. Acad. Dermatol.* **2006**, *54*, 845–854. [CrossRef] [PubMed]
3. Narayanan, D.L.; Saladi, R.N.; Fox, J.L. Ultraviolet radiation and skin cancer. *Int. J. Dermatol.* **2010**, *49*, 978–986. [CrossRef] [PubMed]
4. Hruza, L.L.; Pentland, A.P. Mechanisms of UV-induced inflammation. *J. Investig. Dermatol.* **1993**, *100*, 35S–41S. [CrossRef] [PubMed]
5. Bald, T.; Quast, T.; Landsberg, J.; Rogava, M.; Glodde, N.; Lopez-Ramos, D.; Kohlmeyer, J.; Riesenberg, S.; van den Boorn-Konijnenberg, D.; Hömig-Hölzel, C.; et al. Ultraviolet-radiation-induced inflammation promotes angiotropism and metastasis in melanoma. *Nature* **2014**, *507*, 109–113. [CrossRef] [PubMed]
6. Gilchrest, B.A.; Soter, N.A.; Stoff, J.S.; Mihm, M.C., Jr. The human sunburn reaction: Histologic and biochemical studies. *J. Am. Acad. Dermatol.* **1981**, *5*, 411–422. [CrossRef]
7. Fjellner, B.; Hagermark, O. Histamine release from rat peritoneal mast cells exposed to ultraviolet light. *Acta Dermatovenereol.* **1982**, *62*, 215–220.
8. Danno, K.; Fujii, K.; Tachibana, T.; Toda, K.-I.; Horio, T. Suppressed histamine release from rat peritoneal mast cells by ultraviolet B irradiation: Decreased diacylglycerol formation as a possible mechanism. *J. Investig. Dermatol.* **1988**, *90*, 806–809. [CrossRef] [PubMed]
9. Amano, H.; Kurosawa, M.; Miyachi, Y. Inhibition of substance P-induced histamine release from rat peritoneal mast cells by ultraviolet light B irradiation: Decreased intracellular calcium as a partial mechanism. *Clin. Exp. Allergy* **1997**, *27*, 966–971. [CrossRef] [PubMed]
10. Mio, M.; Yabuta, M.; Kamei, C. Ultraviolet B (UVB) light-induced histamine release from rat peritoneal mast cells and its augmentation by certain phenothiazine compounds. *Immunopharmacology* **1999**, *41*, 55–63. [CrossRef]
11. Smit, A.J. Medicinal and pharmaceutical uses of seaweed natural products: A review. *J. Appl. Phycol.* **2004**, *16*, 245–262. [CrossRef]
12. Vo, T.S.; Ngo, D.H.; Kim, S.K. Marine algae as a potential pharmaceutical source for anti-allergic therapeutics. *Process Biochem.* **2012**, *47*, 386–394. [CrossRef]
13. Wijesekara, I.; Yoon, N.Y.; Kim, S.K. Phlorotannins from *Ecklonia cava* (Phaeophyceae): Biological activities and potential health benefits. *Biofactors* **2010**, *36*, 408–414. [CrossRef] [PubMed]
14. Li, Y.; Lee, S.H.; Le, Q.T.; Kim, M.M.; Kim, S.K. Anti-allergic effects of phlorotannins on histamine release via binding inhibition between IgE and FcεRI. *J. Agric. Food Chem.* **2008**, *56*, 12073–12080. [CrossRef] [PubMed]
15. Le, Q.T.; Li, Y.; Qian, Z.J.; Kim, M.M.; Kim, S.K. Inhibitory effects of polyphenols isolated from marine alga *Ecklonia cava* on histamine release. *Process Biochem.* **2009**, *44*, 168–176. [CrossRef]
16. Shim, S.Y.; Choi, J.S.; Byun, D.S. Inhibitory effects of phloroglucinol derivatives isolated from *Ecklonia stolonifera* on FcεRI expression. *Bioorg. Med. Chem.* **2009**, *17*, 4734–4739. [CrossRef] [PubMed]
17. Heo, S.J.; Ko, S.C.; Cha, S.H.; Kang, D.H.; Park, H.S.; Choi, Y.U.; Kim, D.; Jung, W.K.; Jeon, Y.J. Effect of phlorotannins isolated from *Ecklonia cava* on melanogenesis and their protective effect against photo-oxidative stress induced by UV-B radiation. *Toxicol. In Vitro* **2009**, *23*, 1123–1130. [CrossRef] [PubMed]

18. Arshad, S.H. Does exposure to indoor allergens contribute to the development of asthma and allergy? *Curr. Allergy Asthma Rep.* **2010**, *10*, 49–55. [CrossRef] [PubMed]
19. Nishida, K.; Yamasaki, S.; Ito, Y.; Kabu, K.; Hattori, K.; Tezuka, T.; Nishizumi, H.; Kitamura, D.; Goitsuka, R.; Geha, R.S.; et al. FcεRI-mediated mast cell degranulation requires calcium-independent microtubule-dependent translocation of gran-ules to the plasma membrane. *J. Cell Biol.* **2005**, *170*, 115–126. [CrossRef] [PubMed]
20. Vo, T.S.; Ngo, D.H.; Kang, K.H.; Park, S.J.; Kim, S.K. The role of peptides derived from *Spirulina maxima* in downregulation of FcεRI-mediated allergic responses. *Mol. Nutr. Food Res.* **2014**, *58*, 2226–2234. [CrossRef] [PubMed]
21. Vo, T.S.; Ngo, D.H.; Kim, S.K. Gallic acid-grafted chitooligosaccharides suppress antigen-induced allergic reactions in RBL-2H3 mast cells. *Eur. J. Pharm. Sci.* **2012**, *47*, 527–533. [CrossRef] [PubMed]
22. Galli, S.J.; Tsai, M.; Piliponsky, A.M. The development of allergic inflammation. *Nature* **2008**, *454*, 445–454. [CrossRef] [PubMed]
23. Suzuki, Y.; Yoshimaru, T.; Inoue, T.; Niide, O.; Ra, C. Role of oxidants in mast cell activation. *Chem. Immunol. Allergy* **2005**, *87*, 32–42. [PubMed]
24. Camello-Almaraz, C.; Gomez-Pinilla, P.J.; Pozo, M.J.; Camello, P.J. Mitochondrial reactive oxygen species and Ca^{2+} signaling. *Am. J. Physiol. Cell Physiol.* **2006**, *291*, 1082–1088. [CrossRef] [PubMed]
25. Yoshimaru, T.; Suzuki, Y.; Matsui, T.; Yamashita, K.; Ochiai, T.; Yamaki, M.; Shimizu, K. Blockade of superoxide generation prevents high-affinity immunoglobulin E receptor-mediated release of allergic mediators by rat mast cell line and human basophils. *Clin. Exp. Allergy* **2002**, *32*, 612–618. [CrossRef] [PubMed]
26. Kang, H.S.; Chung, H.Y.; Kim, J.Y.; Son, B.W.; Jung, H.A.; Choi, J.S. Inhibitory phlorotannins from the edible brown alga *Ecklonia stolonifera* on total reactive oxygen species (ROS) generation. *Arch. Pharm. Res.* **2004**, *27*, 194–198. [CrossRef] [PubMed]
27. Shibata, T.; Ishimaru, K.; Kawaguchi, S.; Yoshikawa, H.; Hama, Y. Antioxidant activities of phlorotannins isolated from Japanese Laminariaceae. *J. Appl. Phycol.* **2008**, *20*, 705–711. [CrossRef]
28. Vo, T.S.; Kong, C.S.; Kim, S.K. Inhibitory effects of chitooligosaccharides on degranulation and cytokine generation in rat basophilic leukemia RBL-2H3 cells. *Carbohydr. Polym.* **2011**, *84*, 649–655. [CrossRef]

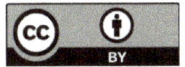

© 2018 by the authors. Licensee MDPI, Basel, Switzerland. This article is an open access article distributed under the terms and conditions of the Creative Commons Attribution (CC BY) license (http://creativecommons.org/licenses/by/4.0/).

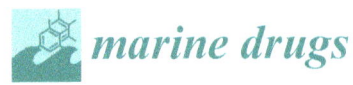

Review

Antioxidative, Anti-Inflammatory, and Anti-Aging Properties of Mycosporine-Like Amino Acids: Molecular and Cellular Mechanisms in the Protection of Skin-Aging

Hakuto Kageyama [1,*] and Rungaroon Waditee-Sirisattha [2,*]

1. Department of Chemistry, Faculty of Science and Technology, Meijo University, 1-501 Shiogamaguchi, Tenpaku-ku, Nagoya, Aichi 468-8502, Japan
2. Department of Microbiology, Faculty of Science, Chulalongkorn University, Phayathai Road, Pathumwan, Bangkok 10330, Thailand
* Correspondence: kageyama@meijo-u.ac.jp (H.K.); Rungaroon.W@chula.ac.th (R.W.-S.); Tel.: +81-52-838-2609 (H.K.); +66-2-2185091 (R.W.-S.)

Received: 8 March 2019; Accepted: 10 April 2019; Published: 12 April 2019

Abstract: Prolonged exposure to ultraviolet (UV) radiation causes photoaging of the skin and induces a number of disorders, including sunburn, fine and coarse wrinkles, and skin cancer risk. Therefore, the application of sunscreen has gained much attention to reduce the harmful effects of UV irradiation on our skin. Recently, there has been a growing demand for the replacement of chemical sunscreens with natural UV-absorbing compounds. Mycosporine-like amino acids (MAAs), promising alternative natural UV-absorbing compounds, are a group of widely distributed, low molecular-weight, water-soluble molecules that can absorb UV radiation and disperse the absorbed energy as heat, without generating reactive oxygen species (ROS). More than 30 MAAs have been characterized, from a variety of organisms. In addition to their UV-absorbing properties, there is substantial evidence that MAAs have the potential to protect against skin aging, including antioxidative activity, anti-inflammatory activity, inhibition of protein-glycation, and inhibition of collagenase activity. This review will provide an overview of MAAs, as potential anti-aging ingredients, beginning with their structure, before moving on to discuss the most recent experimental observations, including the molecular and cellular mechanisms through which MAAs might protect the skin. In particular, we focus on the potential anti-aging activity of mycosporine-2-glycine (M2G).

Keywords: mycosporine-like amino acids; mycosporine-2-glycine; UV-absorbing compound; sunscreen; anti-aging; anti-oxidation; anti-inflammation; anti-protein-glycation activity

1. Introduction

The skin, the largest human organ, is constantly exposed to the external environment. Exposure to a variety of environmental stress factors, particularly ultraviolet (UV) radiation in sunlight, can damage skin. Sunlight can be broken down into three types of nonionizing electromagnetic radiation—infrared (IR) (780–3000 nm), visible (400–780 nm), and UV (100–400 nm). The percentages of energy radiated to the Earth, in the total energy emitted by the Sun, are 53% IR, 39% visible, and 8% UV [1]. On the basis of its physiological and biological effects, UV radiation can be further divided into three main bands—the 315–400 nm band (designated as UV-A), the 280–315 nm band (designated as UV-B), and the 100–280 nm band (designated as UV-C) [2]. Solar UV radiation is drastically diminished as it passes through the ozone layer and the atmosphere; as a result, the proportion of UV rays in the sunlight reaching the Earth's surface, is made up of 95% UV-A and 5% UV-B [1]. Although it comprises only a small portion of the total UV radiation, UV-B is thought to be more harmful than

UV-A, since UV-B is most active in damaging the skin and eyes [3]. UV-A and UV-B are also known to be genotoxic, meaning they can induce photochemical damage in cellular DNA and proteins [4,5]. Consequently, exposure to UV-A and UV-B, stimulates skin photoaging and can be responsible for the induction of skin cancer [6]. Skin photoaging is characterized by the development of pigmentary disorders, such as solar lentigines, fine and coarse wrinkles, and benign, premalignant, and malignant skin tumors on sun-exposed skin [7]. Highly energetic UV-C radiation has no biological significance, because it does not reach the Earth's surface, due to its complete absorption by the ozone layer and the atmosphere [1,3]. The depletion of the ozone layer, over the past few decades, has increased the amount of solar UV radiation reaching the Earth's surface [8], in particular UV-B levels, since UV-A is not absorbed by the ozone layer [9].

Many marine organisms that are exposed to UV radiation have developed photoprotective mechanisms [10]. For example, in cyanobacteria, which dominate the marine environment, UV protection mechanisms have evolved at the molecular, cellular, and behavioral levels [11]. Cyanobacteria can synthesize various types of "sunscreen" compounds, which confer protection against UV radiation. Mycosporine-like amino acids (MAAs), scytonemin, and carotenoids are known to be key compounds in cyanobacteria that can absorb wavelengths in the UV range. These natural products are promising candidate molecules in the field of cosmeceutical compounds discovery [12]. In fact, MAAs have already been commercialized as Helioguard®365. This cosmetic reagent contains the liposomal MAAs, shinorine (SHI), and porphyra-334 (P334), that were originally extracted from the red alga *Porphyra umbilicalis*, and has been successfully commercialized as a natural and safe sunscreen compound [12]. Additionally, MAAs are thought to be multifunctional secondary metabolites, in the cells of producers [13]. Many MAAs are known to act as antioxidants [14], while several recent reports have suggested that MAAs have potential therapeutic applications for reducing skin-aging processes. From this point of view, recently, several review reports with special emphasis on the potential use of MAAs in cosmetic products, have been published [15–17]. In this paper, we review MAAs and their potential as anti-skin-aging ingredients, by describing a basic overview of their structure, before moving on to a detailed account of the most recent experimental observations, accumulated thus far. The mechanisms by which MAAs might act to protect the skin from aging is discussed at, both, the cellular and the molecular level. In particular, the prominent potential anti-aging activity of the MAA mycosporine-2-glycine (M2G), which is biosynthesized by the halotolerant cyanobacterium *Aphanothece halophytica*, is highlighted.

2. Mechanisms of the UV-Induced Skin Aging

UV radiation is important for our health as UV-B exposure can induce the production of a crucial nutrient, vitamin D, in our skin [18]. However, long-term and repeated exposure to UV can promote the skin photoaging process, including skin cancer formation [19]. The mechanisms by which UV-mediated cellular damage is induced are briefly described in this section.

2.1. Cellular DNA Damage

Direct and indirect toxic effects of UV radiation on the DNA molecule, mediate photoaging. Direct absorption of UV-B photons by DNA, can result in the generation of pyrimidine dimers, leading to defects in the DNA strand [20]. UV-B radiation leads mostly to the formation of *cis-syn* cyclobutadipyrimidines (CPDs) and pyrimidine (6-4) pyrimidone photoproducts (6-4PPs). 6-4PPs can be converted into related Dewar valence isomers (DewPPs), upon UV-excitation at 314 nm. Such DNA damage interferes with DNA replication and transcription, and brings various harmful effects to the cell, such as mutation, instability of the chromosome, and cell death. UV-A does not directly alter the structure of DNA as DNA does not strongly absorb radiation in the UV-A range [21]. However, UV-A can damage DNA indirectly, via a photosensitized reaction mediated by generating the radical singlet oxygen ($^1O_2$), resulting in purine base modifications [20]. The singlet oxygen anion oxidizes the guanine moiety, followed by the generation of 8-oxo-7,8-dihydroguanine (8-oxo-G) and

8-oxo-7,8-dihydro-2′-deoxyguanosine (8-oxo-dG). As 8-oxo-G and 8-oxo-dG can associate with adenine instead of cytosine, transition mutations might occur.

2.2. Reactive Oxygen Species Generation

Reactive oxygen species (ROS), initiators of oxidative stress, are oxygen-containing reactive chemical species that include hydrogen peroxide (H_2O_2), hydroxyl radicals ($\cdot OH$), superoxide anion radicals ($\cdot O_2^-$), and $^1O_2$. In our skin, exposure to UV radiation is known to be associated with the generation of ROS. These ROS can activate skin-aging cascades, such as matrix metalloproteinase (MMP)-1-mediated aging and NF-κB-TNF-α-mediated, inflammation-induced aging [22]. The variety of ROS generation mechanism by UV, depend on the UV radiation wavelength range. In addition to $^1O_2$ generation, as mentioned above, it has been reported that UV-A radiation can induce the generation of $\cdot O_2^-$ by the activation of intracellular nicotinamide adenine dinucleotide phosphate (NADPH) oxidase, NOX [23], and association with advanced glycation end-products (AGEs) [24]. Sakurai et al. elucidated that both $^1O_2$ and $\cdot O_2^-$ were generated in the skin of mice exposed to UV-A [25]. H_2O_2, $\cdot O_2^-$, and $\cdot OH$ species might be generated in AGEs, during exposure to UV-A [24]. UV-B is also known to lead to the production of H_2O_2, $\cdot O_2^-$, and $\cdot OH$ [26]. Although the source of these UV-B-induced ROS remains unclear, recently it was reported that NADPH oxidase, NOX1, is associated with UV-B-induced p38/MAPK activation and cytotoxicity, via ROS generation in keratinocytes [26].

To prevent skin damage induced by excess UV-induced ROS and regulate epidermal homeostasis, skin cells possess an antioxidative function that acts as an endogenous defense system [20]. This system mainly consists of six enzymes—superoxide dismutase (SOD), catalase (CAT), glutathione peroxidase (GPX), glutathione reductase (GR), thioredoxin oxidase (TRXR), and peroxiredoxin (PRDX) (Figure 1). SOD and CAT eliminate $\cdot O_2^-$ and H_2O_2, respectively, and ultimately convert $\cdot O_2^-$ to H_2O, whereas GPX, GR, TRXR, and PRDX eliminate H_2O_2, by regulation of the redox conditions of glutathione and thioredoxin. In addition to this enzymatic system, non-enzymatic molecules, such as vitamin C (ascorbic acid), vitamin E (α-tocopherol), glutathione, and ureic acid, play a major role as antioxidants in the skin [27]. These small molecules scavenge and neutralize free radicals, by providing an extra electron to make an electron pair.

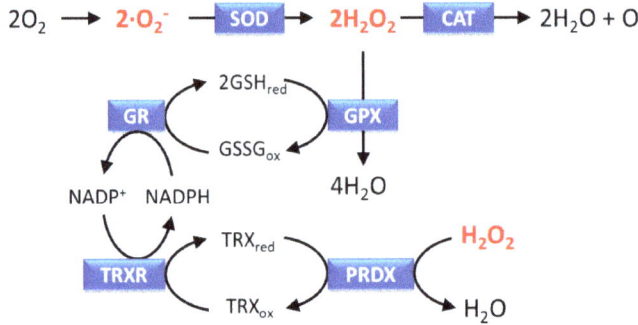

Figure 1. Removal of reactive oxygen species (ROS) by an antioxidant defense system consisting of superoxide dismutase (SOD), catalase (CAT), glutathione peroxidase (GPX), glutathione reductase (GR), thioredoxin oxidase (TRXR), and peroxiredoxin (PRDX). GSHred and GSSGox indicate reduced glutathione and oxidized glutathione, respectively. TRXred and TRXox indicate reduced thioredoxin and oxidized thioredoxin, respectively.

2.3. Inflammatory Responses

Exposure to UV radiation induces inflammation by triggering chemical reactions in the skin. Distinct patterns of inflammation are caused by exposure to specific wavelengths of light. The three groups, UV-A, UV-B, and UV-C, have been classified, based on these different patterns of inflammation [28]. Erythema induced in the skin, following exposure to UV-B radiation is characterized as sunburn. Inflammatory responses induced by UV-B are mostly achieved through a variety of mediators, including nitric oxide (NO), inducible NO synthase (iNOS), prostaglandin E2 (PGE_2), cyclooxygenase-2 (COX-2), tumor necrosis factor-α (TNF-α), and other cytokines, such as interleukin-1 (IL-1) and interleukin-6 (IL-6) (Figure 2). These molecules are predominantly regulated by nuclear factor-kappa B (NF-κB), and mostly produced in keratinocytes, which are the predominant cell type in the epidermis [29]. It has been reported that the expression of the COX-2 protein, which is responsible for PGE_2 production, is upregulated, following exposure to UV-B, in both human skin and in cultured human keratinocytes [30]. ROS are also known to be associated with the inflammatory response, as it has been observed that COX-2 expression was induced by ROS in different cell types [31].

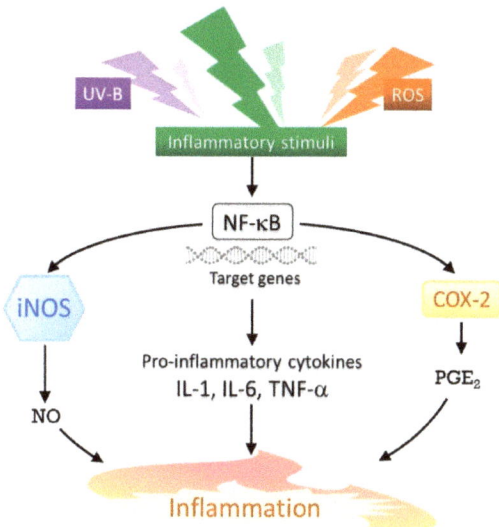

Figure 2. UV-B-induced inflammatory response. Nitric oxide (NO), inducible NO synthase (iNOS), prostaglandin E2 (PGE_2), cyclooxygenase-2 (COX-2), tumor necrosis factor-α (TNF-α), and other cytokines, such as interleukin-1 (IL-1) and interleukin-6 (IL-6), are shown as mediators.

2.4. Induction of Matrix Metalloproteinases

UV radiation upregulates the expression of matrix metalloproteinases (MMPs) in the skin. MMPs, which are known to be responsible for the destruction of extracellular matrix (ECM) proteins, such as collagen, play an important role in maintaining skin homeostasis and skin aging [32]. MMPs are secreted by keratinocytes and dermal fibroblasts, in response to multiple stimuli, including oxidative stress and cytokines, in addition to UV radiation. The repeated induction of these collagen-degrading enzymes, over the long-term, is thought to cause collagen damage, which is one of the reasons for photoaging. Although several MMPs are expressed in the mammalian skin, it has been suggested that MMP-1 is the major collagen-degrading enzyme responsible for collagen destruction, in severely photo-damaged skin [33]. The upregulation of MMP expression is stimulated by the activator protein-1 (AP-1), which is known to be a UV-inducible transcription factor [34]. In fact, AP-1 regulatory element exists in the 5' flanking region of MMP genes. Transforming growth factor-beta (TGF-β) and NF-κB are also known to be involved in the induction of MMPs in the skin [34].

2.5. Induction of Protein Glycation

Protein glycation (non-enzymatic glycosylation), also known as the first step of the Maillard reaction, involves the formation of covalent bonds between proteins and reducing sugars. A condensation reaction between the free amino groups of proteins and the carbonyl groups of sugars, results in the formation of a Schiff base, followed by an Amadori product. Excessive products are oxidized and dehydrated to form stable, molecular, cross-linking products, called advanced glycation end-products (AGEs) [35]. Protein glycation influences the physical and functional properties of a protein, as it causes conformational changes in the protein structure [36]. In skin, it has been reported that glycation of collagen type I is associated with the development of skin dullness and decreased skin elasticity [37]. AGEs are also involved in the generation of ROS. Masaki et al. reported that exposure of AGEs to UV-A irradiation in vitro, resulted in the generation of ROS, such as $\cdot O_2^-$, H_2O_2, and $\cdot OH$, as mentioned above [24]. In humans, skin autofluorescence, a biomarker for AGEs, can function as an endogenous photosensitizer that induces ROS generation, following exposure to UV-A radiation [35]. Thus, a glycation reaction followed by AGE formation is thought to be one of the fundamental mechanisms associated with skin aging, under environmental conditions, especially UV radiation [24].

3. Natural Compounds that Prevent UV radiation (UVR)-Induced Photo-Damage

Wavelength dependency is crucial in determining photobiological effects. Short-wavelength UV-C is the most damaging type of UV, but because it is filtered out by the ozone layer, only UV-B and UV-A are considered to be of biological significance. Considering their impacts, only UV-A causes indirect DNA damage, via the generation of $\cdot O_2^-$, an initiator of important ROS (see Section 2.2). UV-A penetrates deep into the dermis of the skin. Prolonged UV-A exposure can lead to photoaging and suppression of the immune system. Direct DNA damage, however, is caused by UV-B, via the formation of CPDs and 6-4PPs. UV-B also causes skin damage and transformation, for example, by affecting skin structures and causing wrinkling (a sign of photoaging), roughness, and premature aging, and even leading to skin malignancies and fatal diseases, such as skin cancers [38].

To prevent or ameliorate these adverse effects, the blockage of excessive UV or alleviating the cascade of UV-induced photo-damage is crucial. Sunscreen agents (either physical blockers or chemical agents) are often applied to the skin to block excessive UV. Recently, there has been a growing demand for artificial chemical sunscreens to be replaced with natural ones. This is because of the adverse or side effects of artificial chemical sunscreens, and because of environmental concerns. Natural sunscreens and natural compounds that possess properties that resist UV-induced photo-damage are, therefore, of great interest. Some natural compounds can lead to significant improvements in skin health and performance.

Natural compounds that can provide protection against UVR-induced photo-damage can be categorized on the basis of these mechanisms—(1) blockage of UV photons; (2) involvement in the DNA repair system; (3) antioxidant activity; (4) anti-immunomodulatory activity; (5) anti-inflammatory activity; and (6) having inhibitory action on the cellular matrix [39]. In this section, we describe the natural compounds from plant extracts and a class of secondary metabolites which have pharmacological relevance as superior sunscreen compounds, called mycosporine-like amino acids (MAAs).

3.1. Plant Extracts

The database of natural compounds (NCs) contains more than 320,000 compounds, reported in Super Natural II (https://doi.org/10.1093/nar/gku886). Of these, more than 50,000 compounds obtained from plant extracts have been submitted to the database (http://kanaya.aist-nara.ac.jp/KNApSAcK_Family/). The largest class of natural plant extracts which have been shown to have the most relevant activity and the most beneficial effects against UV-B induced photo-damage reported to date, are those which work via inhibitory effects on the signaling pathways (for example, NF-κB, MARK, and AP-1), and biomarker proteins of the target signaling pathways (for example, COX-2 in inflammatory signaling). Inhibitory effects on these signaling pathways further modulate cellular signaling targets and antioxidant properties, to deplete ROS generation. For example, pomegranate fruit extract has been demonstrated to inhibit UV-B-mediated phosphorylation of the NF-κB and MARK pathways, in normal human epidermal keratinocytes (NHEK) [40]. Inhibition of UV-B-induced activation of MARK and NF-κB by proanthocyanidins, a class of polyphenols isolated from grape seeds, polyphenols from green tea, and quercetin from onion, have been reported [41]. Resveratrols, a class of natural phenols obtained from grape skin, cranberries and peanuts, possess the capacity to reduce NF-κB activation [42]. COX-2, a biomarker protein of the inflammatory cascade, is inhibited by phenolic compounds, such as caffeic acid from white grapes [43], kaempferol from grapes [44], and curcumin from turmeric [45]. Comprehensive studies into natural plant agents that can protect against UVB-induced photo-damage have been summarized in previous review papers [46–48].

3.2. Mycosporine-Like Amino Acids

Mycosporine-like amino acids (MAAs) were first discovered in fungi, associated with a physiological role in light-stimulated sporulation. In 1993, a direct effect as a photo-protectant was made evident by the compound's ability to block photons. It was revealed that MAAs could prevent 3 out of 10 photons from hitting a cytoplasmic target in cyanobacteria [49]. This ability has led MAAs to be known as a primary sunscreen.

Accumulating evidence has shown that some MAAs possess additional beneficial functions. Their pronounced photo-protective potential was first noted when they were proved to be ROS scavengers, an ability which arose via their antioxidant ability [14,50]. Further, distinct biological functions have since been proved, including DNA damage-protection, anti-inflammatory activity, and inhibitory action toward AGEs. These multiple beneficial functions make MAAs very interesting biomolecules. More details of these natural compounds will be further reviewed in the next section.

4. Molecular Properties of MAAs

In this section, the current basic understanding of MAAs is summarized in three parts—a general description of MAAs, their chemical structure, and their biosynthetic pathways.

4.1. General Description

'Mycosporine' is a common term used for fungal UV-absorbing metabolites that have been substituted with amino acid residues [51]. Since the 1960s, mycosporine derivatives, grouped as MAAs, have been found and identified from a wide range of organisms, including marine organisms such as red algae, sea stars, corals, dinoflagellates, cyanobacteria, and lichens [12,52]. MAAs comprise a cyclohexenone or cyclohexenimine ring, as their core chromophore ring structure substituted with amino acid residues or imino alcohols, or some further modifications (Figure 3). For example, in the structure of P334, threonine and glycine bind to the C1 and C3 positions of the core chromophore structure, respectively.

MAAs are considered to be the most effective UV-A-absorbing compounds in nature [53]. MAAs exhibit a maximum absorbance within the UV-A and UV-B range (from 310 to 362 nm), with high molar extinction coefficients (ε = 28,100–50,000 $M^{-1}cm^{-1}$). In organisms that accumulate MAAs, these compounds are believed to contribute to the suppression of UV-induced stress, by dissipating excess energy in the form of heat, without generating ROS, after absorbing UV radiation. MAAs are highly water-soluble compounds, due to their zwitterionic properties, derived from their amino acid substitutions, and therefore, they generally accumulate in the cytosolic space. It has been reported that MAAs might act as multifunctional compounds within cells. Besides their UV-protective role, another important biological role of MAAs is their antioxidant properties [14]. Other properties of MAAs, proposed so far, include DNA-protective activity [54], anti-inflammatory activity [55,56], activity to promote osmotic equilibrium [57,58], and involvement in cell–cell interactions [13].

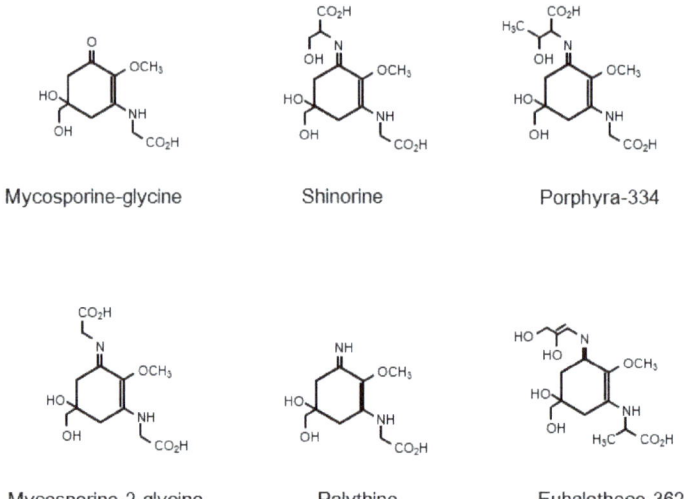

Figure 3. Chemical structures of the selected mycosporine-like amino acids (MAAs)—mycosporine-glycine, shinorine, porphyra-334, mycosporine-2-glycine, palythine, and euhalothece-362.

4.2. Chemical Structure

MAAs can be roughly divided into two groups—mono-substituted MAAs and di-substituted MAAs. In mono-substituted MAAs, the C3 position on the cyclohexenone structure is substituted with an amino compound. One of the mono-substituted MAAs, mycosporine-glycine (MG), which is a common intermediate for the bioproduction of di-substituted MAAs, has been suggested to be an important protectant against sunlight damage in marine organisms, via the elimination of $^1O_2$ [59]. The absorption maximum of MG is reported to be 310 nm. On the other hand, the absorption maxima of di-substituted MAAs, vary from 320 to 362 nm, depending on the type of substituent. For example, the absorption maxima of P334 (C1: Thr; C3: Gly), palythine (C1: $-NH_2$; C3: Gly), and M2G (C1: Gly; C3: Gly) are 334, 320, and 331 nm, respectively [14]. In di-substituted MAAs, a protonated nitrogen atom on the imine group, results in the formation of a zwitterion, followed by conjugation and delocalization of the positive charge on the nitrogen atom, over the core ring structure. This conjugation stimulates UV absorption by MAAs. The extent of resonance delocalization can affect the extinction coefficient and absorption maximum of each MAA [14]. Further modification of the substituents of MAAs by condensation, dehydration, decarboxylation, oxidation, reduction, sulfonation, or glycosylation might also affect them.

To date, more than 30 different MAAs have been identified. To identify and characterize these MAAs, a variety of experimental techniques have been used, such as high-performance liquid chromatography (HPLC) analysis, mass spectrometry (MS) analysis including liquid chromatography (LC)-MS, amino acid analysis, infrared (IR) spectroscopic analysis, nuclear magnetic resonance (NMR) analysis, and gas chromatography (GC)-MS analysis. An appropriate combination of these analytical techniques, along with technological improvements in analytical instruments, has been effective in helping to characterize the structure of MAAs [12]. To prepare MAA materials for analysis, preparative liquid chromatographic techniques have often been used, following the extraction of MAAs from organisms using organic solvents, such as methanol and ethanol [60].

4.3. Biosynthetic Pathways

The molecular factors involved in the biosynthetic pathways of MAAs have so far mainly been identified and analyzed in cyanobacteria. Gene clusters for MAA bioproduction in cyanobacteria, generally consist of four genes. For example, MAA synthetic gene clusters in *Anabaena variabilis* ATCC 29413, *Nostoc punctiforme* ATCC 29133, *Aphanothece halophytica*, and *Microcystis aeruginosa* PCC 7806, contain *Ava_3858* to *Ava_3855*, *NpR5600* to *NpF5597*, *Ap3858* to *Ap3855*, and *mysA* to *mysD*, respectively [13,61,62]. It has been reported that *A. variabilis* ATCC 29413, *N. punctiforme* ATCC 29133, and *M. aeruginosa* PCC 7806, produce mainly SHI, whereas M2G is known as the sole MAA produced by *A. halophytica*. The first two genes encode predicted DHQ synthase (DHQS) and O-methyltransferase (O-MT), respectively. The protein products of these two genes are predicted to synthesize 4-deoxygadusol (4-DG), a common precursor compound for the synthesis of MAAs, from 3-dehydroquinate (DHQ), a shikimate-pathway intermediate, or sedoheptulose-7-phosphate (SHP), an intermediate of the pentose phosphate pathway [10,61]. The protein products of the third genes, which encode the adenosine triphosphate (ATP)-grasp enzyme superfamily, catalyze the imine linkage of 4-DG, with glycine, to produce MG [61]. Finally, the protein products of the fourth genes, which encode a non-ribosomal peptide synthase (NRPS)-like protein or D-Ala-D-Ala ligase, yield di-substituted MAAs, from MG, by the attachment of an additional amino acid moiety. This last step for di-substituted MAA-bioproduction by the fourth protein, might cause the attachment of different amino acid residues, due to differences in substrate specificity. In addition to cyanobacteria (although there is still room for further functional molecular characterization), homologues of these cyanobacterial MAA synthetic genes have been found in fungi, actinobacteria, dinoflagellates, sea anemones, and corals [61,63,64].

Although detailed investigations of the regulatory molecular mechanisms for MAA bioproduction remain to be done, a number of studies have revealed that various environmental factors might affect intracellular MAA accumulation levels in MAA-producing organisms. UV exposure is known to be a typical MAA production-enhancing factor [10]. In addition to UV irradiation, other abiotic stresses, such as salt stress, thermal stress, and nutrient availability, can induce MAA production [12]. For example, salt stress upregulated the expression of M2G synthetic genes and increased M2G production in *A. halophytica*, and a combination of UV-B irradiation and salt stress, resulted in the enhancement of M2G accumulation, compared with UV-B exposure only [62]. In this cyanobacterium, the oversupply of nitrate, glycine, or serine, also induced intracellular M2G accumulation [65]. Enhanced MAA production has been observed in some corals, when simultaneously exposed to UV and thermal stresses, whereas exposure to high solar radiation, which contains both photosynthetically active radiation (PAR) and UV radiation, and thermal stress, was seen to decrease MAA production in the Caribbean coral *Montastraea faveolata* [10]. Thus, it has been suggested that there is complex regulation of MAA bioproduction, in response to these environmental stresses.

5. Potential of Anti-Photoaging and Photo-Protective Activity of MAAs

In this section, experimental observations for understanding the potential of MAAs, in terms of their anti-photoaging and photo-protective activities, are summarized in six parts—DNA damage-protecting activity, anti-oxidative activity, anti-inflammatory activity, anti-protein glycation activity, collagenase inhibitory activity, and other activities.

5.1. DNA Damage-Protecting Activity

DNA damage can be caused both directly by UV-B and indirectly by UV-A, via the formation of ROS. It has been reported that MAAs have the potential to protect DNA against damage from oxidative stress induced by the ROS, H_2O_2 [54]. This study was performed using the A375 human melanoma cell line, a model used for the study of the development of skin cancer. M2G rescued DNA from the damage induced by H_2O_2. Using the comet assay, it was demonstrated that M2G had a somewhat high genoprotective effect, similar to ascorbic acid. This direct in vivo assay, thus, revealed the potential role of M2G in protecting against DNA damage caused by oxidative stress induced by H_2O_2.

The efficacy of protecting against DNA damage by another well-known MAA, P334 (in the form of Helioguard®365), originally isolated from red algae, was evaluated. In this case, the fibroblast cell line IMR-90 was used as the model in the study [66]. Protective activity against DNA damage caused by UV-A was observed in the presence of Helioguard®365. A visible reduction in DNA damage in the presence of Helioguard®365 occurred in a dose-dependent manner. Palythine also exhibited a protective effect against UV-A-induced DNA damage in HaCaT cells [67]. This is a cell line of immortalized human keratinocytes, which has been extensively used to study epidermal homeostasis. The formation of cyclobutane pyrimidine dimers (CPD), 8-oxo-7,8-dihydroguanine (8-oxoGua), and alkali-labile sites (ALS), was drastically reduced in palythine-treated HaCaT cells subjected to UV-A irradiation. Results obtained either from purified MAAs (such as M2G and palythine) and MAAs in formulation (Helioguard®365), indicated the preventive efficacy of MAAs, against DNA damage caused by direct oxidative stress, due to ROS.

5.2. Antioxidant Activity

In biological processes, oxidation is essential for energy metabolism and production. It has long been recognized that energy metabolism is linked to ROS production. The ROS produced can serve as cell signaling molecules, triggering cellular processes, such as cell division, inflammation, immune functions, and stress responses [68]. These molecular and cellular mechanisms are under the tight control of the equilibrium of ROS generation and scavenging. During exposure to UV, or following some oxidative reactions (such as contact with foreign chemicals), ROS can be constantly generated. ROS generation mediated by UV radiation has been shown to stimulate the expression of genes in signaling pathways, which can consequently exert several physiological effects, including inflammation and protein oxidation. To suppress photo-oxidation or scavenging ROS, antioxidant defense mechanisms are vital.

Substantial evidence has revealed that MAAs have potential abilities as antioxidants [14,52,54,60,67,69,70]. Various MAAs have the ability to scavenge such ROS, like hydroxyl radicals, hydroperoxyl radicals, singlet oxygen, and superoxide anions. The antioxidant role of MAAs might have a special significance in scavenging the free radicals propagated by oxidative stress induced by UV radiation or other environmental stresses. Among the 30 MAAs currently known, antioxidant activity has been clearly observed in some of mono-, di-substituted MAAs, and glycosylated MAAs, in both, in vitro and in vivo studies [14,52,54,60,67,69,70]. It should be noted that some MAAs showed indirect evidence for antioxidant capacity, via a slow photodegradation in the presence of a photosynthesizer, or a reaction with singlet oxygen [14]. These observations will not be included in this review. Table 1 summarizes radical scavenging activity of MAAs. IC50 values against organic radical sources, such as DPPH (2,2-diphenyl-1-picryhydrazyl), ABTS (2,2'-azino-bis(3-ethylbenzthiazoline-6-sulphonic acid), and an oxygen radical absorption capacity (ORAC) were reported.

As summarized in Table 1, various research groups performed in vitro analyses to assess antioxidant activity, for example using an organic radical, such as a DPPH assay; an organic cation radical, such as an ABTS assay; and an ORAC assay. The DPPH assay revealed that M2G exhibited the strongest antioxidant properties, followed by MG, while SHI and P334 showed these properties to a lesser extent [54,60,71]. The ABTS assay showed a similar trend to the DPPH assay, with M2G exhibiting the strongest oxygen-radical absorption capacity, followed by SHI and P334 [60]. Glycosylated MAAs seem to display slightly different antioxidant capacities. In some cases, a slow-acting radical scavenging was observed. Among the three glycosylated MAAs, the hexose-bound-P334 [72], 7-O-(β-arabinopyranosyl)-P334 extracted from the cyanobacterium *Nostoc commune* [72,73], and 13-O-β-galactosyl-P334 from *Nostoc sphaericum* [69], the 7-O-(β-arabinopyranosyl)-P334 showed the highest activity. These glycosylated MAAs were derived from P334, and the scavenging activity observed suggested that their glycosylation led to an increase in scavenging activity. Variations in the MAA chemical structure is one of the most interesting features of this class of compounds, particularly with regard to the structure–activity relationships. Structure–activity relationships of the biologically active MAAs have been discussed elsewhere [14,71]. However, the exact mechanisms of these biologically active MAAs are still unknown, and detailed investigations will be a useful direction for future studies. In addition to MAAs, other compounds exhibiting antioxidant activity, such as scytonemins, phenols, isobenzofuranone derivatives, exopolysaccharides, diketopiperazine alkaloids, and dioxopiperazine alkaloids, have been found in various organisms, including marine fungi and bacteria [16]. For the therapeutic application purpose, taking into account that naturally occurring products have been proven to be relatively safer, it could be preferred to utilize these natural antioxidants for human utilization, instead of synthetic ones. Among these natural compounds, scytonemins are a class of well-known natural cyanobacterial UV sunscreen, with basic characteristics such as hydrophobic pigments. The antioxidant property of scytonemins was revealed by an electron spin resonance analysis and ABTS assay. For example, the purified scytonemin from *Nostoc commune* displayed a radical scavenging activity, with an IC50 value of 36 µM, which was comparable with MAAs [11]. Carotenoids, the most common pigments in nature, are also known for their antioxidant activity, as well as light harvesting and photoprotective functions in photosynthetic organisms [11]. Among over 750 carotenoids found so far, astaxanthin is believed to be one of the strongest antioxidants in nature [74]. Recently, Dose et al. estimated the 50% scavenging concentration (SC50) value of astaxanthin, for the DPPH free radical scavenging, to be around 500 µM [75]. On the other hand, Cheewinthamrongrod et al. determined SC50 values of M2G and MG, for DPPH free radical scavenging, as 22 µM and 43 µM, respectively [54]. Although the assays for measurement of DPPH free radical scavenging activities were not identical (electronspin resonance spectroscopy (ESR) method combined with spin trapping for astaxanthin; colorimetric method for M2G and MG), these observations suggest that a certain kind of MAAs are powerful natural antioxidant molecules, derived from marine organisms. It would be desirable that further comprehensive research analyses elucidate the significance of MAAs as antioxidative molecules, by comparing other natural compounds. Apart from the antioxidant capacity obtained from in vitro and in vivo studies, experimental evidence suggests certain MAA, such as M2G and palythine, have the necessary characteristics of biocompatible natural compounds, to protect the human skin [54,67]. M2G is biocompatible with normal human skin fibroblast cells [54]. Palythine significantly reduced a wide range of adverse effects from UV-radiation-induced damage in HaCaT keratinocytes. The combined experimental evidence, either from antioxidant capacity, biocompatibility, or several other lines of evidence, suggest that MAAs have a superior function, compared with other antioxidants.

Oxidative stress can trigger several signaling pathways, and of these, Kelch-like ECH-associated protein 1/nuclear factor erythroid 2-related factor 2/antioxidant response element (Keap1/Nrf2/ARE) signaling, was shown to be the major mechanism in alleviating oxidative stress in human cells, via the regulation of antioxidant and detoxification enzymes [68]. A recent study found that M2G suppressed the expression of the transcription factor Nrf and the antioxidant-associated genes encoding the detoxification enzymes Cu/Zn-superoxide dismutase (*Sod1*), catalase (*Cat*), and heme oxygenase-1 (*Hmox1*) in RAW 264.7 macrophage cells, under oxidative stress induced by H_2O_2. The enzymatic activities of SOD and CAT were also found to be attenuated, in agreement with the transcriptional analysis.

In Keap1/Nrf2/ARE signaling, the transcription factor Nrf2 is generally attached to Keap1, forming a Keap1/Nrf2 complex. This inactivated protein is retained in the cytosol, by the binding of Keap1 with actin or myosin. Activation of the Keap1/Nrf2/ARE pathway only occurs after the detachment of Keap1 and Nrf2. This step is induced by oxidative species and electrophiles. Activated Nrf2 is then localized in the nucleus, where it binds to the basic leucine zipper-musculoaponeurotic fibrosarcoma (bZip-Maf) protein, at the ARE region. Finally, the interaction between heterodimers and the ARE-promotor region, initiates the transcription of antioxidative genes [76–78]. It has been demonstrated that SHI and P334 have the ability to bind with Keap1, associated protein in Keap1/Nrf2/ARE signaling [70]. The ability of MAAs to dissociate Nrf2 from Keap1, was confirmed by the up-regulation of mRNA expression of the Nrf2-targeted genes, which encode oxidative-stress defense proteins in primary skin fibroblasts, prior and post UVR exposure. This molecular evidence suggests that SHI and P334 are activators of the Keap1/Nrf2 signaling pathway, and thus, have beneficial effects for antioxidative gene expression.

Table 1. IC50 values against 2,2-diphenyl-1-picryhydrazyl (DPPH), 2,2′-azino-bis(3-ethylbenzthiazoline-6-sulphonic acid (ABTS), and oxygen radical absorption capacity (ORAC) of mono-, di-substituted MAAs, and glycosylated MAAs.

Mycosporine-like Amino Acids (MAAs)	IC50	References
Mono-Substituted MAAs		
Mycosporine-glycine	3 μM [a] at pH 8.5	[14,52]
	43 μM [b]	[54]
Mycosporine-γ-aminobutyric acid	0.6 mM [a]	[14]
Di-Substituted MAAs		
Mycosporine-2-glycine	45 μM [a]	[54]
	22 μM [b]	[71]
Palythine	21.3 μM [b]	[67]
	714 μM [c]	[67]
Porphyra-334	133 μM [a]	[60]
	185.2 μM [b]	[70]
Shinorine	94 μM [a]	[60]
	399 μM [b]	[70]
Glycosylated MAAs		
Hexose-bound-P334	58 mM [a]	[69]
7-O-(β-arabinopyranosyl)-P334	9.5 mM [a]	[69]
13-O-β-galactosyl-porphyra-334	17 mM [a]	[69]
Standard antioxidants		
Trolox	10 μM [b]	[60]
Ascorbic acid	21.3 μM [b]	[67]
α-Tocopherol	11.1 μM [b]	[67]

[a] Radical scavenging activity measured using ABTS as he organic radical source. [b] Radical scavenging activity measured using DPPH as the organic radical source. [c] Radical scavenging activity measured using the ORAC antioxidant assay kit.

5.3. Anti-Inflammatory Activity

Inflammation is a vital component of the physiological defense process, in response to molecular and cellular damage caused by oxidative stress, irradiation, infection, and exposure to endotoxins, such as lipopolysaccharides (LPS) [79]. Oxidative stress can directly induce inflammation through the canonical pathway [80]. Conversely, UV radiation activates the trigger protein eIF2α, inducing expression of GCN/PERK2 [81].

To date, the anti-inflammatory activities of MAAs have been investigated in human keratinocyte, HaCaT, and RAW 264.7 macrophage models. Suh et al. [56] evaluated the effects of SHI, P334, and MG, on the expression of genes associated with inflammation, using the human fibroblast cell line, HaCaT, in response to UV irradiation. Among these MAAs, only MG suppressed the expression of an inflammation marker gene, COX-2, and in a concentration-dependent manner. An in vitro model comprising RAW 264.7 macrophages was used to evaluate anti-inflammatory effects, in response to stimulation by LPS. Nitric oxide (NO) is an important pro-inflammatory signaling molecule, and is considered to be a good index of inflammation [82,83]. It was shown that M2G exhibited the most potency in reducing NO production, in response to LPS inflammatory stimulation, with effects that were two- to three-fold higher, compared with SHI, P334, and palythine [71]. Another line of anti-inflammatory effects became evident, following the transcriptional analysis. M2G-pre-treatment of RAW 264.7 cells, stimulated by LPS, significantly suppressed the expression of the key inflammatory signaling regulatory genes iNOS and COX-2. The up-regulation of iNOS and COX-2, during inflammation, is controlled by the pro-inflammatory transcription factor NF-κB, therefore, it seems likely that M2G inhibits the production of inflammatory mediators, by suppressing the NF-κB pathway. M2G inhibition of iNOS and COX-2 expression in activated macrophages, is regarded as a potentially interesting tool for the treatment or prevention of inflammation.

5.4. Anti-Protein-Glycation Activity

Glycation of proteins leads to the generation of AGEs, which are linked to the progression of aging and age-related diseases. It was recently reported that MAAs can have inhibitory effects on protein glycation [84]. In that report, the glycation-dependent cross-linking of hen egg white lysozyme (HEWL), which is a structural homologue of human lysozyme, was evaluated with or without addition of M2G, or a mixture of P334 and SHI. Both samples with added MAAs showed inhibitory activity, with M2G isolated from *A. halophytica* showing a greater activity than the mixture of P334 and SHI. The 50% inhibitory concentration (IC50) value for the HEWL dimer formation with M2G, was 1.61 mM. This value was less than that of the aminoguanidine, which is known to be an inhibitor of glycation via reactions with the Amadori carbonyl groups of glycated proteins. These observations suggest that MAAs, and M2G, in particular, can be useful in preventing the formation of AGEs. Further studies using other proteins in addition to HEWL, such as collagen type I, which is known to be associated with skin-aging, will be an interesting avenue for future research. Although detailed investigations are needed to fully understand the glycation-inhibitory activity of MAAs, the antioxidant properties of MAAs, might contribute to this activity, since some antioxidants, including aminoguanidine, inhibit protein glycation, by preventing oxidation of the Amadori product [85]. Taking into account the greater antioxidant activity of M2G, compared with a mixture of P334 and SHI (see above), this hypothesis is reasonable.

5.5. Bacterial Collagenase Inhibitory Activity

Mammalian collagenases that belong to the matrix metalloproteinase (MMP) family are important enzymes for the maintenance of skin homeostasis, through the destruction of ECM proteins; they are involved in the skin-aging process, as described above. On the other hand, bacterial collagenase, which is one of the factors of bacterial virulence, enables the destruction of the extracellular structure, by attacking the collagen helix, and is responsible for part of the pathogenic process in some bacteria, such as *Clostridium* [86]. Thus far, two research groups have reported that MAAs might inhibit bacterial collagenase activity. One group found that SHI, P334, and palythine inhibited *Clostridium histolyticum* collagenase activity [87]. The IC50 values were 104.0, 105.9, and 158.9 µM for SHI, P334, and palythine, respectively. On the other hand, another group showed that both M2G and a mixture of P334 and SHI, inhibited the *C. histolyticum* collagenase activity with IC50 values of 0.47 and more than 10 mM, respectively, in the presence of calcium chloride [84]. Even though the range of IC50 values between these two reports is quite wide, probably due to differences in the assay procedures, these observations indicate that M2G possesses the greatest inhibitory activity among the MAAs tested so far. The inhibitory mechanism of MAAs remains unknown. However, the metal chelating activity of MAAs might play a role in this property because collagenases are metalloproteases. Tarasuntisuk et al. reported that M2G showed a metal chelating activity, when using iron (II) chloride, whereas a mixture of P334 and SHI did not show any remarkable activity [84]. Therefore, the strong inhibitory effect of M2G might be due to the chelation of calcium ions in the reaction system. Besides M2G, euhalothece-362 from the cyanobacterium *Euhalothece* sp. strain LK-1, has also been suggested to be an MAA that acts as an iron chelator [88]. In addition to their effect on bacterial collagenase, the effect of MAAs on mammalian collagenases is also an interesting subject that requires further investigation.

Another protease involved in ECM-degradation is elastase, which is a member of the chymotrypsin-type serine protease family [89]. Elastase can break down an important protein, elastin, within the ECM, and in the absence of metal ions. Degradation of elastin reduces skin elasticity. Our preliminary investigation into elastase from porcine pancreas showed that the purified MAAs tested exhibited no inhibitory activities; M2G, P334, and SHI, were at final concentrations of 4.0, 7.0, and 5.3 mM, respectively. This result again suggests a link between the metal chelating activity and collagenase inhibitory activity in MAAs.

5.6. Other Activity

In addition to the aforementioned anti-photoaging and photo-protective activity of MAAs, in this section we describe our unpublished observations following our testing of the tyrosinase inhibitory activity of MAAs. Melanin, a key pigment that plays an important role in protecting the skin against UV damage, is associated with abnormal pigmentation and melanoma. Overaccumulation of melanin can induce certain types of skin disorder [90]. Tyrosinase is known to be an enzyme involved in melanin biosynthesis. To explore whether tyrosinase activity could be inhibited, the effects of purified M2G, SHI, and P334 were tested with mushroom tyrosinase. None of the MAAs tested affected the tyrosinase activity, at maximum final concentrations of 6.4, 8.4, and 7.5 mM M2G, SHI, and P334, respectively; whereas, 60 µM of a standard inhibitor, kojic acid, inhibited activity by more than 50%. Thus, although there may still be scope for further investigations, the MAAs tested did not show any inhibitory activity toward tyrosinase. As with the research described here, other anti-aging-related activities of MAAs remain to be clarified. For example, an investigation into the possible inhibitory effects of MAAs on hyaluronidase, which can contribute to collagen breakdown in the skin, would be another interesting anti-aging feature of MAAs to characterize. Observations relating to these properties, including negative results, will be important for the future development and application of MAAs as potential therapeutic agents.

6. Concluding Remarks

One of the greatest risk factors for skin-aging is UV radiation. In this review, the protective properties of MAAs were discussed, alongside the challenges for prevention of UV-induced skin-aging. Of the MAAs that were discussed, we highlighted the ability of M2G in particular. M2G exhibits prominent abilities for protecting DNA against UV-related damage, as well as antioxidant, anti-inflammatory, anti-protein-glycation, and collagenase inhibition activities. These observations indicate the potential of M2G for therapeutic applications. However, many promising MAAs, including MAA derivatives, such as glycosylated MAAs, still need to be studied in detail, since the variety of MAAs examined to date is not adequate. In the future, a full understanding of the relationship between the chemical structure of MAAs and their activity, might help to achieve the development and commercialization of MAAs, for multipurpose uses in the cosmeceutical, pharmaceutical, biomedical, and biotechnological fields. In this regard, marine organisms, including cyanobacteria, and green and red macroalgae, are promising candidates as environment-friendly sources of industrially important compounds, like MAAs, because of their photoautotrophic properties, which can convert solar energy and carbon dioxide into useful chemicals.

Author Contributions: R.W.-S. and H.K. had an equal contribution in the consideration of the bibliographic information for the review and in the preparation of the manuscript.

Funding: This research was funded by the Cosmetology Research Foundation (J-18-1).

Conflicts of Interest: The authors declare no conflict of interest.

References

1. Jallad, K.N. Chemical characterization of sunscreens composition and its related potential adverse health effects. *J. Cosmet. Dermatol.* **2017**, *16*, 353–357. [CrossRef] [PubMed]
2. Gao, Q.; Garcia-Pichel, F. Microbial ultraviolet sunscreens. Nature reviews. *Microbiology* **2011**, *9*, 791–802. [CrossRef] [PubMed]

3. Gruber, F.; Peharda, V.; Kastelan, M.; Brajac, I. Occupational skin diseases caused by UV radiation. *Acta Dermatovenerol. Croat. ADC* **2007**, *15*, 191–198. [PubMed]
4. Ikehata, H. Mechanistic considerations on the wavelength-dependent variations of UVR genotoxicity and mutagenesis in skin: The discrimination of UVA-signature from UV-signature mutation. *Photochem. Photobiol. Sci.* **2018**, *17*, 1861–1871. [CrossRef]
5. Browne, N.; Donovan, F.; Murray, P.; Saha, S. Cyanobacteria as bio-factories for production of UV-screening compounds. *OA Biotechnol.* **2014**, *3*, 6.
6. Oyamada, C.; Kaneniwa, M.; Ebitani, K.; Murata, M.; Ishihara, K. Mycosporine-like amino acids extracted from scallop (Patinopecten yessoensis) ovaries: UV protection and growth stimulation activities on human cells. *Mar. Biotechnol.* **2008**, *10*, 141–150. [CrossRef] [PubMed]
7. Ichihashi, M.; Ando, H. The maximal cumulative solar UVB dose allowed to maintain healthy and young skin and prevent premature photoaging. *Exp. Dermatol.* **2014**, *23*, 43–46. [CrossRef]
8. Rastogi, R.P.; Incharoensakdi, A. Analysis of UV-absorbing photoprotectant mycosporine-like amino acid (MAA) in the cyanobacterium *Arthrospira* sp. CU2556. *Photochem. Photobiol. Sci.* **2014**, *13*, 1016–1024. [CrossRef]
9. Nguyen, K.H.; Chollet-Krugler, M.; Gouault, N.; Tomasi, S. UV-protectant metabolites from lichens and their symbiotic partners. *Natl. Prod. Rep.* **2013**, *30*, 1490–1508. [CrossRef]
10. Rosic, N.N.; Dove, S. Mycosporine-like amino acids from coral dinoflagellates. *Appl. Environ. Microbiol.* **2011**, *77*, 8478–8486. [CrossRef] [PubMed]
11. Kageyama, H.; Waditee-Sirisattha, R. Cyanobacterial UV sunscreen: Biosynthesis, regulation, and application. In *Sunscreens: Source, Formulations, Efficacy and Recommendations*; Rastogi, R.P., Ed.; Nova Science Publishers, Inc.: Hauppauge, NY, USA, 2018; pp. 1–28.
12. Kageyama, H.; Waditee-Sirisattha, R. Mycosporine-like amino acids as multifunctional secondary metabolites in cyanobacteria: From biochemical to application aspects. In *Studies in Natural Products Chemistry*; Elsevier: Amsterdam, The Netherlands, 2019; Volume 59, pp. 153–194.
13. Hu, C.; Voller, G.; Sussmuth, R.; Dittmann, E.; Kehr, J.C. Functional assessment of mycosporine-like amino acids in *Microcystis aeruginosa* strain PCC 7806. *Environ. Microbiol.* **2015**, *17*, 1548–1559. [CrossRef]
14. Wada, N.; Sakamoto, T.; Matsugo, S. Mycosporine-like amino acids and their derivatives as natural antioxidants. *Antioxidants* **2015**, *4*, 603. [CrossRef]
15. Chrapusta, E.; Kaminski, A.; Duchnik, K.; Bober, B.; Adamski, M.; Bialczyk, J. Mycosporine-like amino acids: potential health and beauty ingredients. *Mar. Drugs* **2017**, *15*, 326. [CrossRef]
16. Corinaldesi, C.; Barone, G.; Marcellini, F.; Dell'Anno, A.; Danovaro, R. Marine microbial-derived molecules and their potential use in cosmeceutical and cosmetic products. *Mar. Drugs* **2017**, *15*, 118. [CrossRef]
17. Brunt, E.G.; Burgess, J.G. The promise of marine molecules as cosmetic active ingredients. *Int. J. Cosmet. Sci.* **2018**, *40*, 1–15. [CrossRef]
18. Nair, R.; Maseeh, A. Vitamin D: The "sunshine" vitamin. *J. Pharmacol. Pharm.* **2012**, *3*, 118–126. [CrossRef]
19. Bernstein, E.F.; Chen, Y.Q.; Kopp, J.B.; Fisher, L.; Brown, D.B.; Hahn, P.J.; Robey, F.A.; Lakkakorpi, J.; Uitto, J. Long-term sun exposure alters the collagen of the papillary dermis. Comparison of sun-protected and photoaged skin by northern analysis, immunohistochemical staining, and confocal laser scanning microscopy. *J. Am. Acad. Dermatol.* **1996**, *34*, 209–218. [CrossRef]
20. Panich, U.; Sittithumcharee, G.; Rathviboon, N.; Jirawatnotai, S. Ultraviolet radiation-induced skin aging: the role of DNA Damage and oxidative stress in epidermal stem cell damage mediated skin aging. *Stem Cells Int.* **2016**, *2016*, 7370642. [CrossRef]
21. Cadet, J.; Sage, E.; Douki, T. Ultraviolet radiation-mediated damage to cellular DNA. *Mutat. Res.* **2005**, *571*, 3–17. [CrossRef]
22. Subedi, L.; Lee, T.H.; Wahedi, H.; Baek, S.-H.; Kim, S. Resveratrol-Enriched Rice Attenuates UVB-ROS-Induced Skin Aging via Downregulation of Inflammatory Cascades. *Oxid. Med. Cell. Longev.* **2017**, 1–15. [CrossRef]
23. Valencia, A.; Kochevar, I.E. Nox1-based NADPH oxidase is the major source of UVA-induced reactive oxygen species in human keratinocytes. *J. Investig. Dermatol.* **2008**, *128*, 214–222. [CrossRef]
24. Masaki, H.; Okano, Y.; Sakurai, H. Generation of active oxygen species from advanced glycation end-products (AGEs) during ultraviolet light A (UVA) irradiation and a possible mechanism for cell damaging. *Biochim. Biophys. Acta* **1999**, *1428*, 45–56. [CrossRef]

25. Sakurai, H.; Yasui, H.; Yamada, Y.; Nishimura, H.; Shigemoto, M. Detection of reactive oxygen species in the skin of live mice and rats exposed to UVA light: a research review on chemiluminescence and trials for UVA protection. *Photochem. Photobiol. Sci.* **2005**, *4*, 715–720. [CrossRef]
26. Glady, A.; Tanaka, M.; Moniaga, C.S.; Yasui, M.; Hara-Chikuma, M. Involvement of NADPH oxidase 1 in UVB-induced cell signaling and cytotoxicity in human keratinocytes. *Biochem. Biophys. Rep.* **2018**, *14*, 7–15. [CrossRef]
27. Shindo, Y.; Witt, E.; Han, D.; Epstein, W.; Packer, L. Enzymic and non-enzymic antioxidants in epidermis and dermis of human skin. *J. Investig. Dermatol.* **1994**, *102*, 122–124. [CrossRef]
28. Hruza, L.L.; Pentland, A.P. Mechanisms of UV-induced inflammation. *J. Investig. Dermatol.* **1993**, *100*, 35s–41s. [CrossRef]
29. Radhiga, T.; Agilan, B.; Muzaffer, U.; Karthikeyan, R.; Kanimozhi, G.; Paul, V.I.; Prasad, N. Phytochemicals as modulators of ultraviolet-B radiation induced cellular and molecular events: A Review. *J. Radiat. Cancer Res.* **2016**, *7*, 2–12.
30. Bowden, G.T. Prevention of non-melanoma skin cancer by targeting ultraviolet-B-light signalling. *Nat. Rev. Cancer* **2004**, *4*, 23–35. [CrossRef]
31. Onodera, Y.; Teramura, T.; Takehara, T.; Shigi, K.; Fukuda, K. Reactive oxygen species induce Cox-2 expression via TAK1 activation in synovial fibroblast cells. *FEBS Open Bio* **2015**, *5*, 492–501. [CrossRef]
32. Pittayapruek, P.; Meephansan, J.; Prapapan, O.; Komine, M.; Ohtsuki, M. Role of matrix metalloproteinases in photoaging and photocarcinogenesis. *Int. J. Mol. Sci.* **2016**, *17*, 868. [CrossRef]
33. Brennan, M.; Bhatti, H.; Nerusu, K.C.; Bhagavathula, N.; Kang, S.; Fisher, G.J.; Varani, J.; Voorhees, J.J. Matrix metalloproteinase-1 is the major collagenolytic enzyme responsible for collagen damage in UV-irradiated human skin. *Photochem. Photobiol.* **2003**, *78*, 43–48. [CrossRef]
34. Pillai, S.; Oresajo, C.; Hayward, J. Ultraviolet radiation and skin aging: roles of reactive oxygen species, inflammation and protease activation, and strategies for prevention of inflammation-induced matrix degradation—A review. *Int. J. Cosmet. Sci.* **2005**, *27*, 17–34. [CrossRef]
35. Gkogkolou, P.; Bohm, M. Advanced glycation end products: Key players in skin aging? *Dermato Endocrinol.* **2012**, *4*, 259–270. [CrossRef]
36. Ghosh, S.; Pandey, N.K.; Singha Roy, A.; Tripathy, D.R.; Dinda, A.K.; Dasgupta, S. Prolonged glycation of hen egg white lysozyme generates non amyloidal structures. *PLoS ONE* **2013**, *8*, e74336. [CrossRef]
37. Hori, M.; Yagi, M.; Nomoto, K.; Shimode, A.; Ogura, M.; Yonei, Y. Inhibition of advanced glycation end product formation by herbal teas and its relation to anti-skin aging. *J. Anti-Aging Med.* **2012**, *9*, 135–148.
38. Mohania, D.; Chandel, S.; Kumar, P.; Verma, V.; Digvijay, K.; Tripathi, D.; Choudhury, K.; Mitten, S.K.; Shah, D. Ultraviolet radiations: Skin defense-damage mechanism. *Adv. Exp. Med. Biol.* **2017**, *996*, 71–87. [CrossRef]
39. Bosch, R.; Philips, N.; Suárez-Pérez, J.A.; Juarranz, A.; Devmurari, A.; Chalensouk-Khaosaat, J.; González, S. Mechanisms of photoaging and cutaneous photocarcinogenesis, and photoprotective strategies with phytochemicals. *Antioxidants* **2015**, *4*, 248–268. [CrossRef]
40. Syed, D.N.; Malik, A.; Hadi, N.; Sarfaraz, S.; Afaq, F.; Mukhtar, H. Photochemopreventive effect of pomegranate fruit extract on UVA-mediated activation of cellular pathways in normal human epidermal keratinocytes. *Photochem. Photobiol.* **2006**, *82*, 398–405. [CrossRef]
41. Sharma, S.D.; Meeran, S.M.; Katiyar, S.K. Dietary grape seed proanthocyanidins inhibit UVB-induced oxidative stress and activation of mitogen-activated protein kinases and nuclear factor-kappaB signaling in in vivo SKH-1 hairless mice. *Mol. Cancer Ther.* **2007**, *6*, 995–1005. [CrossRef]
42. Adhami, V.M.; Afaq, F.; Ahmad, N. Suppression of ultraviolet B exposure-mediated activation of NF-κB in normal human keratinocytes by resveratrol. *Neoplasia* **2003**, *5*, 74–82. [CrossRef]
43. Kang, N.J.; Lee, K.W.; Shin, B.J.; Jung, S.K.; Hwang, M.K.; Bode, A.M.; Heo, Y.S.; Lee, H.J.; Dong, Z. Caffeic acid, a phenolic phytochemical in coffee, directly inhibits Fyn kinase activity and UVB-induced COX-2 expression. *Carcinogenesis* **2009**, *30*, 321–330. [CrossRef] [PubMed]
44. Lee, K.M.; Lee, K.W.; Jung, S.K.; Lee, E.J.; Heo, Y.S.; Bode, A.M.; Lubet, R.A.; Lee, H.J.; Dong, Z. Kaempferol inhibits UVB-induced COX-2 expression by suppressing Src kinase activity. *Biochem. Pharmacol.* **2010**, *80*, 2042–2049. [CrossRef] [PubMed]

45. Cho, J.; Park, K.; Ryang Kweon, G.; Jang, B.-C.; Baek, W.; Suh, M.; Kim, C.-W.; Lee, K.-S.; Suh, S.-I. Curcumin inhibits the expression of COX-2 in UVB-irradiated human keratinocytes (HaCaT) by inhibiting activation of AP-1: p38 MAP kinase and JNK as potential upstream targets. *Exp. Mol. Med.* **2005**, *37*, 186–192. [CrossRef] [PubMed]
46. Afaq, F. Natural agents: Cellular and molecular mechanisms of photoprotection. *Arch. Biochem. Biophys.* **2011**, *508*, 144–151. [CrossRef] [PubMed]
47. Cavinato, M.; Waltenberger, B.; Baraldo, G.; Grade, C.V.C.; Stuppner, H.; Jansen-Durr, P. Plant extracts and natural compounds used against UVB-induced photoaging. *Biogerontology* **2017**, *18*, 499–516. [CrossRef] [PubMed]
48. Cefali, L.C.; Ataide, J.A.; Moriel, P.; Foglio, M.A.; Mazzola, P.G. Plant-based active photoprotectants for sunscreens. *Int. J. Cosmet. Sci.* **2016**, *38*, 346–353. [CrossRef]
49. Garcia-Pichel, F.; Castenholz, R.W. Occurrence of UV-absorbing, Mycosporine-like compounds among cyanobacterial isolates and an estimate of their screening capacity. *Appl. Environ. Microbiol.* **1993**, *59*, 163–169. [PubMed]
50. Lawrence, K.P.; Long, P.F.; Young, A.R. Mycosporine-like amino acids for skin photoprotection. *Curr. Med. Chem.* **2018**, *25*, 5512–5527. [CrossRef] [PubMed]
51. Bhatia, S.; Garg, A.; Sharma, K.; Kumar, S.; Sharma, A.; Purohit, A.P. Mycosporine and mycosporine-like amino acids: A paramount tool against ultra violet irradiation. *Pharm. Rev.* **2011**, *5*, 138–146. [CrossRef]
52. De la Coba, F.; Aguilera, J.; Figueroa, F.L.; de Gálvez, M.V.; Herrera, E. Antioxidant activity of mycosporine-like amino acids isolated from three red macroalgae and one marine lichen. *J. Appl. Phycol.* **2009**, *21*, 161–169. [CrossRef]
53. Daniel, S.; Cornelia, S.; Fred, Z. UV-A sunscreen from red algae for protection against premature skin aging. *Cosmet. Toilet. Manuf. Worldw* **2004**, 139–143.
54. Cheewinthamrongrod, V.; Kageyama, H.; Palaga, T.; Takabe, T.; Waditee-Sirisattha, R. DNA damage protecting and free radical scavenging properties of mycosporine-2-glycine from the Dead Sea cyanobacterium in A375 human melanoma cell lines. *J. Photochem. Photobiol. B Biol.* **2016**, *164*, 289–295. [CrossRef]
55. Ryu, J.; Park, S.J.; Kim, I.H.; Choi, Y.H.; Nam, T.J. Protective effect of porphyra-334 on UVA-induced photoaging in human skin fibroblasts. *Int. J. Mol. Med.* **2014**, *34*, 796–803. [CrossRef]
56. Suh, S.S.; Hwang, J.; Park, M.; Seo, H.H.; Kim, H.S.; Lee, J.H.; Moh, S.H.; Lee, T.K. Anti-inflammation activities of mycosporine-like amino acids (MAAs) in response to UV radiation suggest potential anti-skin aging activity. *Mar. Drugs* **2014**, *12*, 5174–5187. [CrossRef]
57. Oren, A. Mycosporine-like amino acids as osmotic solutes in a community of halophilic cyanobacteria. *Geomicrobiol. J.* **1997**, *14*, 231–240. [CrossRef]
58. Patipong, T.; Hibino, T.; Waditee-Sirisattha, R.; Kageyama, H. Efficient bioproduction of mycosporine-2-glycine, which functions as potential osmoprotectant, using *Escherichia coli* cells. *Natl. Prod. Commun.* **2017**, *12*, 1593–1594. [CrossRef]
59. Suh, H.J.; Lee, H.W.; Jung, J. Mycosporine glycine protects biological systems against photodynamic damage by quenching singlet oxygen with a high efficiency. *Photochem. Photobiol.* **2003**, *78*, 109–113. [CrossRef]
60. Ngoennet, S.; Nishikawa, Y.; Hibino, T.; Waditee-Sirisattha, R.; Kageyama, H. A method for the isolation and characterization of mycosporine-like amino acids from cyanobacteria. *Methods Protocols* **2018**, *1*, 46. [CrossRef]
61. Balskus, E.P.; Walsh, C.T. The genetic and molecular basis for sunscreen biosynthesis in cyanobacteria. *Science* **2010**, *329*, 1653–1656. [CrossRef]
62. Waditee-Sirisattha, R.; Kageyama, H.; Sopun, W.; Tanaka, Y.; Takabe, T. Identification and upregulation of biosynthetic genes required for accumulation of Mycosporine-2-glycine under salt stress conditions in the halotolerant cyanobacterium *Aphanothece halophytica*. *Appl. Environ. Microbiol.* **2014**, *80*, 1763–1769. [CrossRef]
63. Shinzato, C.; Shoguchi, E.; Kawashima, T.; Hamada, M.; Hisata, K.; Tanaka, M.; Fujie, M.; Fujiwara, M.; Koyanagi, R.; Ikuta, T.; et al. Using the *Acropora digitifera* genome to understand coral responses to environmental change. *Nature* **2011**, *476*, 320. [CrossRef]
64. Micallef, M.L.; D'Agostino, P.M.; Sharma, D.; Viswanathan, R.; Moffitt, M.C. Genome mining for natural product biosynthetic gene clusters in the Subsection V cyanobacteria. *BMC Genom.* **2015**, *16*, 669. [CrossRef]

65. Waditee-Sirisattha, R.; Kageyama, H.; Fukaya, M.; Rai, V.; Takabe, T. Nitrate and amino acid availability affects glycine betaine and mycosporine-2-glycine in response to changes of salinity in a halotolerant cyanobacterium *Aphanothece halophytica*. *FEMS Microbiol. Lett.* **2015**, *362*, fnv198. [CrossRef]
66. Schmid, D.; Schürch, C.; Zülli, F. Mycosporine-like amino acids from red algae protect against premature skin-aging. *Euro Cosmet.* **2006**, *9*, 1–4.
67. Lawrence, K.P.; Gacesa, R.; Long, P.F.; Young, A.R. Molecular photoprotection of human keratinocytes in vitro by the naturally occurring mycosporine-like amino acid palythine. *Br. J. Dermatol.* **2018**, *178*, 1353–1363. [CrossRef]
68. Ma, Q. Role of nrf2 in oxidative stress and toxicity. *Annu. Rev. Pharmacol. Toxicol.* **2013**, *53*, 401–426. [CrossRef]
69. Ishihara, K.; Watanabe, R.; Uchida, H.; Suzuki, T.; Yamashita, M.; Takenaka, H.; Nazifi, E.; Matsugo, S.; Yamaba, M.; Sakamoto, T. Novel glycosylated mycosporine-like amino acid, 13-*O*-(β-galactosyl)-porphyra-334, from the edible cyanobacterium *Nostoc sphaericum*-protective activity on human keratinocytes from UV light. *J. Photochem. Photobiol. B* **2017**, *172*, 102–108. [CrossRef]
70. Gacesa, R.; Lawrence, K.P.; Georgakopoulos, N.D.; Yabe, K.; Dunlap, W.C.; Barlow, D.J.; Wells, G.; Young, A.R.; Long, P.F. The mycosporine-like amino acids porphyra-334 and shinorine are antioxidants and direct antagonists of Keap1-Nrf2 binding. *Biochimie* **2018**, *154*, 35–44. [CrossRef]
71. Tarasuntisuk, S.; Palaga, T.; Kageyama, H.; Waditee-Sirisattha, R. Mycosporine-2-glycine exerts anti-inflammatory and antioxidant effects in lipopolysaccharide (LPS)-stimulated RAW 264.7 macrophages. *Arch. Biochem. Biophys.* **2019**, *662*, 33–39. [CrossRef]
72. Nazifi, E.; Wada, N.; Yamaba, M.; Asano, T.; Nishiuchi, T.; Matsugo, S.; Sakamoto, T. Glycosylated porphyra-334 and palythine-threonine from the terrestrial cyanobacterium *Nostoc commune*. *Mar. Drugs* **2013**, *11*, 3124–3154. [CrossRef]
73. Matsui, K.; Nazifi, E.; Kunita, S.; Wada, N.; Matsugo, S.; Sakamoto, T. Novel glycosylated mycosporine-like amino acids with radical scavenging activity from the cyanobacterium *Nostoc commune*. *J. Photochem. Photobiol. B Biol.* **2011**, *105*, 81–89. [CrossRef]
74. Biswal, S. Oxidative stress and astaxanthin: the novel supernutrient carotenoid. *Int. J. Health Allied Sci.* **2014**, *3*, 147–153. [CrossRef]
75. Dose, J.; Matsugo, S.; Yokokawa, H.; Koshida, Y.; Okazaki, S.; Seidel, U.; Eggersdorfer, M.; Rimbach, G.; Esatbeyoglu, T. Free radical scavenging and cellular antioxidant properties of astaxanthin. *Int. J. Mol. Sci.* **2016**, *17*, 103. [CrossRef]
76. Zhang, H.; Davies, K.J.A.; Forman, H.J. Oxidative stress response and Nrf2 signaling in aging. *Free Radic. Biol. Med.* **2015**, *88*, 314–336. [CrossRef]
77. Ahmed, S.M.; Luo, L.; Namani, A.; Wang, X.J.; Tang, X. Nrf2 signaling pathway: Pivotal roles in inflammation. *Biochimica et biophysica acta. Mol. Basis Dis.* **2017**, *1863*, 585–597. [CrossRef]
78. Krajka-Kuzniak, V.; Paluszczak, J.; Baer-Dubowska, W. The Nrf2-ARE signaling pathway: An update on its regulation and possible role in cancer prevention and treatment. *Pharmacol. Rep. PR* **2017**, *69*, 393–402. [CrossRef]
79. Newton, K.; Dixit, V.M. Signaling in innate immunity and inflammation. *Cold Spring Harb. Perspect. Biol.* **2012**, *4*. [CrossRef]
80. Siomek, A. NF-kappaB signaling pathway and free radical impact. *Acta Biochim. Polonica* **2012**, *59*, 323–331. [CrossRef]
81. Mitchell, S.; Vargas, J.; Hoffmann, A. Signaling via the NFkappaB system. *Wiley interdisciplinary reviews. Syst. Biol. Med.* **2016**, *8*, 227–241. [CrossRef]
82. Chun, K.S.; Cha, H.H.; Shin, J.W.; Na, H.K.; Park, K.K.; Chung, W.Y.; Surh, Y.J. Nitric oxide induces expression of cyclooxygenase-2 in mouse skin through activation of NF-kappaB. *Carcinogenesis* **2004**, *25*, 445–454. [CrossRef] [PubMed]
83. Murakami, A.; Ohigashi, H. Targeting NOX, INOS and COX-2 in inflammatory cells: chemoprevention using food phytochemicals. *Int. J. Cancer* **2007**, *121*, 2357–2363. [CrossRef]
84. Tarasuntisuk, S.; Patipong, T.; Hibino, T.; Waditee-Sirisattha, R.; Kageyama, H. Inhibitory effects of mycosporine-2-glycine isolated from a halotolerant cyanobacterium on protein glycation and collagenase activity. *Lett. Appl. Microbiol.* **2018**, *67*, 314–320. [CrossRef]
85. Peyroux, J.; Sternberg, M. Advanced glycation endproducts (AGEs): Pharmacological inhibition in diabetes. *Pathol. Biol.* **2006**, *54*, 405–419. [CrossRef]

86. Duarte, A.S.; Correia, A.; Esteves, A.C. Bacterial collagenases—A review. *Crit. Rev. Microbiol.* **2016**, *42*, 106–126. [CrossRef]
87. Hartmann, A.; Gostner, J.; Fuchs, J.E.; Chaita, E.; Aligiannis, N.; Skaltsounis, L.; Ganzera, M. Inhibition of collagenase by mycosporine-like amino acids from marine sources. *Planta Med.* **2015**, *81*, 813–820. [CrossRef]
88. Volkmann, M.; Gorbushina, A.A.; Kedar, L.; Oren, A. Structure of euhalothece-362, a novel red-shifted mycosporine-like amino acid, from a halophilic cyanobacterium (*Euhalothece* sp.). *FEMS Microbiol. Lett.* **2006**, *258*, 50–54. [CrossRef]
89. Thring, T.S.; Hili, P.; Naughton, D.P. Anti-collagenase, anti-elastase and anti-oxidant activities of extracts from 21 plants. *BMC Complement. Altern. Med.* **2009**, *9*, 27. [CrossRef]
90. Di Petrillo, A.; González-Paramás, A.M.; Era, B.; Medda, R.; Pintus, F.; Santos-Buelga, C.; Fais, A. Tyrosinase inhibition and antioxidant properties of *Asphodelus microcarpus* extracts. *BMC Complement. Altern. Med.* **2016**, *16*, 453. [CrossRef]

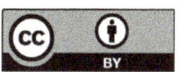

© 2019 by the authors. Licensee MDPI, Basel, Switzerland. This article is an open access article distributed under the terms and conditions of the Creative Commons Attribution (CC BY) license (http://creativecommons.org/licenses/by/4.0/).

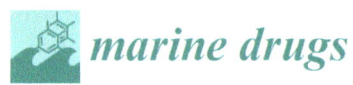

Review

Beneficial Effects of Marine Algae-Derived Carbohydrates for Skin Health

Ji Hye Kim [1,2], Jae-Eun Lee [1], Kyoung Heon Kim [3,*] and Nam Joo Kang [1,*]

1. School of Food Science and Biotechnology, Kyungpook National University, Daegu 41566, Korea; friend8201@naver.com (J.H.K.); lju1033@naver.com (J.-E.L.)
2. Korean Medicine Application Center, Korea Institute of Oriental Medicine, Daegu 41566, Korea
3. Department of Biotechnology, Graduate School, Korea University, Seoul 02841, Korea
* Correspondence: khekim@korea.ac.kr (K.H.K.); njkang@knu.ac.kr (N.J.K.); Tel.: +82-2-3290-3028 (K.H.K.); +82-53-950-5753 (N.J.K.)

Received: 31 October 2018; Accepted: 17 November 2018; Published: 21 November 2018

Abstract: Marine algae are considered to be an abundant sources of bioactive compounds with cosmeceutical potential. Recently, a great deal of interest has focused on the health-promoting effects of marine bioactive compounds. Carbohydrates are the major and abundant constituent of marine algae and have been utilized in cosmetic formulations, as moisturizing and thickening agents for example. In addition, marine carbohydrates have been suggested as promising bioactive biomaterials for their various properties beneficial to skin, including antioxidant, anti-melanogenic and skin anti-aging properties. Therefore, marine algae carbohydrates have potential skin health benefits for value-added cosmeceutical applications. The present review focuses on the various biological capacities and potential skin health benefits of bioactive marine carbohydrates.

Keywords: marine algae; carbohydrates; oligosaccharides; monosaccharides; skin health; cosmeceuticals

1. Introduction

Cosmeceuticals can be defined as cosmetic products with biologically active ingredients purporting to exert pharmaceutical effects on the skin. Recently, great interest has been shown by consumers in novel bioactive compounds from natural sources, instead of synthetic ingredients, thanks to their perceived beneficial effects [1]. Therefore, there are numerous efforts to develop biologically active ingredients from natural organisms [2]. Most studies have been based on terrestrial sources; however, it has been shown that natural compounds isolated from marine sources show higher biological activity than those isolated from terrestrial sources, and as a result, there is a lot of interest in the studies of ingredients using natural marine sources [3,4]. In particular, oceans account for about 70% of the earth's surface and their biodiversity makes them an excellent reservoir of sources for natural products [5]. Among various natural organisms, marine algae, which grow much faster than terrestrial plants, are considered to be abundant and essential sources of numerous constituents beneficial for human skin health [2,6].

Algae are photosynthetic organisms with a complex and controversial taxonomy [7]. To date, more than 20,000 species of algae have been identified, and there are two kinds of algae depending on size [6]. Macroalgae (seaweeds) are defined as multicellular marine plants that live in coastal areas and have simpler structures than terrestrial plants [6]. Marine macroalgae are classified into three species according to their pigments: *Phaeophyceae* (brown macroalgae, *Chromophyta*), *Chlorophyta* (green macroalgae) and *Rhodophyta* (red macroalgae) [6,8]. In contrast, microalgae are small unicellular or simple multicellular species and are found in various environments [6,7].

Marine algae are composed of various substances including carbohydrates, lipids, proteins, amino acids, minerals and flavonoids [9]. Among the various ingredients, carbohydrates are the most abundant constituents of marine algae [1,10,11]. Based on degrees of polymerization (DPs), carbohydrates, also called saccharides, exist in marine algae as various forms of monosaccharides, disaccharides, oligosaccharides and polysaccharides [1]. Marine carbohydrates have been utilized in cosmeceutical industries due to their chemical and physical properties [12,13]. Fucoidans/alginate from brown algae, ulvans from green algae and carrageenans/agar from red algae are used as gelling, thickening and stabilizing agents [2,6,12,14]. In addition, accumulating reports suggest that marine carbohydrates have been proven to exhibit potential benefits for skin [2,12]. The biological activities of marine carbohydrates are known to be linked with their structure as determined by DPs ormolecular weights, the presence of sulfate groups and types of sugars [15]. Therefore, in this review, we discuss the skin health cosmetic effects of carbohydrates extracted from marine algae, which are considered to be sources of excellent carbohydrates.

2. Bioactive Effects and Potential Health Benefits of Marine Algae

2.1. Biological Activities of Marine Algal Extracts

Table 1 shows the beneficial effects of marine algal extracts, including macroalgae and microalgae, for skin health.

Table 1. Bioactive functions of marine algal extracts.

Species	Solvent	Function	Mechanism	Ref.
Endarachne binghamiae Sargassum siliquastrum Ecklonia cava	A	Anti-melanogenesis	In vitro (B16F10 cells) Mushroom TYR activity ($\downarrow$) Melanin content ($\downarrow$) Cellular TYR activity (-)	[16]
S. siliquastrum E. cava			In vivo (Zebrafish) Melanin content ($\downarrow$) TYR activity ($\downarrow$)	
Ishige okamurae Yendo	A	Anti-melanogenesis	In vitro (B16F10 cells) Mushroom TYR activity ($\downarrow$) Melanin content ($\downarrow$)	[17]
Sargassum polycystum Padina tenuis	E, H	Anti-melanogenesis	In vitro (HEMs) Mushroom TYR activity ($\downarrow$) In vivo (Guinea pigs) Melanin content ($\downarrow$)	[18]
Schizymenia dubyi	A	Anti-melanogenesis	In vitro (B16F10 cells) Mushroom TYR activity ($\downarrow$) Melanin content ($\downarrow$)	[16]
Sargassum wightii Padina gymnospora	M, C, EAc, A	Antioxidant	In vitro DPPH radical ($\downarrow$) Ferrous ion chelation	[19]
Caulerpa peltata				
Gelidiella acerosa				
Fucus vesiculosus (Bladder wrack)	A	Skin anti-aging	In vivo (human cheek skin) Thickness ($\uparrow$) Elasticity ($\uparrow$)	[20]

Table 1. Cont.

Species	Solvent	Function	Mechanism	Ref.
Blue Lagoon coccoid Filamentous	PBS w/o Mg and Ca (pH 7)	Skin anti-aging Skin barrier function	In vitro (HEKs, HDFs) Gene expression of INV, LOR, TGM-1, FLG (↑) UVA-induced expression of MMP-1 (↓) type 1 collagen (↑)	[21]
			In vivo (Human skin) UVA-induced expression of MMP-1 (↓) type 1 collagen (↑) level of TEWL (↓)	
Botryococcus braunii	A	Antioxidant	In vitro (NIH3T3 cells) ORAC (↑), ROS level (↓) DNA damage (↓)	[22]
		Skin anti-aging	In vitro (HaCaT cells) Expression of AQP3, FLG, INV and type 1 and 3 pro-collagen (↑)	
		Anti-inflammation	In vitro (RAW 264.7 cells) iNOS expression (↓) NO production (↓)	
Chlorella vulgaris	A	Anti-atopic dermatitis	In vivo (NC/Nga mice) DFE-induced AD (↓) Epidermal thickness (↓) Skin hydration (↑) Infiltration of eosinophil and mast cell (↓) Serum chemokine levels of TARC and MDC (↓) mRNA level of IL-4, IFN-γ (↓)	[23]
Chlorella sorokiniana (ROQUETTE Chlorella sp.)	Spring water	Anti-skin inflammation	In vivo (hairless Skh-1 mice) TPA-induced skin inflammation (↓) macroscopic score (↓)	[24]
Chlorella vulgaris		Anti-skin cancer	In vivo DMBA-induced skin papillomagenesis (↓) Tumor burden (↓) Cumulative number of skin papillomas (↓) Percent incidence of mice bearing skin papillomas (↓)	[25]
Schizochytrium (ROQUETTE Schizochytrium sp.)	Spring water	Anti-skin inflammation	In vivo (hairless Skh-1 mice) TPA-induced skin inflammation (↓) Macroscopic score (↓)	[26]
Porphyra yezoensis (laver)	M	UV protection	In vitro (HaCaT cells) Cell viability (↑) Apoptosis (↓) Activation of JNK, ERK (↓)	[27]

Table 1. *Cont.*

Species	Solvent	Function	Mechanism	Ref.
Porphyra umbilicalis Vitamins, *Ginkgo biloba*	A	UV protection	In vivo (HRS/J-hairless mice) UVA/UVB-induced DNA damage (↓), erythema (↓), level of p53, caspase-3 (↓)	[28]
Furcellaria lumbricalis *Fucus vesiculosus*	A	Skin anti-aging	In vitro (HDFs) Expression of type 1 pro-collagen (↑)	[29]
Spirulina maxima *Ulva lactuca* *Lola implexa* with other compounds		Skin anti-aging	In vivo (Human skin) Skin hydrating (↑) Skin firming effects (↑)	[30]

A: aqueous extract, **AD**: atopic dermatitis, **AQP3**: aquaporin-3, **C**: chloroform extract, **Ca**: calcium, **DFE**: *Dermatophagoides farinae* extract, **DMBA**: 7,12-dimethylbenz [a] anthracene, **DPPH**: 2,2-diphenyl-1-picrylhydrazyl, **E**: ethanol extract, **EAc**: ethyl acetate extract, **ERK**: extracellular signal–regulated kinase, **FLG**: filaggrin, **H**: hexane extract, **HaCaT cells**: immortalized human keratinocytes, **HDFs**: human dermal fibroblasts, **HEKs**: human epidermal keratinocytes, **HEMs**: human epidermal melanocytes, **IFN-γ**: interferon-gamma, **IL-4**: interleukin-4, **iNOS**: inducible nitric oxide synthase, **INV**: involucrin, **JNK**: c-Jun N-terminal kinase, **LOR**: loricrin, **M**: methanol extract, **MDC**: macrophage-derived chemokine, **Mg**: magnesium, **MMP-1**: matrix metalloproteinase-1, **NIH3T3 cells**: mouse embryo fibroblast cells, **NO**: nitric oxide, **ORAC**: oxygen radical absorbance capacity, **PBS**: phosphate-buffered saline, **TARC**: thymus- and activation-regulated chemokine, **TEWL**: transepidermal water loss, **TGM-1**: transglutaminase-1, **TPA**: 12-O-tetradecanoylphorbol-13-acetate, **TYR**: tyrosinase, **UVA**: ultraviolet A, **UVB**: ultraviolet B, **w/o**: without.

2.1.1. Macroalgal Extracts

Cha et al. screened 43 indigenous marine algae for new skin-whitening agents [16]. The aqueous extracts from brown algae *Endarachne binghamiae*, *Sargassum silquastrum*, *Ecklonia cava* and red algae *Schizymenia dubyi* exhibited potent mushroom tyrosinase (TYR) inhibitory activity. Both *E. cava* and *S. silquastrum* reduced cellular melanin synthesis and TYR activity in a murine cell model and zebrafish model at non-toxic concentrations. Heo et al. recently screened 21 species of marine algae for effects on melanogenesis using mushroom TYR activity [17]. Extracts of *Ishige okamurae* Yendo inhibited mushroom TYR activity and melanin synthesis in murine melanoma B16F10 cells.

According to Quah et al., ethanol or hexane extract of brown algae, including *Sargassum polycystum* and *Padina tenuis*, significantly reduced mushroom TYR activity and melanin content in human epidermal melanocytes (HEMs) [18]. Topical application with ethanol or hexane extract of *S. polycystum* attenuated melanin production in guinea pigs in dermal irritation tests and de-pigmentation assessments. Hexane extract of *S. polycystum* was the most potent without toxicity for in vitro and in vivo models.

Murugan et al. reported the antioxidant activity of extracts of brown, green and red marine algae. In vitro 2,2-diphenyl-1-picrylhydrazyl (DPPH) radical scavenging assay and ferrous ion chelation were performed with methanol (M), chloroform (C), ethyl acetate (EAc), and aqueous (A) extracts of *Sargassum wightii* (brown algae), *Padina gymnospora* (brown algae), *Caulerpa peltata* (green algae) and *Gelidiella acerosa* (red algae) [19]. Non-polar C and EAc extracts showed higher DPPH radical-scavenging. However, A extracts (polar extracts) showed higher ferrous ion chelation. These results suggest that the antioxidant activity of marine algal extracts may relieve skin aging and skin inflammation processes that are affected by oxidative stress [31].

In 2002, Fujimura's group found that topical application of brown algae *Fucus vesiculosus* (Bladder wrack) aqueous extracts improved the thickness and elasticity of human cheek skin [20]. These results suggest that the *F. vesiculosus* extract possesses anti-aging activities and may be useful for a variety of cosmetics [20].

Previous study has shown the photoprotective effects of cosmetic formulations containing ultraviolet (UV) filters, vitamins, *Ginkgo biloba* and red algae *Porphyra umbilicalis* extracts for in vitro and in vivo models [28]. Topical formulations including F (sunscreen formulation containing only UV filters), FA (sunscreen formulation with red algae extract) and FVGA (sunscreen formulation with red algae extract, *G. biloba* and vitamins A, C and E) were applied on hairless mice. Extracts from the red algae *P. umbilicalis* could be considered effective ingredients for use in sunscreen formulations. The combination of vitamins A, E, C and *G. biloba* along with red algae extracts can significantly improve the performance of the sunscreens, preventing UV-induced DNA damage and inflammation. Al-Bader et al. reported the potential of skin anti-aging cosmetic ingredients containing red algae *Furcellaria lumbricalis* (black carrageen) and brown algae *Fucus vesiculosus* [29]. A mixture of *F. vesiculosus* and *F. lumbricalis* extracts induced expression of type 1 pro-collagen in aged human dermal fibroblasts (HDFs). Another clinical study demonstrated the skin anti-aging effects of *Spirulina maxima* (blue algae), *Ulva lactuca* (green algae) and *Lola implexa* (green algae) with other compounds [30]. Marine algal mixtures enhanced the skin hydrating and skin firming effects on human skin, suggesting the utilization of marine algae in cosmeceuticals.

2.1.2. Microalgal Extracts

Skin anti-aging and skin barrier functions of microalgae extracts were assessed in vitro and in vivo [21]. Green-blue microalgae, *Blue Lagoon coccoid Filamentous*, were extracted with phosphate-buffered saline (PBS) without magnesium (Mg) and calcium (Ca). In human epidermal keratinocytes (HEKs), green-blue microalgae extracts increased the expression genes of the transcriptional level of involucrin (INV), loricrin (LOR), transglutaminase-1 (TGM-1) and filaggrin (FLG) which are major markers for skin barrier function [32]. UV radiation upregulates collagen degradation through the increase of matrix metalloproteinase-1 (MMP-1) expression in HDFs. *Blue Lagoon* extracts suppressed MMP-1 upregulation and type 1 pro-collagen downregulation stimulated by ultraviolet A (UVA). Topical treatment with *Blue Lagoon* extracts (0.25% and 2.5%) consistently reduced levels of transepidermal water loss (TEWL) in human skin. Collectively, *Blue Lagoon* extracts improved skin barrier function and showed a capacity to prevent premature skin aging.

Buono et al. demonstrated that aqueous extracts of *Botryococcus braunii* exhibited antioxidant, skin anti-aging and anti-inflammatory capacities in various cell-based models [22]. Skin aging is driven by oxidative stress in skin caused by intrinsic and extrinsic factors [31]. Oxygen radical absorbance capacity (ORAC) assay and COMET assay showed that intracellular reactive oxygen species (ROS) levels and DNA damage were decreased by *B. braunii* extracts in NIH3T3 mouse embryo fibroblasts. Decreased levels of aquaporin-3 (AQP3) and FLG, INV and pro-collagen were observed in aged skin [33,34]. *B. braunii* extract treatment increased expression of AQP3, FLG, INV and type 1 and 3 pro-collagen in HaCaT cells, indicating potential skin anti-aging activity. Antioxidant activity is also closely related to anti-inflammatory processes [31]. During inflammation, some pro-inflammatory cytokines and endotoxins induce the expression of an inducible nitric oxide synthase (iNOS), leading to the generation of nitric oxide (NO) in macrophages. Data revealed that *B. braunii* extracts significantly reduced lipopolysaccharide (LPS)-induced iNOS expression and NO production in murine macrophage RAW 264.7 cells. These results asserted that *B. braunii* water extract had been proved to exert biological activities consistent with skin health maintenance.

Several studies described diverse beneficial effects of aqueous extracts of green microalgae *Chlorella* for skin health. Kang et al. reported *Chlorella vulgaris* attenuates *Dermatophagoides Farinae* (DFE)-induced atopic dermatitis (AD) in NC/Nga mice [23]. Hidalgo-Lucas et al. reported that oral and topical administration of *Chlorella sorokiniana* (ROQUETTE *Chlorella* sp.) extracts improved skin inflammation induced by 12-O-tetradecanoylphorbol-13-acetate (TPA) in hairless Skh-1 mice [24]. A previous study assessed the chemopreventive potential of *C. vulgaris* against murine skin papillomagenesis [25]. Topical application of *C. vulgaris* (500 mg/kg b.w./day) significantly attenuated 12-dimethylbenz [a] anthracene (DMBA)-induced tumor size and number by upregulating the sulfhydryl (-SH) and glutathione S-transferase (GST) levels in skin tissues. The results indicated that marine algae could be utilized as preventive and therapeutic agents for various inflammatory skin diseases.

Recently, spring water extracts of *Schizochytrium* (ROQUETTE *Schizochytrium* sp.) were reported to exert skin anti-inflammatory potential in vivo [26]. TPA-induced skin inflammation was significantly attenuated by oral administration (125, 250 and 500 mg/kg) and cutaneous application (2.5%, 5% and 10%) with *Schizochytrium* extracts in Skh-1 hairless mice. However, further studies are required to examine the active ingredients and to understand details of the molecular mechanism(s) and direct target(s).

Kim et al. reported the modulatory ability of 80% methanol extract of *Porphyra yezoensis* (laver) on ultraviolet B (UVB)-induced cell death in immortalized human keratinocyte, HaCaT cells [27]. The *P.yezoensis* extract can modulate cell viability and apoptosis of UVB-exposed cells via activating c-Jun N-terminal kinase (JNK) and extracellular signal–regulated kinase (ERK) signaling pathways, in which the modulation of redox status and content of glutathione by the extract. The results indicate that *P.yezoensis* extract can protect skin cells from UVB damage, contributing to improved skin health.

2.2. Biological Activities of Polysaccharides from Marine Algae

Marine algae are abundant in polysaccharides, such as fucoidans in brown algae, ulvans in green algae and carrageenans in red algae [35]. The beneficial effects on skin of polysaccharides from marine algae are summarized in Table 2 along with the species, biological function and mechanism of action.

Table 2. Bioactive functions of marine algal polysaccharides.

Species	Saccharides	Function	Mechanism	Ref.
	Fucoidan	Anti-melanogenesis	In vitro (Mel-Ab cells) Activation of ERK ($\downarrow$) Melanin content ($\downarrow$)	[36]
Sargassum tenerrimum *Turbinaria conoides*	Fucoidan	Antioxidant	In vitro DPPH radical ($\downarrow$) Superoxide radical ($\downarrow$) High total antioxidant and FRAP ability	[37–40]
Costaria costata	Fucoidan	Skin anti-aging	In vitro (HS68 cells) UVB-induced mRNA and pro-tein expression of MMP-1 ($\downarrow$) type 1 pro-collagen ($\uparrow$) Activation of ERK, JNK ($\downarrow$)	[41,42]
	Fucoidan		In vitro (HaCaT cells) Expression of MMP-1 ($\downarrow$) type 1 pro-collagen ($\uparrow$)	[43]
Mekabu	Fucoidan		In vivo UVB-induced edema ($\downarrow$) Thickness of prickle cell layer ($\downarrow$) MMP-1 activity & expression, IFN-γ ($\downarrow$)	[44]
Ascophyllum nodosum	Fucoidan (16 kDa) by acidic hydrolysis		In vitro (HDFs) IL-1β-induced MMP-9, MMP-3 expression/secretion ($\downarrow$) TIMP-1 ($\uparrow$)	[45]
			Ex vivo (human skin) Elastic fiber degradation ($\downarrow$) Leukocyte elastase activity ($\downarrow$)	

Table 2. Cont.

Species	Saccharides	Function	Mechanism	Ref.
Laminaria cichorioides	Fucoidan	Anti-atopic dermatitis	In vivo (Nc/Nga mice) DNCB-induced AD (↓) Clinical severity scores (↓) Scratching counts (↓) Epidermis thickness (↓) Mast cell count (↓) Infiltration of mast cells (↓) Serum histamine (↓) Total IgE (↓)	[46]
			in vitro (Human keratinocytes) AD-associated chemokines TARC, MDC, RANTES (↓)	
	Fucoidan		Ex vivo IgE production in PBMC from patients with AD (↓) Immunoglobulin germline transcripts of B cells (↓) IgE-secreting cells count (↓)	[47]
Saccharina japonica	Fucoidan	Moisturizing	Higher moisture-absorption and moisture-retention ability than HA	[48]
Laminaria cichorioides	Fucoidan (water soluble)	Anti-skin cancer	In vitro (JB6 Cl41 cells) EGF or TPA-induced neoplastic cell transformation (↓) Binding of EGF and EGFR (↓)	[49]
Saccharina longicruris	Laminaran	Skin anti-aging	In vivo (Kunming SPF mice) UVA+UVB-induced skin dermal thickness (↓) Hyp content (↑) Serum or mRNA level of MMP-1 (↓), TIMP-1 (↑)	[50]
		Dermal tissue-engineered production	Deposition of matrix (↑)	[51]
Ulva pertusa	Ulvans	Antioxidant	In vitro Superoxide (↓) Hydroxyl radicals (↓) Reducing power (↑) Metal chelating ability (↑)	[52]
	Acetylated and benzoylated ulvans			[53]
Ulva sp.	Crude ulvans (57 kDa) LMW ulvan (4 kDa)	Skin anti-aging	In vitro (HDFs) Hyaluronan production Collagen release (-)	[54]
Porphyra sp.	Porphyran		In vitro Ferrous ion chelating Reducing power (↑) DPPH radical (↓) Superoxide (↓)	[55]
Porphyra haitanensis	Porphyran fraction F1 fraction F2	Antioxidant	In vivo (Kumming mice) Antioxidant enzyme activity such as MDA (↓), SOD (↑), GSH-Px (↑) lipid peroxidation (↓) TAOC in different organs (↑)	[56,57]
	Porphyran with different MW		In vitro DPPH radical (↓) Reducing power (↑)	[58]
	LMW Porphyran SD, AD, PD, BD		In vitro DPPH radical (↓) Hydroxyl radicals (↓) Superoxide (↓)	[59]

Table 2. Cont.

Species	Saccharides	Function	Mechanism	Ref.
Porphyra yezoensis	Porphyran	Anti-inflammation	In vitro (RAW264.7 cells) LPS-induced NO, iNOS level, NF-κB activation, TNF-α, nuclear translocation of p65, phosphorylation and degradation of IκB-α (↓)	[60,61]
Porphyridium	Carrageenan	Anti-melanogenesis	In vivo (Guinea pig) Level of melanosome (↓)	[62]
Commercial	ι(II)-Carrageenan	Antioxidant Photoprotective	In vitro (HaCaT cells) UVB-induced cell death (↓) DCF-DA: Intracellular ROS (↓) DPPH radical (↓)	[63]
Eucheuma spinosum (*Eucheuma denticulatum*)	ι(V)-Carrageenan			
Commercial	λ-Carrageenan			
Eucheuma cottonii (*Kappaphycus alvarezii*)	κ(III)-Carrageenan			
Commercial	ι(II)-Carrageenan			
	κ-COSs (37.7 kDa)	Antioxidant	In vitro Superoxide radical (↓) Hydroxyl radical (↓) DPPH radical (↓) Reducing power (↑)	[64]
	κ-COSs (1.2 kDa) SD (0.8 kDa) LAD (1.2 kDa) HAD (1.4 kDa) PD (1.1 kDa)		In vitro Superoxide (↓) Hydroxyl radical (↓) DPPH radical (↓) Reducing power (↑) Iron ion chelation (↑) Total antioxidant activity (↑)	[65,66]
	κ-COSs with CP	Photo-protective	In vitro (HaCaT cells, MEFs) UVB-induced damage (↓)	[67]

AD: atopic dermatitis, **BD**: benzoylated derivatives, **COSs**: carrageenan oligosaccharides, **CP**: collagen peptide, **DCF-DA**: 2′,7′-dichlorofluorescin diacetate, **DNCB**: 2,4-dinitrochlorobenzene, **DPPH**: 2,2-diphenyl-1-picrylhydrazyl, **EGF**: epidermal growth factor, **EGFR**: epidermal growth factor receptor, **ERK**: extracellular signal–regulated kinase, **FRAP**: ferric reducing antioxidant power, **GSH-Px**: glutathione peroxidase, **HA**: hyaluronic acid, **HaCaT cells**: immortalized human keratinocytes, **HDFs**: human dermal fibroblasts, **HS68 cells**: human foreskin fibroblast, **Hyp**: hydroxyproline, **IgE**: immunoglobulin E, **IκB-α**: inhibitor of kappa B, **IL-1β**: interleukin-1β, **IFN-γ**: interferon-gamma, **iNOS**: inducible nitric oxide synthase, **iota 2 [ι(II)], iota 5 [ι (V)]**, **JB6 cells**: mouse epidermal cells, **JNK**: c-Jun N-terminal kinase, **kappa (κ), lambda (λ) kappa [κ(III)]**, **LMW**: low molecular weight, **LPS**: lipopolysaccharide, **MDA**: malondialdehyde, **MDC**: macrophage-derived chemokine, **MEF**: mouse embryonic fibroblasts, **Mel-Ab cells**: immortalized murine melanocyte cell line, **MMP-1**: matrix metalloproteinase-1, **MMP-3**: matrix metalloproteinase-3, **MMP-9**: matrix metalloproteinase-9, **MW**: molecular weight, **NF-κB**: nuclear factor kappa B, **NO**: nitric oxide, **PBMC**: peripheral blood mononuclear cell, **PD**: phosphorylated derivatives, **RANTES**: regulated upon activation, normal T-cell expressed and secreted chemokine, **ROS**: reactive oxygen species, **SD**: sulfated derivatives, **SOD**: superoxide dismutase, **SPF**: specific pathogen free, **TAOC**: total antioxidant capacity, **TARC**: thymus- and activation-regulated chemokine, **TIMP-1**: tissue inhibitor of metalloproteinases inhibitor 1, **TNF**: tumor necrosis factor, **TPA**: 12-O-tetradecanoylphorbol-13-acetate, **UVA**: ultraviolet A, **UVB**: ultraviolet B.

2.2.1. Fucoidans

Fucoidans are major sulfated polysaccharides (SPs) found in the cell wall of some brown algae [10]. Numerous studies have reported the benefits of fucoidans for diverse skin disorders including pigmentation, skin aging, atopic dermatitis and skin carcinogenesis.

Anti-Melanogenic Activity

Song et al. reported that fucoidan reduced melanin content by activating the ERK pathway in Mel-Ab Cells [36]. While fucoidan treatment did not directly decrease TYR activity, it downregulated the microphthalmia-associated transcription factor (MITF) and TYR protein expression.

Antioxidant Activity

In vitro antioxidant capacities of fucoidan from *Sargassum tenerrimum* were analyzed with DPPH, superoxide radical scavenging and total antioxidant assays [40]. The antioxidant activity of SPs depends on their structural properties such as the level or distribution of sulfate groups, MW, sugar composition, and stereochemistry [35]. It has been consistently documented that fucoidan from brown algae *Laminaria japonica* possesses high superoxide radical and hydroxyl radical scavenging assays according to sulfate content [38,39]. Fucoidans from *Fucus vesiculosus* exhibited considerable ferric reducing antioxidant power (FRAP) [37] and superoxide radical scavenging property [68].

Skin Anti-Aging Activity

A study conducted by Moon et al. reported that fucoidan from *Costaria costata* showed skin anti-aging activity in human foreskin fibroblast HS68 cells [41,42] and HaCaT cells [43].

Fucoidan suppressed mRNA and protein expression of MMP-1 upregulation and type 1 pro-collagen downregulation stimulated by UVB via inactivation of ERK and JNK. Additionally, fucoidan from *Mekabu* inhibited Interleukin-1β (IL-1β)-induced secretion of MMP-9, -3 and degradation of tissue inhibitor of metalloproteinases inhibitor 1 (TIMP-1) in HDFs [45]. In addition, positive correlations reported for UVB-induced edema, thickness of the prickle cell layer, MMP-1 activation and interferon (IFN)-γ were attenuated by fucoidan treatment on the skin of mice [44]. Senni et al. demonstrated that fucoidan (16 kDa) from *Ascophyllum nodosum*, using acidic hydrolysis, exhibited skin anti-aging potential in human skin via preventing elastic fiber degradation and leukocyte elastase activity [45]. These results indicate that fucoidans present skin anti-aging potential with varied mechanisms of action.

Anti-Atopic Dermatitis Activity

Fucoidan from *Laminaria cichorioides* alleviated 2,4-dinitrochlorobenzene (DNCB)-induced AD in vitro and in vivo [46]. AD-associated chemokines including thymus- and activation-regulated chemokine (TARC), macrophage-derived chemokine (MDC) and regulated upon activation, normal T-cell expressed and secreted chemokine (RANTES), were inhibited by fucoidan treatment in human keratinocytes. Another study reported anti-atopic dermatitis effects ex vivo whereby fucoidan inhibited IgE production in peripheral blood mononuclear cells (PBMC) from patients with AD, as well as immunoglobulin germline transcripts of B cells and the IgE-secreting cell count [47]. Thus, fucoidan could contribute to the development of preventive and therapeutic agents for inflammatory diseases such as AD.

Moisturizing Activity

Previously, *Saccharina japonica* extracts from brown algae showed a profound moisture retention ability, greater than that of other kinds of algae [6]. In particular, *S. japonica* polysaccharides were identified as a better humectant than hyaluronic acid (HA, or hyaluronan), which has the ability to retain a large amount of water [48], followed by red macroalgae extracts. Other extracts from green algae showed lower water retention capacity than HA. Therefore, SPs from marine algae, especially fucoidan, have potential as humectants to protect against skin dehydration.

Anti-Skin Cancer Activity

The chemopreventive activity and the underlying molecular mechanisms of fucoidan from *Laminaria cichorioides* was elucidated by Lee et al. in 2008. Treatments with water-soluble fucoidan from *L. cichorioides* up to 100 μg/mL were not cytotoxice in JB6Cl41 mouse epidermal cells. Fucoidan inhibited the epidermal growth factor (EGF), or TPA-induced neoplastic cell transformation, through preventing the binding of EGF to its cell surface receptor (EGFR) [49]. This evidence suggests an anti-skin carcinogenic molecular mechanism action of fucoidan with potential application for chemopreventive agents.

2.2.2. Laminaran

Laminaran (also known as laminarin) is one of the major non-SPs found in brown algae. The biological activities of fucoidans have been well-studied, while those of laminaran have been poorly understood to date. Laminaran from the brown algae *Saccharina longicruris* has been reported to show skin anti-aging induced by UVA/UVB in an in vivo model [50]. The Kumming mouse is an experimental animal model reflecting age-related decline characteristics of female fertility in humans [69]. UV irradiation facilitates the process of extrinsic aging as well as intrinsic aging. Intraperitoneal (IP) injection of laminaran (1 or 5 mg/kg) attenuated UVA/UVB-induced skin dermal thickness by downregulating MMP-1 and upregulating TIMP-1 and hydroxyproline (Hyp) content. Ayoub et al. demonstrated that laminaran from *Saccharina longicruris* prevented matrix deposition [51]. Considering these results, laminaran may help prevent the progression of skin aging.

2.2.3. Ulvans

Ulvans are sulfated heteropolysaccharides extracted from the cell wall of green algae *Ulva pertusa* [52]. Ulvans are water-soluble sulfated polysaccharides and their main constituents are rhamnose, xylose, glucose, uronic acid and sulfate. It has also been identified that glucuronic acid and rhamnose occur mainly in the form of the aldobiouronic acid, 4-O-β-D-glucuronosyl-l-rhamnose [70]. Due to the high recalcitrance of ulvans, related to their complex chemical structure, their biological functions have been less exploited.

Radical scavenging assay revealed that the antioxidant, reducing activity and ferrous ion chelating ability of ulvans were proportionate to sulfate content [52]. High sulfate content showed more profound antioxidant properties [52]. A follow-up study reported that low molecular weight (LMW) and high sulfate content derivatives of ulvans showed enhanced antioxidant activities [35]. In addition, the antioxidant activity of acetylated and benzoylated ulvans was stronger than that of natural ulvan [53]. Recently, SPs including crude ulvans (57 kDa) and LMW ulvan (4 kDa) were isolated from *Ulva* sp. and their skin anti-aging activities were evaluated [54]. HA production was significantly upregulated by SPs from *Ulva* sp. in HDFs. Crude ulvans (57 kDa) showed stronger stimulatory activity of HA production than LMW ulvan (4 kDa). These findings revealed the biological activities of ulvans and may account for the development of ingredients beneficial to skin from marine algae.

2.2.4. Porphyran

Red algae *Porphyra* is an edible seaweed well-known as laver, gim (Korean) or nori (Japanese). Porphyra is mainly composed of porphyran, which is the sulfated polysaccharide comprising the hot-water soluble portion of the cell wall [58]. Porphyran is related to agarose in that it contains disaccharide units consisting of 3-linked β-d-galactosyl residues alternating with 4-linked 3,6-anhydro-α-L-galactose, but differs in that some residues occur as 6-sulfate [57].

Antioxidant Activity

Porphyran has been reported to scavenge oxidative radicals in vitro [55], and to increase antioxidant enzyme activity and antioxidant capacity in aging mice [56,57].

Porphyran from *Porphyra* sp. aqueous extract showed significant ferrous ion chelating capacity and reducing power [55]. In addition, DPPH radicals and superoxide radicals were dose-dependently quenched by porphyran treatment. Zhao et al. [58] found that the porphyrans from *Porphyra haitanensis* with different MWs showed different antioxidant activities. Assays including DPPH radical and reducing power indicated that porphyrans with lower MW exhibited higher antioxidant activities. According to a follow-up study, LMW porphyran and its different derivatives determined the relationship between antioxidant activity and chemical modifications [59]. Sulfated (SD), acetylated (AD), phosphorylated (PD) and benzoylated (BD) derivatives of porphyran from *P. haitanensis* showed higher antioxidant activities in vitro than those of LMW porphyran. Among the diverse derivatives, BD exerted the best antioxidant activities in DPPH radical, hydroxyl radical and superoxide scavenging assays. These results also support the conclusion that the antioxidant activity of polysaccharide is closely related to several structural elements such as MW, degree of substitution (DS) and functional groups [59].

In vivo antioxidant activity of porphyran fraction F1 [57] and F2 [56] derived from *P. haitanensis* has been assessed in aging mice (Kumming mouse) [35,69]. Malondialdehyde (MDA) is a main marker of endogenous lipid peroxidation. With aging, the organs showed significantly increased levels of MDA indicating that peroxidative damage increases with the aging process [56,57]. IP administration of porphyran fractions F1 (50, 100 and 200 mg/kg) and F2 (100, 200 and 400 mg/kg) significantly decreased the MDA level in aging mice, indicating a prevention effect of lipid peroxidation. Superoxide dismutase (SOD) is an intracellular antioxidant enzyme that protects against oxidative processes initiated by the superoxide anion [57]. Glutathione peroxidase (GSH-Px) is an enzymatic antioxidant defense system to protect against oxidative damage, while total antioxidant capacity (TAOC) reflects the capacity of the non-enzymatic antioxidant defense system [57]. Porphyran fractions F1 and F2 both increased the TAOC and upregulated activity of SOD and GSH-Px in Kumming aging mice suggesting their significant in vivo antioxidant activity [56,57].

Skin Anti-Inflammatory Activity

Porphyran from *Porphyra yezoensis* showed the anti-inflammation activity in LPS-stimulated macrophages [60]. Porphyran suppressed LPS-induced NO production and iNOS level by blocking nuclear factor kappa B (NF-κB) activation in RAW264.7 cells. Porphyran reduced LPS-induced NF-κB activation by inhibiting nuclear translocation of p65, phosphorylation and degradation of inhibitor of kappa B (IκB)-α in RAW264.7 cells. Meanwhile, porphyran showed a moderate inhibitory effect on LPS-induced tumor necrosis factor (TNF)-α production in RAW264.7 cells. These results suggest that porphyran blocked LPS-induced NO production via inactivation of NF-κB in murine macrophage cells.

2.2.5. Carrageenan

Carrageenan from red algae is linear SP composed of 3,6-anhydro-D-galactose (D-AHG) and D-galactose. Carrageenan has been utilized in cosmetic products as a stabilizer, emulsifier and moisturizer due to its chemical and physical properties. In addition, carrageenan is known to exhibit various beneficial effects on skin health as summarized in Table 2.

Anti-Melanogenic Activity

Carrageenan from red microalgae *Porphyridium*, has been reported as being a macrophage toxic substance [62]. The injection of carrageenan effectively degraded and eliminated dermal melanosomes/melanin from the dermis of guinea pigs indicating the skin-whitening potential of carrageenan.

Antioxidant Activity

Thevanayagam et al. assessed the photoprotective and antioxidative activities of various isoforms of carrageenan in HaCaT cells [63]. The types of carrageenan are iota 2 [ι (II)] iota 5 [ι (V)] from

Eucheuma spinosum, and lambda (λ) and kappa (κ) type III from *Eucheuma cottonii*. Commonly, all types of carrageenan can scavenge free radicals, however, in vitro antioxidant capability did not correlate with the amount of sulfur moieties in the different isomers. Although κ-carrageenan contained the least sulfate content compared to ι- and λ-carrageenan, κ-carrageenan exhibited the highest radical scavenging activity. The DPPH reducing capability of carrageenan followed the order: λ < ι < κ. This evidence indicates that the increase in the oxidative property with irradiation dose can be attributed mainly to the depolymerization of the carrageenan with a corresponding increase in reducing sugar. In addition, the presence of the hydrophobic 3,6-anhydrogalatose could affect the antioxidant activity of carrageenan.

Other studies investigated the antioxidant capacity of κ-carrageenan, κ-carrageenan oligosaccharides (κ-COSs) and their chemically modified derivatives including oversulfated (SD, 0.8 kDa), lowly acetylated (LAD, 1.2 kDa), highly acetylated (HAD, 1.4 kDa) and phosphorylated (PD, 1.1 kDa) [64–66]. An in vitro antioxidant activity assay was performed reducing power, iron ion chelation, and total antioxidant activity. Generally, chemical modification of COSs can enhance their antioxidant activity in vitro as follows: PD > SD > LAD > HAD [66]. In this study, sulfate contents seemed to be related to antioxidant activity. Taken together, these investigations indicate that the antioxidant properties of carrageenans have are closely related to sulfate content structure as well as with the type of sugar unit and DPs according to MW.

Photoprotective Activity

Ren et al. reported the anti-oxidative and photoprotective effects of a complex of κ-COSs and collagen peptide (CP) in HaCaT cells and mouse embryonic fibroblasts (MEFs) [67]. A complex of κ-COSs and CP (100 μg/mL) could significantly attenuate UV-induced cell death and apoptosis in HaCaT and MEF through reduction of the intracellular ROS level. A complex of κ-COSs and CP mostly inhibited the UV-induced decrease of type 1 pro-collagen and increase in MMP-1 by suppressing the mitogen-activated protein kinases (MAPKs) signaling pathway. Collectively, a complex of κ-COSs and CP may have photoprotective potential against skin aging.

2.3. Biological Activities of Monosaccharides and Oligosaccharides from Red Algae

Agar is the major polysaccharide of red macroalgae. Agar is easily hydrolyzed into oligosaccharides by various chemical and enzymatic methods [71]. Depending on the hydrolysis method, oligosaccharides with different DPs can be generated from agar [72]. Agarose-derived oligosaccharides are referred to as agarooligosaccharides (AOSs). There are two forms of AOSs, namely, neo-form and agaro-form. Neo-form AOSs are called neoagarooligosaccharides (NAOSs) and have repeating neoagarobiose units composed of D-galactose at the non-reducing end and 3,6-anhydro-L-galactose (L-AHG) at the reducing end. Table 3 shows the beneficial effects of monosaccharides and oligosaccharides from red algae.

Table 3. Bioactive functions of marine algal monosaccharides and oligosaccharides.

DP	Name	Mode of Linkage	Function	Mechanism	Ref.
1	D-Glucose	-	Anti-melanogenesis	In vitro (B16 cells) TYR activity (↓) Melanin content (-)	[73]
	L-AHG	-		In vitro (B16F10 cells or HEMs) Melanin content (↓), TYR activity (-)	[74,75]
	D-AHG	-	Anti-inflammation	In vitro (Raw264.7 cells) LPS-induced NO level (↓)	[75]
	D-Galactose	-	Melanogenesis	In vitro (B16 cells) Melanin content (-) TYR activity (↑)	[73,75]

Table 3. Cont.

DP	Name	Mode of Linkage	Function	Mechanism	Ref.
2	Agarobiose	Gal$_{\beta 1}$→$_4$AHG	Antioxidant	In vitro DPPH radical (↓)	[76]
			Anti-inflammation	In vitro (RAW264.7 cell) LPS-induced level of NO, PGE2 (↓) Expression of HO-1 (↑) Protein level of iNOS (↓)	[77]
				In vitro (Human Monocytes) LPS-induced Cytokines TNF-α, IL-1b, IL-6 (↓)	
				In vitro (Human Monocytes) LPS-induced NO level (↓) mRNA level of COX-2, mPGES-1 (↓)	[78]
	Neoagarobiose	AHG$_{\alpha 1}$→$_3$Gal	Anti-melanogenesis	In vitro (B16 cells) Melanin content (↓) Cellular TYR activity (↓)	[79,80]
			Moisturizing	Higher moisture-absorption and moisture-retention ability than HA	
3	Agarotriose	Gal$_{\beta 1}$→$_4$AHG$_{\alpha 1}$→$_3$Gal	N.a.	-	-
	Neoagarotriose	AHG$_{\alpha 1}$→$_3$Gal$_{\beta 1}$→$_4$AHG	N.a.	-	-
4	Agarotetraose	Gal$_{\beta 1}$→$_4$AHG$_{\alpha 1}$→$_3$Gal$_{\beta 1}$→$_4$AHG	Antioxidant	In vitro DPPH radical (↓)	[76]
			Anti-inflammation	In vitro (RAW264.7 cell) LPS-induced level of NO (↓)	[77]
	Neoagarotetraose	AHG$_{\alpha 1}$→$_3$Gal$_{\beta 1}$→$_4$AHG$_{\alpha 1}$→$_3$Gal	Anti-melanogenesis	In vitro (B16 cells or HEMs) Melanin content (↓) Cellular TYR activity (↓)	[74,81]
5	Agaropentaose	Gal$_{\beta 1}$→$_4$AHG$_{\alpha 1}$→$_3$Gal$_{\beta 1}$→$_4$AHG$_{\alpha 1}$→$_3$Gal	N.a.	-	-
	Neoagaropentaose	AHG$_{\alpha 1}$→$_3$Gal$_{\beta 1}$→$_4$AHG$_{\alpha 1}$→$_3$Gal$_{\beta 1}$→$_4$AHG	N.a.	-	-
6	Agarohexaose	Gal$_{\beta 1}$→$_4$AHG$_{\alpha 1}$→$_3$Gal$_{\beta 1}$→$_4$AHG$_{\alpha 1}$→$_3$Gal$_{\beta 1}$→$_4$AHG	Antioxidant	In vitro DPPH radical (↓)	[76]
			Anti-inflammation	In vitro (RAW264.7 cell) LPS-induced level of NO (↓)	[77]
				In vitro (Human Monocytes) LPS-induced NO level (↓) mRNA level of COX-2, mPGES-1 (↓)	[78]
	Neoagarohexaose	AHG$_{\alpha 1}$→$_3$Gal$_{\beta 1}$→$_4$AHG$_{\alpha 1}$→$_3$Gal$_{\beta 1}$→$_4$AHG$_{\alpha 1}$→$_3$Gal	Anti-melanogenesis	In vitro (B16 cells or HEMs) Melanin content (↓) Cellular TYR activity (↓)	[74,81,82]
7	Agaroheptaose	Gal$_{\beta 1}$→$_4$AHG$_{\alpha 1}$→$_3$Gal$_{\beta 1}$→$_4$AHG$_{\alpha 1}$→$_3$Gal$_{\beta 1}$→$_4$AHG$_{\alpha 1}$→$_3$Gal	N.a.	-	-
	Neoagaroheptaose	AHG$_{\alpha 1}$→$_3$Gal$_{\beta 1}$→$_4$AHG$_{\alpha 1}$→$_3$Gal$_{\beta 1}$→$_4$AHG$_{\alpha 1}$→$_3$Gal$_{\beta 1}$→$_4$AHG	N.a.	-	-
8	Agarooctaose	Gal$_{\beta 1}$→$_4$AHG$_{\alpha 1}$→$_3$Gal$_{\beta 1}$→$_4$AHG$_{\alpha 1}$→$_3$Gal$_{\beta 1}$→$_4$AHG$_{\alpha 1}$→$_3$Gal$_{\beta 1}$→$_4$AHG	Antioxidant	In vitro DPPH radical (↓)	[76]
	Neoagarooctaose	AHG$_{\alpha 1}$→$_3$Gal$_{\beta 1}$→$_4$AHG$_{\alpha 1}$→$_3$Gal$_{\beta 1}$→$_4$AHG$_{\alpha 1}$→$_3$Gal$_{\beta 1}$→$_4$AHG$_{\alpha 1}$→$_3$Gal	N.a.	-	-

Table 3. Cont.

DP	Name	Mode of Linkage	Function	Mechanism	Ref.
9	Agarononaose	Gal$_{\beta1}$→$_4$AHG$_{\alpha1}$→$_3$Gal$_{\beta1}$→$_4$AHG$_{\alpha1}$→$_3$Gal$_{\beta1}$→$_4$AHG$_{\alpha1}$→$_3$Gal$_{\beta1}$→$_4$AHG$_{\alpha1}$→$_3$Gal	N.a.	-	-
	Neoagarononaose	AHG$_{\alpha1}$→$_3$Gal$_{\beta1}$→$_4$AHG$_{\alpha1}$→$_3$Gal$_{\beta1}$→$_4$AHG$_{\alpha1}$→$_3$Gal$_{\beta1}$→$_4$AHG$_{\alpha1}$→$_3$Gal$_{\beta1}$→$_4$AHG	N.a.	-	-
10	Agarodecaose	Gal$_{\beta1}$→$_4$AHG$_{\alpha1}$→$_3$Gal$_{\beta1}$→$_4$AHG$_{\alpha1}$→$_3$Gal$_{\beta1}$→$_4$AHG$_{\alpha1}$→$_3$Gal$_{\beta1}$→$_4$AHG$_{\alpha1}$→$_3$Gal$_{\beta1}$→$_4$AHG	Antioxidant	In vitro DPPH radical (↓)	[76]
	Neoagarodecaose	AHG$_{\alpha1}$→$_3$Gal$_{\beta1}$→$_4$AHG$_{\alpha1}$→$_3$Gal$_{\beta1}$→$_4$AHG$_{\alpha1}$→$_3$Gal$_{\beta1}$→$_4$AHG$_{\alpha1}$→$_3$Gal$_{\beta1}$→$_4$AHG$_{\alpha1}$→$_3$Gal	N.a.	-	-
-	Mixture of AOSs with DP 2, 4, 6 and 8	[Gal$_{\beta1}$→$_4$AHG]$_n$	Anti-melanogenesis	In vitro (B16 cells) Melanin content (↓) Cellular TYR activity (↓)	[82]
			Anti-skin cancer	In vivo (ICR mice) DMBA/TPA-induced tumor incidence (↓), number of papilloma (↓), TPA-induced ear edema (↓) TPA-induced PGE2 (↓)	[78]
			Anti-inflammation	In vitro (Human monocytes) LPS-induced NO level (↓)	

AOSs: agaro-oligosaccharides, **B16(F10) cells**: mouse melanoma B16(F10) cells, **COX-2**: cyclooxygenase-2, **D-AHG**: 3,6-anhydro-D-galactose, **DMBA**: 12-dimethylbenz [a] anthracene, **DP**: degree of polymerization, **DPPH**: 2,2-diphenyl-1-picrylhydrazyl, **HA**: hyaluronan, **HEMs**: human epidermal melanocytes, **HO-1**: heme oxygenase-1, **IL**: interleukin, **iNOS**: liducible nitric oxide synthase, **L-AHG**: 3,6-anhydro-L-galactose, **LPS**: lipopolysaccharides, **mPGES-1**: microsomal prostaglandin E synthase-1, **N.a.**: not applicable, **NO**: nitric oxide, **PGE2**: prostaglandin E2, **TNF**: tumor necrosis factor, **TPA**: 12-O-tetradecanoylphorbol-13-acetate, **TYR**: tyrosinase, **(-)**: not effective.

2.3.1. Anti-Melanogenic Activity

Previous studies have reported that NAOSs with different DPs, including neoagarobiose (NeoDP2), neoagarotetraose (NeoDP4) and neoagarohexaose (NeoDP6), had a whitening effect and inhibited TYR activity in murine melanoma B16F10 cells [80–82]. NAOSs with different DPs were not cytotoxic to B16F10 up to 100 µg/mL, showing that their skin-whitening effect was not derived from affecting cell viability. In addition, NeoDP4 and NeoDP6 reduced extracellular melanin contents in B16F10 cells and pigmentation evaluated by Fontana-Masson staining in HEMs, whereas agarotriose (DP3), agaropentaose (DP5) and agaroheptaose (DP7) did not reduce melanin production [74].

Recent studies have reported that oligosaccharides from agarose showed anti-melanogenic activity according to the DP of the galactosyl groups [83]. D-glucose and D-galactose are common mono-saccharides of marine algae. L-AHG is major component of agar, while D-AHG is a major monomeric sugar unit of carrageenan from red macroalgae. Previously, effects of monosaccharides including L-AHG, D-AHG and D-galactose on α-MSH-induced melanin production in B16F10 melanoma cells have been reported [74,75]. The melanin level was significantly suppressed by 100 µg/mL of L-AHG. D-AHG also showed an inhibitory effect on melanin production only at 100 µg/mL, but its effect was slightly lower than that of L-AHG. Another monomeric sugar, D-galactose, did not exert any significant reduction in melanin production in B16F10 cells. In addition, a previous study reported that TYR activity was promoted by D-galactose, but it seems likely to be decreased in the presence of glucose [73]. D-glucose also did not affect melanin content in murine melanoma cells [73]. Furthermore, a recent study has demonstrated that L-AHG suppresses melanogenic proteins via inhibiting cyclic adenosine monophosphate/cyclic adenosine monophosphate-dependent protein kinase, MAPK, and Akt signaling pathways in HEMs [84]. Collectively, red macroalgal sugars, such as

L-AHG and D-AHG, showed anti-melanogenic activity and are considered to be active components of red macroalgae for skin-whitening activity.

2.3.2. Skin Anti-Inflammatory Activity

An effect of L-AHG on LPS-induced NO production in RAW264.7 cells has been reported [75]. To our knowledge, this was the first report on the biological activity of L-AHG. Nitrite production was significantly suppressed by 100 and 200 μg/mL of L-AHG. D-AHG showed a nitrite-suppressing effect only at 200 μg/mL, but its effect was significantly lower than that of L-AHG. Other saccharides, such as NeoDP2 and D-galactose, did not induce any significant reduction in the nitrite production of RAW264.7 cells.

Enoki et al. reported the anti-inflammatory activities of AOSs including agarobiose (DP2), agarotetraose (DP4) and agarohexaose (DP6), which have L-AHG at the reducing end. Agarobiose (DP2), agarotetraose (DP4) and agarohexaose (DP6) dose-dependently suppressed NO production in RAW264.7 cells [77]. Meanwhile, neo-agarohexaose (DP6), which has D-galactose at the reducing end, had no inhibitory effect on nitrite production. Agarobiose (DP2) suppressed LPS-induced prostaglandin E2 (PGE2), and pro-inflammatory cytokine levels in activated monocytes/macrophages via heme oxygenase-1 (HO-1) induction.

A later study conducted by Enoki et al. demonstrated the anti-inflammatory effects of AOSs mixed with DP 2, 4, 6 and 8 in human monocytes [78]. The AOS mixture attenuated LPS-induced NO levels in human monocytes. Agarobiose (DP2) and agarohexaose (DP6) decreased LPS-induced mRNA levels of COX-2, mPGES-1 in human monocytes. However, it is currently unclear whether AOSs can elicit anti-inflammatory activity in vivo by contacting activated monocytes/machrophages at an inflammation site, since a high dose of AOSs was needed to inhibit the release of pro-inflammatory mediators in an in vitro study.

2.3.3. Antioxidant Activity

Ajisaka et al. compared the antioxidative potency of various carbohydrates including fucoidan and AOSs [85]. In a DPPH assay, fucoidan showed remarkable radical scavenging activity, although lower than ascorbic acid, but AOSs showed almost no DPPH radical scavenging activity up to 20 mM. Notably, the SOD activity assay revealed that AOS had high antioxidant activity, showing almost half of the antioxidant activity of ascorbic acid.

Chen et al. evaluated the antioxidant activity of AOSs with different DPs in cell-based systems [76]. An in vitro DPPH assay revealed that agarohexaose showed the highest radical scavenging capacity. Intracellular ROS levels were investigated using the dichlorofluorescein (DCF) assay in L-02 human liver cells. Agarohexaose at 1 mg/mL significantly reduced H_2O_2-induced oxidants up to 50%, showing the highest scavenging capability. In conclusion, AOSs may be novel antioxidants which could protect against cell damage caused by ROS, especially agarohexaose which exhibited excellent effects.

2.3.4. Moisturizing Activity

Previously, NeoDP2 has been reported to show not only whitening effects but also moisturizing effects [80]. NeoDP2 showed a higher hygroscopic ability than glycerol or HA, typical moisturizing reagents, indicating that algae-derived saccharides could be used as a moisturizer in cosmetics.

2.3.5. Anti-Skin Cancer Activity

The ability of AOSs from red macroalgae to prevent tumor promotion in the two-stage mouse skin carcinogenesis model has been reported previously [78]. AOS feeding led to delayed DMBA/TPA-induced tumor incidence and tumor number in Institute of Cancer Research (ICR)mice. PGE2 production was also suppressed by AOS intake in a TPA-induced ear edema model. AOSs downregulated cyclooxygenase-2 (COX-2) and microsomal PGE synthase-1 (mPGES-1), rate-limiting enzymes in PGE2 production, in human monocytes. Consequently, AOSs are expected to prevent tumor promotion by inhibiting PGE2 elevation in chronic inflammation sites.

3. Concluding Remarks

In this review, we have presented evidence that various biological activities of marine algae extracts and marine algal carbohydrates act as novel cosmeceuticals. Marine algae extracts and carbohydrates were categorized by source (species), structural parameters, bioactive functions and mechanism. Numerous in vitro and in vivo studies showed that marine algae extracts and algal carbohydrates showed various biological activities against skin disorders including hyperpigmentation, wrinkles, dry skin disorders, skin inflammation and skin cancer. However, although diverse biological activities of marine carbohydrates have been determined, their detailed molecular mechanisms and target proteins are not fully understood. Therefore, further investigations to elicit the precise molecular basis for the biological activity of marine algal compounds should be undertaken. Recently, bioinformatics has been used to screen functional materials derived from natural resources more rapidly and to predict the mechanisms of biological actions [86–88]. Thus, using a bioinformatics approach will be a good strategy for finding and understanding more effective marine algal compounds, which will contribute to the development of novel cosmeceuticals.

Author Contributions: J.H.K., K.H.K. and N.J.K. conceived and designed the structure of the review. J.H.K., J.E.L. and N.J.K. wrote the manuscript. All the authors read and approved the final version of the manuscript.

Funding: The Basic Research Laboratory Program (2018R1A4A1022589) and the C1 Gas Refinery Program (2016M3D3A1A01913268) through the National Research Foundation of Korea funded by the MSIT and the National Coordinating Centre for Global Cosmetics R&D (NCR) grant (HN14C0097).

Acknowledgments: This study was financially supported by the Basic Research Laboratory Program (2018R1A4A1022589) and the C1 Gas Refinery Program (2016M3D3A1A01913268) through the National Research Foundation of Korea funded by the MSIT , and by the National Coordinating Centre for Global Cosmetics R&D (NCR) grant (HN14C0097) funded by the Ministry of Health and Welfare. This study was performed at the Institute of Biomedical and Food Safety at CJ Food Safety Hall, Korea University.

Conflicts of Interest: The authors declare no conflicts of interest.

References

1. Ruocco, N.; Costantini, S.; Guariniello, S.; Costantini, M. Polysaccharides from the marine environment with pharmacological, cosmeceutical and nutraceutical potential. *Molecules* **2016**, *21*, 551. [CrossRef] [PubMed]
2. Thomas, N.V.; Kim, S.K. Beneficial effects of marine algal compounds in cosmeceuticals. *Mar. Drugs* **2013**, *11*, 146–164. [CrossRef] [PubMed]
3. Molinski, T.F.; Dalisay, D.S.; Lievens, S.L.; Saludes, J.P. Drug development from marine natural products. *Nat. Rev. Drug Discov.* **2009**, *8*, 69–85. [CrossRef] [PubMed]
4. Munro, M.H.; Blunt, J.W.; Dumdei, E.J.; Hickford, S.J.; Lill, R.E.; Li, S.; Battershill, C.N.; Duckworth, A.R. The discovery and development of marine compounds with pharmaceutical potential. *J. Biotechnol.* **1999**, *70*, 15–25. [CrossRef]
5. Snelgrove, P.V. An Ocean of Discovery: Biodiversity Beyond the Census of Marine Life. *Planta Med.* **2016**, *82*, 790–799. [CrossRef] [PubMed]
6. Wang, H.M.D.; Chen, C.C.; Huynh, P.; Chang, J.S. Exploring the potential of using algae in cosmetics. *Bioresour. Technol.* **2015**, *184*, 355–362. [CrossRef] [PubMed]
7. Zia, K.M.; Tabasum, S.; Nasif, M.; Sultan, N.; Aslam, N.; Noreen, A.; Zuber, M. A review on synthesis, properties and applications of natural polymer based carrageenan blends and composites. *Int. J. Biol. Macromol.* **2016**, *96*, 282–301. [CrossRef] [PubMed]
8. De Jesus Raposo, M.F.; de Morais, A.M.; de Morais, R.M. Marine polysaccharides from algae with potential biomedical applications. *Mar. Drugs* **2015**, *13*, 2967–3028. [CrossRef] [PubMed]
9. Hamed, I.; Ozogul, F.; Ozogul, Y.; Regenstein, J.M. Marine bioactive compounds and their health benefits: A Review. *Compr. Rev. Food Sci. Food Saf.* **2015**, *14*, 446–465. [CrossRef]

10. Kang, H.K.; Seo, C.H.; Park, Y. The effects of marine carbohydrates and glycosylated compounds on human health. *Int. J. Mol. Sci.* **2015**, *16*, 6018–6056. [CrossRef] [PubMed]
11. Wei, N.; Quarterman, J.; Jin, Y.S. Marine macroalgae: An untapped resource for producing fuels and chemicals. *Trends Biotechnol.* **2013**, *31*, 70–77. [CrossRef] [PubMed]
12. Laurienzo, P. Marine polysaccharides in pharmaceutical applications: An Overview. *Mar. Drugs* **2010**, *8*, 2435–2465. [CrossRef] [PubMed]
13. Cunha, L.; Grenha, A. Sulfated seaweed polysaccharides as multifunctional materials in drug delivery applications. *Mar. Drugs* **2016**, *14*, 42. [CrossRef] [PubMed]
14. Ahmed, A.B.; Adel, M.; Karimi, P.; Peidayesh, M. Pharmaceutical, cosmeceutical, and traditional applications of marine carbohydrates. *Adv. Food Nutr. Res.* **2014**, *73*, 197–220. [PubMed]
15. Melo, M.R.S.; Feitosa, J.P.A.; Freitas, A.L.P.; de Paula, R.C.M. Isolation and characterization of soluble sulfated polysaccharide from the red seaweed Gracilaria cornea. *Carbohydr. Polym.* **2002**, *49*, 491–498. [CrossRef]
16. Cha, S.H.; Ko, S.C.; Kim, D.; Jeon, Y.J. Screening of marine algae for potential tyrosinase inhibitor: Those inhibitors reduced tyrosinase activity and melanin synthesis in zebrafish. *J. Dermatol.* **2011**, *38*, 343–352. [CrossRef]
17. Heo, S.J.; Ko, S.C.; Kang, S.M.; Cha, S.H.; Lee, S.H.; Kang, D.H.; Jung, W.K.; Affan, A.; Oh, C.; Jeon, Y.J. Inhibitory effect of diphlorethohydroxycarmalol on melanogenesis and its protective effect against UV-B radiation-induced cell damage. *Food Chem. Toxicol.* **2010**, *48*, 1355–1361. [CrossRef] [PubMed]
18. Quah, C.C.; Kim, K.H.; Lau, M.S.; Kim, W.R.; Cheah, S.H.; Gundamaraju, R. Pigmentation and dermal conservative effects of the astonishing algae *Sargassum polycystum* and *Padina tenuis* on guinea pigs, human epidermal melanocytes (HEM) and Chang cells. *Afr. J. Tradit. Complement. Altern. Med.* **2014**, *11*, 77–83. [CrossRef] [PubMed]
19. Murugan, K.; Iyer, V.V. Differential growth inhibition of cancer cell lines and antioxidant activity of extracts of red, brown, and green marine algae. *In Vitro Cell. Dev. Biol. Anim.* **2013**, *49*, 324–334. [CrossRef] [PubMed]
20. Fujimura, T.; Tsukahara, K.; Moriwaki, S.; Kitahara, T.; Sano, T.; Takema, Y. Treatment of human skin with an extract of *Fucus vesiculosus* changes its thickness and mechanical properties. *J. Cosmet. Sci.* **2002**, *53*, 1–9. [PubMed]
21. Grether-Beck, S.; Muhlberg, K.; Brenden, H.; Felsner, I.; Brynjolfsdottir, A.; Einarsson, S.; Krutmann, J. Bioactive molecules from the *Blue Lagoon*: In vitro and in vivo assessment of silica mud and microalgae extracts for their effects on skin barrier function and prevention of skin ageing. *Exp. Dermatol.* **2008**, *17*, 771–779. [CrossRef] [PubMed]
22. Buono, S.; Langellotti, A.L.; Martello, A.; Bimonte, M.; Tito, A.; Carola, A.; Apone, F.; Colucci, G.; Fogliano, V. Biological activities of dermatological interest by the water extract of the microalga *Botryococcus braunii*. *Arch. Dermatol. Res.* **2012**, *304*, 755–764. [CrossRef] [PubMed]
23. Kang, H.; Lee, C.H.; Kim, J.R.; Kwon, J.Y.; Seo, S.G.; Han, J.G.; Kim, B.G.; Kim, J.E.; Lee, K.W. Chlorella vulgaris attenuates dermatophagoides Farinae-induced atopic dermatitis-like symptoms in NC/Nga mice. *Int. J. Mol. Sci.* **2015**, *16*, 21021–21034. [CrossRef] [PubMed]
24. Hidalgo-Lucas, S.; Bisson, J.F.; Duffaud, A.; Nejdi, A.; Guerin-Deremaux, L.; Baert, B.; Saniez-Degrave, M.H.; Rozan, P. Benefits of oral and topical administration of ROQUETTE *Chlorella* sp. on skin inflammation and wound healing in mice. *Anti-Inflamm. Anti-Allergy Agents Med. Chem.* **2014**, *13*, 93–102. [CrossRef]
25. Singh, A.; Singh, S.P.; Bamezai, R. Inhibitory potential of *Chlorella vulgaris* (E-25) on mouse skin papillomagenesis and xenobiotic detoxication system. *Anticancer Res.* **1999**, *19*, 1887–1891. [PubMed]
26. Hidalgo-Lucas, S.; Rozan, P.; Guerin-Deremaux, L.; Violle, N.; Baert, B.; Saniez-Degrave, M.H.; Bisson, J.F. Oral and topical administration of ROQUETTE *Schizochytrium* sp. alleviate skin inflammation and improve wound healing in mice. *Anti-Inflamm. Anti-Allergy Agents Med. Chem.* **2015**, *13*, 154–164. [CrossRef]
27. Kim, S.; You, D.H.; Han, T.; Choi, E.M. Modulation of viability and apoptosis of UVB-exposed human keratinocyte HaCaT cells by aqueous methanol extract of laver (*Porphyra yezoensis*). *J. Photochem. Photobiol. B* **2014**, *141*, 301–307. [CrossRef] [PubMed]
28. Mercurio, D.G.; Wagemaker, T.A.L.; Alves, V.M.; Benevenuto, C.G.; Gaspar, L.R.; Campos, P.M. In vivo photoprotective effects of cosmetic formulations containing UV filters, vitamins, Ginkgo biloba and red algae extracts. *J. Photochem. Photobiol. B* **2015**, *153*, 121–126. [CrossRef] [PubMed]

29. Al-Bader, T.; Byrne, A.; Gillbro, J.; Mitarotonda, A.; Metois, A.; Vial, F.; Rawlings, A.V.; Laloeuf, A. Effect of cosmetic ingredients as anticellulite agents: Synergistic action of actives with *in vitro* and in vivo efficacy. *J. Cosmet. Dermatol.* **2012**, *11*, 17–26. [CrossRef] [PubMed]
30. Xhauflaire-Uhoda, E.; Fontaine, K.; Pierard, G.E. Kinetics of moisturizing and firming effects of cosmetic formulations. *Int. J. Cosmet. Sci.* **2008**, *30*, 131–138. [CrossRef] [PubMed]
31. Rinnerthaler, M.; Bischof, J.; Streubel, M.K.; Trost, A.; Richter, K. Oxidative stress in aging human skin. *Biomolecules* **2015**, *5*, 545–589. [CrossRef] [PubMed]
32. Rinnerthaler, M.; Streubel, M.K.; Bischof, J.; Richter, K. Skin aging, gene expression and calcium. *Exp. Gerontol.* **2015**, *68*, 59–65. [CrossRef] [PubMed]
33. Takahashi, M.; Tezuka, T. The content of free amino acids in the stratum corneum is increased in senile xerosis. *Arch. Dermatol. Res.* **2004**, *295*, 448–452. [CrossRef] [PubMed]
34. Li, J.; Tang, H.; Hu, X.; Chen, M.; Xie, H. Aquaporin-3 gene and protein expression in sun-protected human skin decreases with skin ageing. *Australas. J. Dermatol.* **2010**, *51*, 106–112. [CrossRef] [PubMed]
35. Ngo, D.H.; Kim, S.K. Sulfated polysaccharides as bioactive agents from marine algae. *Int. J. Biol. Macromol.* **2013**, *62*, 70–75. [CrossRef] [PubMed]
36. Song, Y.S.; Balcos, M.C.; Yun, H.Y.; Baek, K.J.; Kwon, N.S.; Kim, M.K.; Kim, D.S. ERK activation by fucoidan leads to inhibition of melanogenesis in Mel-Ab Cells. *Korean J. Physiol. Pharmacol.* **2015**, *19*, 29–34. [CrossRef] [PubMed]
37. Ruperez, P.; Ahrazem, O.; Leal, J.A. Potential antioxidant capacity of sulfated polysaccharides from the edible marine brown seaweed *Fucus vesiculosus*. *J. Agric. Food Chem.* **2002**, *50*, 840–845. [CrossRef] [PubMed]
38. Wang, J.; Zhang, Q.; Zhang, Z.; Li, Z. Antioxidant activity of sulfated polysaccharide fractions extracted from *Laminaria japonica*. *Int. J. Biol. Macromol.* **2008**, *42*, 127–132. [CrossRef] [PubMed]
39. Wang, J.; Wang, F.; Zhang, Q.B.; Zhang, Z.S.; Shi, X.L.; Li, P.C. Synthesized different derivatives of low molecular fucoidan extracted from *Laminaria japonica* and their potential antioxidant activity *in vitro*. *Int. J. Biol. Macromol.* **2009**, *44*, 379–384. [CrossRef] [PubMed]
40. Marudhupandi, T.; Kumar, T.T.; Senthil, S.L.; Devi, K.N. *In vitro* antioxidant properties of fucoidan fractions from *Sargassum tenerrimum*. *Pak. J. Biol. Sci.* **2014**, *17*, 402–407. [CrossRef] [PubMed]
41. Moon, H.J.; Lee, S.R.; Shim, S.N.; Jeong, S.H.; Stonik, V.A.; Rasskazov, V.A.; Zvyagintseva, T.; Lee, Y.H. Fucoidan inhibits UVB-induced MMP-1 expression in human skin fibroblasts. *Biol. Pharm. Bull.* **2008**, *31*, 284–289. [CrossRef] [PubMed]
42. Moon, H.J.; Lee, S.H.; Ku, M.J.; Yu, B.C.; Jeon, M.J.; Jeong, S.H.; Stonik, V.A.; Zvyagintseva, T.N.; Ermakova, S.P.; Lee, Y.H. Fucoidan inhibits UVB-induced MMP-1 promoter expression and down regulation of type I procollagen synthesis in human skin fibroblasts. *Eur. J. Dermatol.* **2009**, *19*, 129–134. [PubMed]
43. Moon, H.J.; Park, K.S.; Ku, M.J.; Lee, M.S.; Jeong, S.H.; Imbs, T.I.; Zvyagintseva, T.N.; Ermakova, S.P.; Lee, Y.H. Effect of *Costaria costata* fucoidan on expression of matrix metalloproteinase-1 promoter, mRNA, and protein. *J. Nat. Prod.* **2009**, *72*, 1731–1734. [CrossRef] [PubMed]
44. Maruyama, H.; Tamauchi, H.; Kawakami, F.; Yoshinaga, K.; Nakano, T. Suppressive effect of dietary fucoidan on proinflammatory immune response and MMP-1 expression in UVB-irradiated mouse skin. *Planta Med.* **2015**, *81*, 1370–1374. [PubMed]
45. Senni, K.; Gueniche, F.; Foucault-Bertaud, A.; Igondjo-Tchen, S.; Fioretti, F.; Colliec-Jouault, S.; Durand, P.; Guezennec, J.; Godeau, G.; Letourneur, D. Fucoidan a sulfated polysaccharide from brown algae is a potent modulator of connective tissue proteolysis. *Arch. Biochem. Biophys.* **2006**, *445*, 56–64. [CrossRef] [PubMed]
46. Yang, J.H. Topical application of fucoidan improves atopic dermatitis symptoms in NC/Nga mice. *Phytother. Res.* **2012**, *26*, 1898–1903. [CrossRef] [PubMed]
47. Iwamoto, K.; Hiragun, T.; Takahagi, S.; Yanase, Y.; Morioke, S.; Mihara, S.; Kameyoshi, Y.; Hide, M. Fucoidan suppresses IgE production in peripheral blood mononuclear cells from patients with atopic dermatitis. *Arch. Dermatol. Res.* **2011**, *303*, 425–431. [CrossRef] [PubMed]
48. Wang, J.; Jin, W.; Hou, Y.; Niu, X.; Zhang, H.; Zhang, Q. Chemical composition and moisture-absorption/retention ability of polysaccharides extracted from five algae. *Int. J. Biol. Macromol.* **2013**, *57*, 26–29. [CrossRef] [PubMed]
49. Lee, N.Y.; Ermakova, S.P.; Choi, H.K.; Kusaykin, M.I.; Shevchenko, N.M.; Zvyagintseva, T.N.; Choi, H.S. Fucoidan from *Laminaria cichorioides* inhibits AP-1 transactivation and cell transformation in the mouse epidermal JB6 cells. *Mol. Carcinog.* **2008**, *47*, 629–637. [CrossRef] [PubMed]

50. Li, J.; Xie, L.; Qin, Y.; Liang, W.H.; Mo, M.Q.; Liu, S.L.; Liang, F.; Wang, Y.; Tan, W.; Liang, Y. Effect of laminarin polysaccharide on activity of matrix metalloproteinase in photoaging skin. *China J. Chin. Mater. Med.* **2013**, *38*, 2370–2373.
51. Ayoub, A.; Pereira, J.M.; Rioux, L.E.; Turgeon, S.L.; Beaulieu, M.; Moulin, V.J. Role of seaweed laminaran from *Saccharina longicruris* on matrix deposition during dermal tissue-engineered production. *Int. J. Biol. Macromol.* **2015**, *75*, 13–20. [CrossRef] [PubMed]
52. Qi, H.; Zhang, Q.; Zhao, T.; Chen, R.; Zhang, H.; Niu, X.; Li, Z. Antioxidant activity of different sulfate content derivatives of polysaccharide extracted from *Ulva pertusa* (*Chlorophyta*) in vitro. *Int. J. Biol. Macromol.* **2005**, *37*, 195–199. [CrossRef] [PubMed]
53. Qi, H.; Zhang, Q.; Zhao, T.; Hu, R.; Zhang, K.; Li, Z. *In vitro* antioxidant activity of acetylated and benzoylated derivatives of polysaccharide extracted from *Ulva pertusa* (*Chlorophyta*). *Bioorg. Med. Chem. Lett.* **2006**, *16*, 2441–2445. [CrossRef] [PubMed]
54. Adrien, A.; Bonnet, A.; Dufour, D.; Baudouin, S.; Maugard, T.; Bridiau, N. Pilot production of ulvans from *Ulva* sp. and their effects on hyaluronan and collagen production in cultured dermal fibroblasts. *Carbohydr. Polym.* **2017**, *157*, 1306–1314. [CrossRef] [PubMed]
55. Kuda, T.; Tsunekawa, M.; Goto, H.; Araki, Y. Antioxidant properties of four edible algae harvested in the Noto Peninsula, Japan. *J. Food Compos. Anal.* **2005**, *18*, 625–633. [CrossRef]
56. Zhang, Q.; Li, N.; Zhou, G.; Lu, X.; Xu, Z.; Li, Z. In vivo antioxidant activity of polysaccharide fraction from *Porphyra haitanesis* (*Rhodephyta*) in aging mice. *Pharmacol. Res.* **2003**, *48*, 151–155. [CrossRef]
57. Zhang, Q.; Li, N.; Liu, X.; Zhao, Z.; Li, Z.; Xu, Z. The structure of a sulfated galactan from *Porphyra haitanensis* and its in vivo antioxidant activity. *Carbohydr. Res.* **2004**, *339*, 105–111. [CrossRef] [PubMed]
58. Zhao, T.; Zhang, Q.; Qi, H.; Zhang, H.; Niu, X.; Xu, Z.; Li, Z. Degradation of porphyran from *Porphyra haitanensis* and the antioxidant activities of the degraded porphyrans with different molecular weight. *Int. J. Biol. Macromol.* **2006**, *38*, 45–50. [CrossRef] [PubMed]
59. Zhang, Z.S.; Zhang, Q.B.; Wang, J.; Zhang, H.; Niu, X.Z.; Li, P.C. Preparation of the different derivatives of the low-molecular-weight porphyran from *Porphyra haitanensis* and their antioxidant activities *in vitro*. *Int. J. Biol. Macromol.* **2009**, *45*, 22–26. [CrossRef] [PubMed]
60. Jiang, Z.; Hama, Y.; Yamaguchi, K.; Oda, T. Inhibitory effect of sulphated polysaccharide porphyran on nitric oxide production in lipopolysaccharide-stimulated RAW264.7 macrophages. *J. Biochem.* **2012**, *151*, 65–74. [CrossRef] [PubMed]
61. Isaka, S.; Cho, K.; Nakazono, S.; Abu, R.; Ueno, M.; Kim, D.; Oda, T. Antioxidant and anti-inflammatory activities of porphyran isolated from discolored nori (*Porphyra yezoensis*). *Int. J. Biol. Macromol.* **2015**, *74*, 68–75. [CrossRef] [PubMed]
62. Takematsu, H.; Seiji, M. Effect of macrophages on elimination of dermal melanin from the dermis. *Arch. Dermatol. Res.* **1984**, *276*, 96–98. [CrossRef] [PubMed]
63. Thevanayagam, H.; Mohamed, S.M.; Chu, W.L. Assessment of UVB-photoprotective and antioxidative activities of carrageenan in keratinocytes. *J. Appl. Phycol.* **2014**, *26*, 1813–1821. [CrossRef]
64. Sun, Y.J.; Yang, B.Y.; Wu, Y.M.; Liu, Y.; Gu, X.; Zhang, H.; Wang, C.J.; Cao, H.Z.; Huang, L.J.; Wang, Z.F. Structural characterization and antioxidant activities of kappa-carrageenan oligosaccharides degraded by different methods. *Food Chem.* **2015**, *178*, 311–318. [CrossRef] [PubMed]
65. Yuan, H.M.; Song, J.M.; Zhang, W.W.; Li, X.G.; Li, N.; Gao, X.L. Antioxidant activity and cytoprotective effect of kappa-carrageenan oligosaccharides and their different derivatives. *Bioorg. Med. Chem. Lett.* **2006**, *16*, 1329–1334. [CrossRef] [PubMed]
66. Yuan, H.M.; Zhang, W.W.; Li, X.G.; Lu, X.X.; Li, N.; Gao, X.L.; Song, J.M. Preparation and *in vitro* antioxidant activity of kappa-carrageenan oligosaccharides and their oversulfated, acetylated, and phosphorylated derivatives. *Carbohydr. Res.* **2005**, *340*, 685–692. [CrossRef] [PubMed]
67. Ren, S.W.; Li, J.; Wang, W.; Guan, H.S. Protective effects of kappa-ca3000+CP against ultraviolet-induced damage in HaCaT and MEF cells. *J. Photochem. Photobiol. B* **2010**, *101*, 22–30. [CrossRef] [PubMed]
68. Ferreres, F.; Lopes, G.; Gil-Izquierdo, A.; Andrade, P.B.; Sousa, C.; Mouga, T.; Valentao, P. Phlorotannin Extracts from Fucales Characterized by HPLC-DAD-ESI-MSn: Approaches to Hyaluronidase Inhibitory Capacity and Antioxidant Properties. *Mar. Drugs* **2012**, *10*, 2766–2781. [CrossRef] [PubMed]
69. Cui, L.B.; Zhou, X.Y.; Zhao, Z.J.; Li, Q.; Huang, X.Y.; Sun, F.Z. The Kunming mouse: As a model for age-related decline in female fertility in human. *Zygote* **2013**, *21*, 367–376. [CrossRef] [PubMed]

70. Lahaye, M.; Robic, A. Structure and functional properties of ulvan, a polysaccharide from green seaweeds. *Biomacromolecules* **2007**, *8*, 1765–1774. [CrossRef] [PubMed]
71. Yun, E.J.; Choi, I.G.; Kim, K.H. Red macroalgae as a sustainable resource for bio-based products. *Trends Biotechnol.* **2015**, *33*, 247–249. [CrossRef] [PubMed]
72. Chen, H.; Yan, X.; Zhu, P.; Lin, J. Antioxidant activity and hepatoprotective potential of agaro-oligosaccharides *in vitro* and in vivo. *Nutr. J.* **2006**, *5*, 31. [CrossRef] [PubMed]
73. Nakayasu, M.; Saeki, H.; Tohda, H.; Oikawa, A. Effects of sugars on melanogenesis in cultured melanoma cells. *J. Cell. Physiol.* **1977**, *92*, 49–55. [CrossRef] [PubMed]
74. Kim, J.H.; Yun, E.J.; Yu, S.; Kim, K.H.; Kang, N.J. Different Levels of Skin Whitening Activity among 3,6-Anhydro-l-galactose, Agarooligosaccharides, and Neoagarooligosaccharides. *Mar. Drugs* **2017**, *15*, 321. [CrossRef] [PubMed]
75. Yun, E.J.; Lee, S.; Kim, J.H.; Kim, B.B.; Kim, H.T.; Lee, S.H.; Pelton, J.G.; Kang, N.J.; Choi, I.G.; Kim, K.H. Enzymatic production of 3,6-anhydro-L-galactose from agarose and its purification and *in vitro* skin whitening and anti-inflammatory activities. *Appl. Microbiol. Biotechnol.* **2013**, *97*, 2961–2970. [CrossRef] [PubMed]
76. Chen, H.M.; Yan, X.J. Antioxidant activities of agaro-oligosaccharides with different degrees of polymerization in cell-based system. *Biochim. Biophys. Acta* **2005**, *1722*, 103–111. [CrossRef] [PubMed]
77. Enoki, T.; Okuda, S.; Kudo, Y.; Takashima, F.; Sagawa, H.; Kato, I. Oligosaccharides from agar inhibit pro-inflammatory mediator release by inducing heme oxygenase 1. *Biosci. Biotechnol. Biochem.* **2010**, *74*, 766–770. [CrossRef] [PubMed]
78. Enoki, T.; Tominaga, T.; Takashima, F.; Ohnogi, H.; Sagawa, H.; Kato, I. Anti-tumor-promoting activities of agaro-oligosaccharides on two-stage mouse skin carcinogenesis. *Biol. Pharm. Bull.* **2012**, *35*, 1145–1149. [CrossRef] [PubMed]
79. Bin, B.H.; Kim, S.T.; Bhin, J.; Lee, T.R.; Cho, E.G. The development of sugar-based anti-melanogenic agents. *Int. J. Mol. Sci.* **2016**, *17*, 583. [CrossRef] [PubMed]
80. Kobayashi, R.; Takisada, M.; Suzuki, T.; Kirimura, K.; Usami, S. Neoagarobiose as a novel moisturizer with whitening effect. *Biosci. Biotechnol. Biochem.* **1997**, *61*, 162–163. [CrossRef] [PubMed]
81. Jang, M.K.; Lee, D.G.; Kim, N.Y.; Yu, K.H.; Jang, H.J.; Lee, S.W.; Jang, H.J.; Lee, Y.J.; Lee, S.H. Purification and characterization of neoagarotetraose from hydrolyzed agar. *J. Microbiol. Biotechnol.* **2009**, *19*, 1197–1200. [PubMed]
82. Lee, D.G.; Jang, M.K.; Lee, O.H.; Kim, N.Y.; Ju, S.A.; Lee, S.H. Over-production of a glycoside hydrolase family 50 beta-agarase from *Agarivorans* sp. JA-1 in *Bacillus subtilis* and the whitening effect of its product. *Biotechnol. Lett.* **2008**, *30*, 911–918. [CrossRef] [PubMed]
83. Ariga, O.; Okamoto, N.; Harimoto, N.; Nakasaki, K. Purification and characterization of alpha-neoagarooligosaccharide hydrolase from Cellvibrio sp OA-2007. *J. Microbiol. Biotechnol.* **2014**, *24*, 48–51. [CrossRef] [PubMed]
84. Kim, J.H.; Kim, D.H.; Cho, K.M.; Kim, K.H.; Kang, N.J. Effect of 3,6-anhydro-l-galactose on alpha-melanocyte stimulating hormone-induced melanogenesis in human melanocytes and a skin-equivalent model. *J. Cell. Biochem.* **2018**, *119*, 7643–7656. [CrossRef] [PubMed]
85. Ajisaka, K.; Agawa, S.; Nagumo, S.; Kurato, K.; Yokoyama, T.; Arai, K.; Miyazaki, T. Evaluation and comparison of the antioxidative potency of various carbohydrates using different methods. *J. Agric. Food Chem.* **2009**, *57*, 3102–3107. [CrossRef] [PubMed]
86. Villaverde, J.J.; Sevilla-Moran, B.; Lopez-Goti, C.; Alonso-Prados, J.L.; Sandin-Espana, P. Computational Methodologies for the Risk Assessment of Pesticides in the European Union. *J. Agric. Food Chem.* **2017**, *65*, 2017–2018. [CrossRef] [PubMed]
87. Domingo, L.R.; Rios-Gutierrez, M.; Perez, P. Applications of the Conceptual Density Functional Theory Indices to Organic Chemistry Reactivity. *Molecules* **2016**, *21*, 748. [CrossRef] [PubMed]
88. Alice, B.N.; Richard, J.F. Strategies for the discovery and identification of food protein-derived biologically active peptides. *Trends Food Sci. Technol.* **2017**, *69*, 289–305.

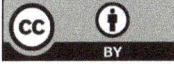

© 2018 by the authors. Licensee MDPI, Basel, Switzerland. This article is an open access article distributed under the terms and conditions of the Creative Commons Attribution (CC BY) license (http://creativecommons.org/licenses/by/4.0/).

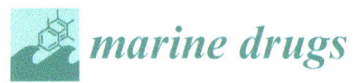

Review

Photoprotective Substances Derived from Marine Algae

Ratih Pangestuti [1], Evi Amelia Siahaan [2] and Se-Kwon Kim [3,*]

1   Research Center for Oceanography, Indonesian Institute of Sciences (LIPI), Jakarta 14430, Indonesia; pangestuti.ratih@gmail.com
2   Research and Development Division of Marine Bio-Industry, Indonesian Institute of Sciences (LIPI), West Nusa Tenggara 83552, Indonesia; eviamelia.siahaan@gmail.com
3   Department of Marine Life Science, College of Ocean Science and Technology, Korea Maritime and Ocean University, Busan 606-791, Korea
*   Correspondence: sknkim@pknu.ac.kr; Tel.: +82-51-629-6870

Received: 4 October 2018; Accepted: 18 October 2018; Published: 23 October 2018

Abstract: Marine algae have received great attention as natural photoprotective agents due to their unique and exclusive bioactive substances which have been acquired as an adaptation to the extreme marine environment combine with a range of physical parameters. These photoprotective substances include mycosporine-like amino acids (MAAs), sulfated polysaccharides, carotenoids, and polyphenols. Marine algal photoprotective substances exhibit a wide range of biological activities such as ultraviolet (UV) absorbing, antioxidant, matrix-metalloproteinase inhibitors, anti-aging, and immunomodulatory activities. Hence, such unique bioactive substances derived from marine algae have been regarded as having potential for use in skin care, cosmetics, and pharmaceutical products. In this context, this contribution aims at revealing bioactive substances found in marine algae, outlines their photoprotective potential, and provides an overview of developments of blue biotechnology to obtain photoprotective substances and their prospective applications.

Keywords: natural; bioactive; marine algae; photoprotective; substances

1. Introduction

The ocean covers more than 70% of the Earth's surface and represents an enormous resource of biodiversity. Marine organisms have adapted excellently to extreme environmental conditions with a range of physical parameters, such as pH, high salt concentration, low or high temperature, high-pressure, low nutrient availability, and low or high sun exposure [1]. The wide diversity in the biochemical composition of marine organisms provides an excellent reservoir to explore functional materials, many of which are rare or absent in other taxonomic groups. Large numbers of studies have demonstrated health-benefit effects of marine-derived functional materials [2,3].

Marine algae are one of the most extensively studied marine organisms. These marine organisms have attracted special interest because they are good sources of nutrients and functional materials. Many studies have reported biological activities, including antioxidant, anti-cancer, anti-hypertension, hepatoprotective, immunomodulatory, and neuroprotective activity. Marine algae are already used in a wide range of foods, supplements, pharmaceuticals, and cosmetics and are often claimed to have beneficial effects on human health. One particular interesting feature in marine algae is their richness in photoprotective substances. Marine algae found in intertidal shores to a depth of 150 m are highly exposed to ultraviolet (UV) radiation. Therefore, to counteract and minimize photodamage induced by high UV radiation, photoprotective substances such as mycosporine-like amino acids (MAAs), sulfated polysaccharides, carotenoids, and polyphenols were synthesized [4]. These substances can be used for photoprotection to provide the skin with adequate protection against ultraviolet B (UVB) and ultraviolet A (UVA)-induced photodamage (Figure 1) [5].

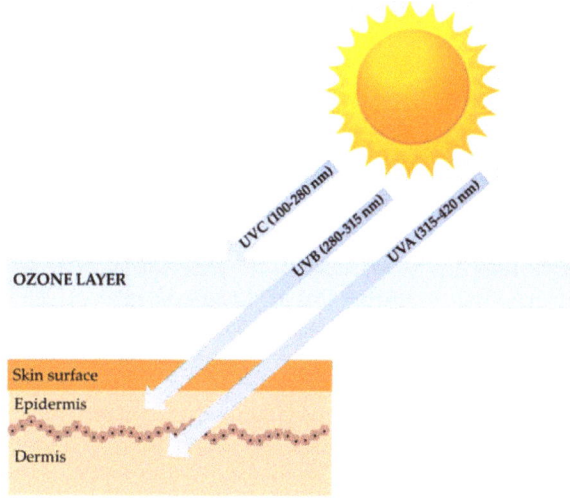

Figure 1. The ultraviolet (UV)-induced photodamage.

Present approaches on the isolation and recovery of photoprotective substances from marine algae have been rapidly developing. Not only limited to organic solvent extraction, novel environmental friendly extraction and separation techniques, such as enzyme-assisted extraction (EAE), ultrasound assisted extraction (UAE), microwave assisted extraction (MAE), supercritical carbon dioxide (SC–CO_2) and subcritical water extraction (SWE), have recently been applied to the development of photoprotective substances derived from marine algae. The recovery yield of photoprotective substances from marine algae depends on the technology applied and the marine algae species. In addition, the isolation process applied also affects photoprotective activity. Hence, this contribution focuses on photoprotective substances reported in marine algae. The most relevant studies on the photoprotective substances found in marine algae as well as their biological roles and photoprotective activity are discussed. Additionally, an overview of the developments of blue biotechnology and potential applications is also provided.

2. Photoprotective Substances Derived from Marine Algae

2.1. Sulfated Polysaccharides

Marine algae are considered as the most important source of non-animal sulfated polysaccharides, and chemical structures of these polymers differ according to class and species of algae [6,7]. Carrageenan and fucoidan are the major sulfated polysaccharides found in red and brown algae, respectively. Carrageenans are widely used in food, pharmacy, dairy, and cosmetic products due to the unique physical functional properties, such as thickening, gelling, emulsifying, and stabilizing properties [8]. These sulfated polysaccharides have been considered as safe additives for many commercial products in many countries. In addition to their unique physical functions, carrageenan composition in cosmetic and skin care products has often been found with antioxidant, tonifying, cleaning, hydrating, and revitalizing bioactivities. Recently, photoprotective effects of carrageenan (kappa, iota and lambda) in UVB-induced human keratinocytes (HaCaT) cells have been reported [9]. Carrageenan has shown significant protection against the detrimental effects of UVB-induced apoptosis in HaCaT cells and has decreased the release of reactive oxygen species (ROS). The accumulation of excess ROS has been related to skin diseases including skin aging and cancers. Therefore, antioxidants are usually viewed as preventive agents against UV-related skin diseases. We assumed that the photoprotective activity of carrageenan may also correlate to their immunomodulatory properties. Carrageenan has been known as an immunomodulator, which induces the expression of cyclooxygenase-2 (COX-2) and the release of prostaglandin-E_2 (PGE_2) [10]. Based on an in vivo experiment in SKH-1 hairless mice, Tripp et al. (2003) suggested that COX-2 expression is an important factor for keratinocyte survival and proliferation after acute UV irradiation. Inhibition of COX-2 expression has been demonstrated to reduce epidermal keratinocytes proliferation [11]. Taken together, it may be hypothesized that immunomulatory activities and ROS scavenging activities of carrageenan might play an important role in their photoprotective mechanisms. The addition of carrageenan to a broad spectrum of skin care and cosmetic products might decrease UV-induced photodamage compared with sunscreen alone.

Fucoidan is the most commonly sulfated polysaccharide isolated from brown algae. In general, these linier polysaccharides have a backbone of α-linked L-fucose residues with various substitutions. Fucoidan structures and bioactivities are different among brown algae species [12]. Recent findings have reported the photoprotective activity of fucoidan isolated from brown algae including *Ecklonia cava*, *Undaria pinnatifida*, *Costaria costata*, and *Fucus evanescens* [13–19]. The photoprotective activity of fucoidan has been determined in UVB-irradiated human dermal fibroblast and mice models. Most studies report that the photoprotective activity of fucoidan is mediated through the suppression of matrix metalloproteinase-1 (MMP-1) activity. MMP-1 is a major enzyme implicated in the collagen damage and photoaging of UV-irradiated human skin. More precisely, these sulfated polysaccharides downregulate the expressions of NF-κB, which, in turn, diminish MMP-1 expression. Recently, it was reported that topical applications of low-molecular-weight fucoidan have stronger photoprotective activity than high-molecular-weight fucoidan [14]. The rationale for this is that low-molecular-weight fucoidan is mostly absorbed before irradiation. This low-molecular-weight fucoidan seems to be involved in photoprotective effects rather than UV filtering effects.

Photoprotective activity in orally administered fucoidan, in addition to topical applications, has been reported. This information on the bioavailability of fucoidan might have stimulated further research on the relationship between the oral administration of fucoidan and their bioavailability, mode of action, and potency in skin care and cosmetic products.

2.2. Carotenoids

Carotenoids are natural pigments found in all photosynthetic organisms (including plants, algae, and cyanobacteria) and some non-photosynthetic archaea, bacteria, fungi, and animals [20]. These photosynthetic pigments consist of two classes of molecules: carotenes and xanthophylls. Carotenoids play an important role in photosynthetic light-harvesting complexes; they absorb the solar spectrum in the blue-green region and transfer the energy to chlorophylls [21]. Furthermore, carotenoids also act as a photoprotector in photosynthetic organisms. Many studies have reported a strong correlation between increased UVB irradiation and carotenoid accumulation in terrestrial and marine plants [22,23]. As an example, Hupel et al. (2011) demonstrated that UVB irradiation increased the carotenoid contents in brown algae *Pelvetia canaliculata*.

Photoprotective effects of fucoxanthin (Figure 2) derived from marine brown algae against UVB-induced photoaging have been reported [24]. Photoprotective activity of fucoxanthin has been determined by various in vitro and in vivo methods such as comet assay, human dermal fibroblast, and hairless mice irradiation. ROS scavenging activity is mainly considered to be a mechanism of action underlying the photoprotective activity of fucoxanthin [25–27]. Carotenoids, including fucoxanthin, are known as a singlet oxygen quencher. These photosynthetic pigments mitigate the harmful effects associated with UV irradiation by dissipating the excess energy as heat and returns to the initial ground state. Recently, fucoxanthin has been demonstrated to stimulate filaggrin promoter activity in UV-induced sunburn [28]. Filaggrin is a UV-sensitive gene that reflects the state of the skin damage.

This stimulation of a UV-sensitive gen promotor by fucoxanthin suggested that other protective mechanisms of fucoxanthin might be exerted by the promotion of skin barrier formation through the induction of UV-sensitive gene expression.

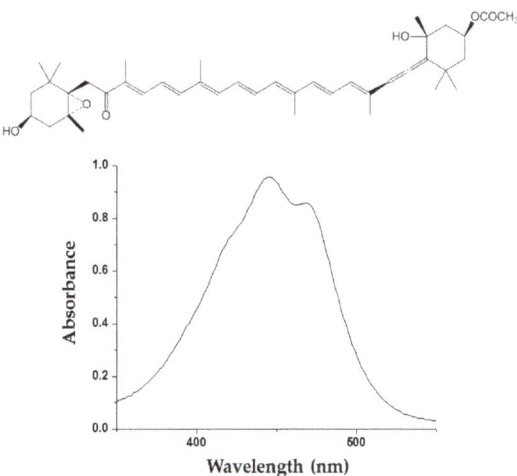

Figure 2. Molecular structure and ultraviolet (UV) absorption spectra of fucoxanthin from brown algae.

Photoprotection mechanisms of fucoxanthin might also be achieved by oral administration. It has been shown that photodamage on the skin or eyes can be protected by biological compounds in tissues, which come from nutritional sources via the bloodstream. Stahl and Sies (2012) reported the concentration of carotenoids in human skin and demonstrated that there are considerable differences in the patterns in each skin layer. As an example, high concentrations of carotenoids are found in the skin of the forehead, the palm of the hand, and dorsal skin. Meanwhile, lower concentrations are found in the skin of the arm and the back of the hand of the human body [29]. In the human body, fucoxanthin absorption strongly depends on a number of factors, including the amount and type of dietary lipids consumed, the stability of the matrix to which the carotenoid is bound, and additional dietary factors such as dietary fiber. The esterified fucoxanthin is likely to be incorporated into the lipid core in chylomicron and carried into a variety of tissues, including the skin [30].

Recently, it has been reported that skimmed milk is an excellent food matrix for fucoxanthin application in terms of stability and bioavailability [31]. An in vivo pharmacokinetic study with a single oral administration of fucoxanrhin fortified in skimmed milk showed the highest absorption of fucoxanthinol and amarouciaxanthin A (two prime metabolites of fucoxanthin). Considering the potency of fucoxanthin as a photoprotective substance, further research studies are needed in order to verify photoprotective mechanisms of fucoxanthin oral consumption and the bioavailability of fucoxanthin (and its derivatives) in human skin.

2.3. Mycosporine Like Amino Acids

Mycosporine-like amino acids (MAAs) are low-molecular-weight, water-soluble molecules with maximum absorption bands in the UV spectrum between 310 and 360 nm. These molecules can be found in cyanobacteria, phytoplankton, lichens, gorgonians, cnidarians, sponges, shrimp, sea urchins, starfish, clams, ascidians, and marine algae. Most of the MAA-producing marine algae are red algae, followed by brown and green algae, respectively [32]. The type and accumulation of MAAs in marine algae varied based on season, climate, depth, and environmental variables (i.e., salinity, temperature, and nutrient availability) [33]. Unlike photosynthetic pigments, MAAs were invoked to function as passive shielding substances by dissipating the absorbed radiation energy in the form of harmless heat without generating photochemical reactions. In the organisms, MAAs not only function as "nature's sunscreen compounds" but also serve as antioxidant molecules scavenging toxic oxygen radicals [34]. Up to now, more than 30 different chemical structures of MAAs have been elucidated. Table 1 present major MAAs identified from marine red algae.

Table 1. Mycosporines-like amino acids (MAAs) identified in marine algae.

Mycosporine-Like Amino Acids	Marine Algae	Reference
Shinorine	*Gloiopeltis fucatas*; *Mazzaella* sp.; *Gracilaria vermiculophylla*; *Palmaria palmata*; *Porphyra* sp.; *Porphyra umbilicalis*	[35–37]
Palythine	*Gloiopeltis fucatas*; *Mazzaella* sp.; *Gracilaria vermiculophylla*; *Palmaria palmata*; *Porphyra* sp.; *Porphyra umbilicalis*	[35–38]
Porphyra-334	*Gracilaria vermiculophylla*; *Palmaria palmata*; *Porphyra* sp.; *Porphyra umbilicalis*; *Poprphyra yezoensis*; *Porphyra vietnamensis*	[35,37–41]
Asterina-330	*Gracilaria vermiculophylla*	[35,38]
Mycosporine-glycine	*Mazzaella laminarioides*	[38]

MAAs have been reported as the strongest UVA-absorbing compounds in nature [42]. These low-molecular-weight molecules have gained considerable attention as highly active photoprotective candidates. Among other MAAs, porphyra-334 has been extensively studied. Daniel et al. (2004) reported that cream with 0.005% MAAs containing porphyra-334 can neutralize photodamage of UVA as efficiently as a cream with 1% synthetic UVA filters and 4% UVB filters [42]. In addition, porphyra-334 has been demonstrated to suppress ROS formation and downregulate the expression of MMP-1 and -13 on human dermal fibroblast following UVA irradiation. No adverse side effects have been reported from the treatment of porphyra-334 at concentration $\leq$200 µM on human skin fibroblasts. The formulation of porphyra-334 has been reported to increase photoprotective activity of sunscreen formula [41]. MAAs protect the skin cell due to their ability to disperse the harmful UV into heat that dissipates into the surroundings without forming reactive photoproducts. In addition, MAAs have also been reported as strong antioxidant molecules [40]. Hence, MAAs derived from marine algae can be recommended as photoprotective materials for skin care products.

2.4. Polyphenolic Compounds

Polyphenolic compounds are a class of secondary metabolites with diverse biological functions. These bioactive substances are divided into several classes according to the number of phenol rings and structural elements that bind these rings to one another [43]. The three main groups of polyphenols are phenolic acids, flavonoids, and tannins. Marine algae-derived polyphenols have been investigated for their photoprotective activities. Dieckol, phloroglucinol, fucofuroeckol-A, and triphlorethol-A (Figure 3) isolated from marine brown algae exhibited prominent protective effect against photodamage induced by UVB radiation, as demonstrated in many studies [44–48]. In order to understand the cellular and molecular photoprotective mechanisms of phloroglucinol, Piao and his colleagues developed it in UVB-irradiated mice and a HaCaT cell model. Phloroglucinol (10 µM) scavenged free radical and protects macromolecules damage in UVB-irradiated HaCaT cells [49]. In addition, phloroglucinol treatment significantly inhibited the UVB-induced upregulation of MMP-1 and phosphorylation of mitogen-activated protein kinases (MAPK) and activator protein-1 (AP-1) binding to the MMP-1 promoter [50]. Phloroglucinol has been demonstrated to be safe and effective when applied in the mouse skin irradiated with UVB [51]. Photoprotective activity of phloroglucinol is shown in Figure 4. The findings confirm the effectiveness of phloroglucinol as potential cosmeceutical leads for the formulations of sun-protective lotions and creams.

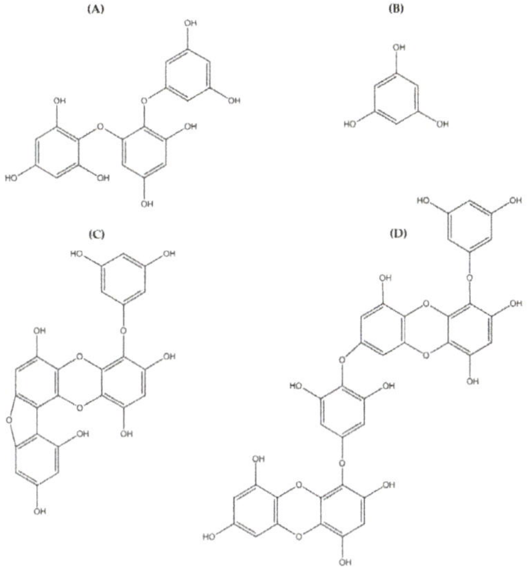

Figure 3. Chemical structure photoprotective polyphenol isolated from marine brown algae. Triphlorethol-A (**A**), phloroglucinol (**B**), fucofuroeckol-A (**C**), and dieckol (**D**).

Polyphenols are bioactive substances characterized by the presence of more than one phenolic group (a hydroxyl group bound to an aromatic ring). Based on several reports, we assumed that their photoprotection activity is strongly correlated with their radical scavenging activity. The hydroxyl (–OH) group bound to the aromatic ring acts as an electron donor, giving it to a free radical or other reactive species. This underlies the inhibition of ROS and ROS-mediated damage on macromolecules, which in turn inhibit the activation of the signal transduction pathways such as the MAPK signaling pathway.

As mentioned in the many scientific reports, polyphenolic compounds represent an interesting class of active substance in the protection of UV-light-induced skin damage. Up to a certain concentration, marine algal-polyphenol did not exert any toxic effect, anticipating its potential use as a safe photoprotector that can be utilized in skin care products.

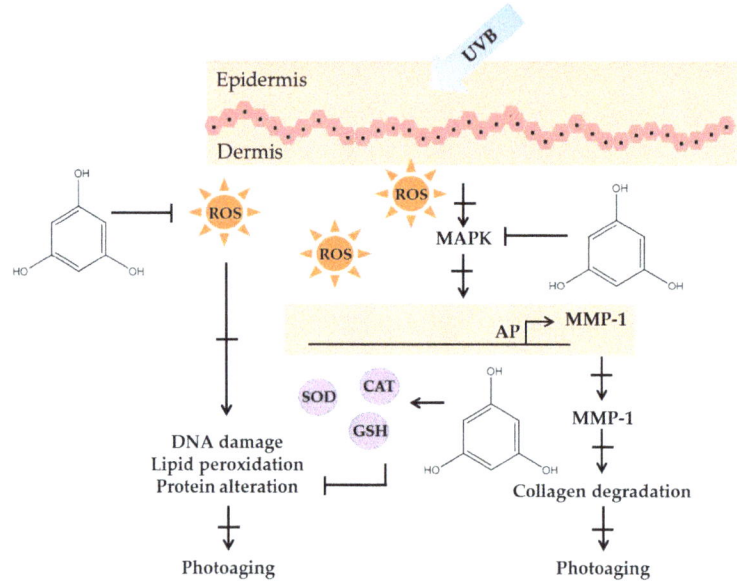

Figure 4. The photoprotective mechanism of phloroglucinol derived from marine algae.

2.5. Marine Algae Extracts and Fractions

Extraction of active components from plant materials is the first and most important step in the development of photoprotective substances. Marine algae have been extracted with various solvents and investigated for their photoprotective effects (Table 2). Guinea et al. (2012) investigated the photoprotective potential of 21 commercial marine red and brown algae originated from Chile, Spain, South Africa, Argentina, Ireland, and Tonga. Compared to other extracts, two marine red algae *Macrocystis pyrifera* and *Porphyra columbina* exhibited the highest photoprotective activity [52]. Many studies have reported that certain species of marine algae can protect the skin against UVB-induced photoaging and damage due to antioxidant properties and their UV absorbing capacity. In addition, the photoprotection of marine algae extract has been correlated with MAAs and polyphenol constituents. As an example, *Porphyra yezoensis* extract showed photoprotective activity on the UVB-exposed HaCaT cells and human keratinocytes. The *Porphyra yezoensis* extract showed absorbance spectrum characteristics of MAAs in red algae and contained high phenolic compounds [53]. Polyphenolic compounds are generally more soluble in polar organic solvents, so organic solvents such as ethanol and methanol can be considered as effective extractants of polyphenolic components from marine algae. Supporting this hypothesis, aqueous extract of marine green algae (*Halimeda incrassate*) and red algae (*Bryothamnion triquetrum*) showed no photoprotective activity in UVC-irradiated plasmids [54].

Synthetic UV filters are used in skin care products to prevent photodamage and skin cancer. However, UV filters still have to be complemented by other compounds to make sun protection skin care more efficient to photodamage and skin photoaging. The combination of *Porphyra umbilicalis* extracts and *Ginkgo biloba* has been demonstrated to improve the photoprotective performance of sunscreens, which then prevent UV-induced photodamage [55]. Thus, marine algae can be considered potent materials for an effective photoprotective formulation with anti-aging properties. Photoprotective activity of marine red and brown algae have been characterized in many studies; however, up to now very little attention has been given to unraveling photoprotective substances from marine green algae.

Table 2. Summary of photoprotective effects of marine algae extracts.

Class	Species	Origin	Extract/Fraction	Activity	Reference
Red algae	Solieria chordalis	France	MeOH extract/CPC fractionation	UVB absorption & free radical scavenging activity	[56]
	Porphyra umbilicalis	France	n-heptane/EtOAc//MeOH/dW (19/1/19/1; v/v) Cosmetic formula (5% extract)	Protect UV-radiated skin from erythema	[55]
	Porphyra yezoensis	Korea	EtOH extract (80%)/chloroform/MeOH/dW (2/1/0.9)	Modulate viability of UVB-exposed HaCaT	[53]
	Gelidium amansii	Korea	MeOH extract and fermentation	Protect skin photoaging in Hairless Mice induced by UVB	[57]
	Polyopes affinis	Korea	EtOH extract	Inhibit UVB-induced ROS in HaCaT	[58]
	Solieria chordalis	France	EtOAc extract	Protect synthetic chlorophyll solution from UVB	[59]
	Polysiphonia morrowii	Korea	EtOH extract (80%)	Protect HaCaT from UVB-induced cell damage	[60]
	Chondracanthus tenellus	Korea	EtOH extract (80%)	Protect HaCaT from UVB-induced cell damage	[61]
	Bonnemaisonia hamifera	Korea	EtOH extract (80%)	Protect HaCaT from UVB-induced cell damage and inhibit ROS	[62]
	Lomentaria hakodatensis	Korea	EtOH extract (80%)	Protect HaCaT from UVB-induced cell damage	[63]
	Macrocystis pyrifera	Argentina	Ace extract	UVB protection on zebrafish embryo	[52]
	Porphyra columbina	Argentina	Ace extract	UVB protection on zebrafish embryo	[52]
Brown algae	Sargassum muticum	Korea	EtOAc fraction	Inhibits wrinkle formation in UVB-induced mice (in vivo)	[64]
	Sargassum muticum	Korea	EtOAc fraction	UVB irradiated human keratinocytes (in vitro)	[65]
	Undaria crenata	Korea	EtOH extract (80%)	Protect HaCaT from UVB-induced cell damage	[15]
	Lessonia vadosa	Argentina	Ace extract	UVB protection on zebrafish embryo	[52]
	Lessonia nigrescens	Chile	Ace extract	UVB protection on zebrafish embryo	[52]
	Ecklonia maxima	South Africa	Ace extract	UVB protection on zebrafish embryo	[52]
	Durvillaea antarctica	Chile	Ace extract	UVB protection on zebrafish embryo	[52]
	Fucus vesiculosus	Spain	Ace extract	UVB protection on zebrafish embryo	[52]
	Saccharina latissima	Spain	Ace extract	UVB protection on zebrafish embryo	[52]
	Ascophyllum nodosum	Ireland	Ace extract	UVB protection on zebrafish embryo	[52]

3. The Development of Photoprotective Compounds-Derived from Marine Algae

Organic solvent extraction is the most common technique to isolate photoprotective substances from marine algae. Extraction conditions, such as temperature, sample-to-solvent ratios, and extraction time, must then be adjusted in order to optimize the extraction process. Organic solvent such as ethanol, methanol, acetone, and ethyl acetate can be used for the extraction of photoprotective substances [15]. However, in the last few decades, the volume of solvents used in the chemical process is extremely concerning. Organic solvents are a major contributor to the overall toxicity potential associated with many industrial processes and to the waste generation of chemical industries. The disposal of excessive solvent to the environment significantly contributes to the release of greenhouse gases and other emissions [66]. Both academic and industrial researchers have therefore focused on minimizing solvent consumption through the development of solvent-free processes. Environmentally friendly "blue biotechnologies" such as EAE, UAE, MAE, SC–CO_2, and SWE have been demonstrated as potential technologies to obtain photoprotective compounds from marine algae. Table 3 shows advantages and disadvantages of blue biotechnologies to obtain photoprotective substances from marine algae.

Table 3. Technologies for the recovery of photoprotective substances from marine algae.

Techniques	Advantage	Disadvantage	Target Photoprotective Substances
Organic solvent	Easy to operate	Environmental waste Cost of organic solvent Clean up step needed	Carotenoids, Phenolics, MAAs, Sulfated Polysaccharides, Extracts
EAE	No harmful solvents High yield Mild process	Extracted substances required further process Cost of the enzymes Optimization of enzymatic process Clean up step needed	Extracts, Sulfated Polysaccharides
UAE & MAE	Reduce extraction time Low solvent	High power consumption Scaling up is difficult Clean up step needed	Sulfated Polysaccharides
SC–CO_2	Reduce extraction time Simple process Environmental friendly Low operating temperatures (40–60 °C) Clean final product Low solvent	Cost of the installations Required special manpower Optimization process	Carotenoids (i.e., fucoxanthin);
SWE	Reduce extraction time Simple process Environmental friendly High yield Low solvent	Cost of the installations Clean up step needed Elevated temperatures	Sulfated polysaccharides (i.e., carrageenan; fucoidan); polyphenols

3.1. Enzyme-Assisted Extraction

The EAE technique has been widely used to improve the extraction efficiency of bioactive substances from terrestrial plants. On the contrary, the application of the EAE method to extract photoprotective substances from marine algae has rarely been reported. The EAE allows preparation of bioactive substances from marine green, brown, and red algae [67]; however, physico-chemical conditions of the reaction media, such as temperature, pH of the protein solution, and enzyme ratios, must then be adjusted in order to optimize the activity of the enzyme. Proteolytic enzymes from different sources such as microbes, plants, and animals can be used for the hydrolysis process of marine algae [68]. Crude polysaccharide from the brown algae *Ecklonia cava* has been recovered by using EAE. Lyophilized *E. cava* was ground and sieved to obtain a smaller particle size, and this produced higher extraction yields. Hence, in addition to physic-chemical conditions of reaction media, surface areas of the sample is another important factor in the EAE process [69]. Recently, it was reported that the EAE process increases antioxidant activity of fucoidan from marine brown algae *Cystoseira trinodis* [70]. Alternative extraction conditions such as EAE can be successfully employed in order to degrade marine algae tissues on the basis of the recovery of bioactive compounds with a considerably high yield.

3.2. Ultrasound Assisted Extraction and Microwave Assisted Extraction

The established extraction technology that can be used to isolate photoprotective substances from marine algae is MAE and UAE. Both are energy input-assisted extraction methods and have been used to isolate bioactive substance from terrestrial plant material for many years [71]. MAE involves the heating process of a solution in contact with a sample using microwave energy. Different from classical heating, microwaves heat the sample simultaneously without heating the vessel. Therefore, the solution reaches its boiling point very rapidly, leading to very short extraction times [72]. The high recovery of fucoidans derived from *Ascophyllum nodosum* by MAE has been reported [73]. The MAE of fucoidan from *Ascophyllum nodosum* at 90 °C has a similar composition, molecular weight, and reducing power than native fucoidan extracted by the conventional method. It is assumed that the sulfate contents were only affected to the extraction temperature of fucoidan. In addition to MAE, UAE has also been reported to improve the yield of fucoidan with antioxidant activities from marine brown algae, *Sargassum muticum* [74]. The UAE principle is based on the waves migrating through a medium inducing pressure variations. Notably, considering that the energy input of MAE and UAE can exceed the energy level required for the cleavage of the sulfate esters, it is recommended that the necessary energy input be temporarily exerted during the extraction process to avoid any structural alterations to the sulfated polysaccharide [72].

3.3. Supercritical Carbon Dioxide

Recently, scientists and industrialists have paid a great deal of attention to the application of SC–CO_2 fluid (Figure 5), a hydrophobic and environmentally friendly medium, as an alternative to conventional organic solvent extraction [75]. SC–CO_2 is a promising method for the recovery of photoprotective substances from marine algae, which can be carried out under mild operating conditions. The SC–CO_2 process offers new opportunities for the solution of separation problems as it is a nontoxic, nonflammable, inexpensive, and clean solvent [76]. The higher carotenoids yield from *Saccharina japonica* and *Sargassum horneri* obtained by SC–CO_2 as compared to the conventional extraction has been reported [77]. The solvating capacity of SC–CO_2 fluid can be controlled by manipulating pressure and temperature to give suitable selectivity. Therefore, the temperature and pressure applied greatly affected the carotenoids solvating power of SC–CO_2 and hence the yield of carotenoids. Co-solvent has also been demonstrated to increase the yield of bioactive substances from marine algae [78,79]. As an example, Roh et al. (2008) and Conde et al. (2014) reported that the use of ethanol as co-solvent in the SC–CO_2 process increases phenolic and fucoxanthin yield from marine brown algae, *Undaria pinnatifida*, and *Sargassum muticum*, respectively. More recently, sunflower oil has been shown to improve the extraction yield of carotenoids and fucoxanthin from *Saccharina japonica* [80].

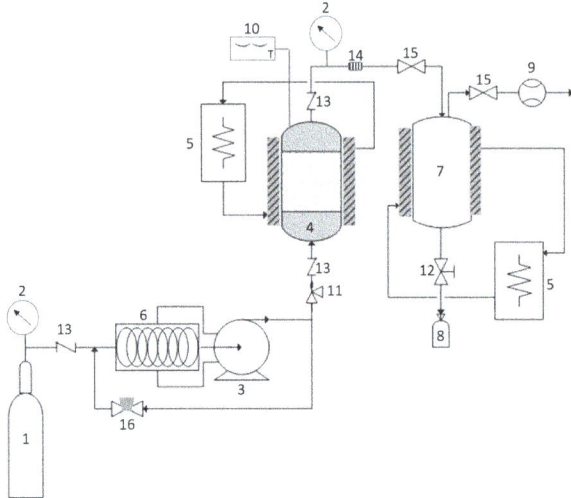

Figure 5. Schematic diagram of SC–CO_2. The CO_2 tank (1); pressure gauge (2); high pressure pump (3); extractor (4); heat exchanger (5); chiller (6); separator (7); sample collector (8); flow meter (9); digital thermometer (10); safety valve (11); needle valve (12); check valve (13); filter (14); metering valve (15); back pressure regulator (16).

3.4. Subcritical Water Extraction

The SWE process is an environmentally clean technique that can be used to recover photoprotective substances from marine algae. During SWE, water is maintained in the subcritical state, between its boiling point (100 °C and 0.10 MPa) and critical point (374 °C and 22 MPa), where it remains as a liquid due to the high pressure [81]. High yield of fucoidan and carrageenan extracted by SWE has been demonstrated [82,83]. Generally, the SWE process increases the yield of bioactive substances and their biological activities. However, lower physical properties such as gelling and viscosity were also observed; these might be due to the degradation of polysaccharidea in higher temperature. The SWE process can be used, in addition to recovering photoprotective substances, to modify the structure of those substances. Meillisa et al. (2015) demonstrated structure modification of alginate from *Saccharina japonica* by SWE. Considering the blue extraction technique, SCE exhibits a number of advantages over conventional organic solvent extraction. The important advantages of this method include its simplicity, reduced extraction time, lower cost of the extracting agent, and its environmental friendliness.

4. Conclusions and Future Prospects of Photoprotective Substances from Marine Algae

Marine algae are the subject of increasing interest for their potential as a source of bioactive substances in cosmetics industries for several reasons. First, these marine organisms are considered as the fastest growing organisms on Earth. Extensively available marine areas are potential areas for marine algae aquaculture. Moreover, marine algae aquaculture techniques of commercial species (i.e., *Eucheuma cottonii*, *Laminaria japonica*, *Ecklonia cava*, *Gracilaria* sp.) have developed rapidly in the last decades. Marine algae can be found from tropical, cold-temperate areas to polar areas. This great number of biodiversity can be seen as a potential field for the blue exploration of marine algae. In addition, marine algae have exhibited unique chemical structures unlike those found in terrestrial counterparts. These organisms are viewed as "natural and healthy" by many people, and this promotes a positive response for consumers, who often regard natural and nontoxic entities. Many species of marine algae have been used as extracts in cosmetics, and there is no restriction for cosmetic use. Hence, marine algae may be considered a consumer-friendly source of skin care and cosmetic products that may be used for photoprotection. However, the health claims of photoprotective substances derived from marine algae that have been reported by many studies are mostly acquired only through in vitro and in vivo studies, so comprehensive studies on the mode of photoprotective action, biological consequences, and possible side effects have to be conducted in order to use those functional materials as skin care and cosmetic products. Photoprotective activity of orally administered bioactive substances from marine algae has also been reported. These findings reveal the potential of the development of photoprotective supplements and/or pharmaceuticals derived from marine algae.

The use of blue biotechnologies to recover photoprotective substances is becoming very important since the volume of solvents used in the chemical process is extremely concerning. Further, advances in molecular biology and aquaculture technologies such as Integrated Multi Trophic Aquaculture (IMTA) and Recirculating Aquaculture systems (RAS) are important to bridge the gap between the challenges pertaining to the exploitation of marine algae. Particularly, the aquaculture techniques of many brown algae species still remains a challenge and are necessary for the sustainable use of marine algal metabolites and for reduced production cost. Collectively, we predict that extensive application of marine algae in skin care, cosmetics, and pharmaceuticals with advanced photoprotective benefits is not a distant prospect.

Author Contributions: Design and writing—review and editing: R.P., E.A.S. and S.-K.K.

Funding: This article received no external funding.

Acknowledgments: The authors would like to thank National Research Foundation (NRF) Republic of Korea and Indonesian Institute of Science (LIPI) Republic of Indonesia for the LIPI-NRF Postdoctoral Fellowship Award (2017–2018). The authors also acknowledge the Research Center for Oceanography LIPI, Pukyong National University, and Marine Bioprocess Research Centers for all the support.

Conflicts of Interest: The authors declare no conflict of interest.

References

1. Kim, S.K.; Mendis, E. Bioactive compounds from marine processing byproducts-a review. *Food Res. Int.* **2006**, *39*, 383–393. [CrossRef]
2. Pangestuti, R.; Kim, S.-K. Bioactive peptide of marine origin for the prevention and treatment of non-communicable diseases. *Mar. Drugs* **2017**, *15*, 67. [CrossRef] [PubMed]
3. Siahaan, E.A.; Pangestuti, R.; Munandar, H.; Kim, S.-K. Cosmeceuticals properties of sea cucumbers: Prospects and trends. *Cosmetics* **2017**, *4*, 26. [CrossRef]
4. Pallela, R.; Na-Young, Y.; Kim, S.-K. Anti-photoaging and photoprotective compounds derived from marine organisms. *Mar. Drugs* **2010**, *8*, 1189–1202. [CrossRef] [PubMed]
5. Kim, S.-K.; Pangestuti, R. *Biological Properties of Cosmeceuticals Derived from Marine Algae*; CRC Press: Boca Raton, FL, USA, 2011; pp. 191–200.
6. Costa, L.; Fidelis, G.; Cordeiro, S.; Oliveira, R.; Sabry, D.; Câmara, R.; Nobre, L.; Costa, M.; Almeida-Lima, J.; Farias, E. Biological activities of sulfated polysaccharides from tropical seaweeds. *Biomed. Pharmacother.* **2010**, *64*, 21–28. [CrossRef] [PubMed]
7. Wijesekara, I.; Pangestuti, R.; Kim, S.-K. Biological activities and potential health benefits of sulfated polysaccharides derived from marine algae. *Carbohydr. Polym.* **2010**, *84*, 14–21. [CrossRef]
8. Pangestuti, R.; Kim, S.-K. Biological activities of carrageenan. *Adv. Food Nutr. Res.* **2014**, *72*, 113–124. [PubMed]
9. Thevanayagam, H.; Mohamed, S.M.; Chu, W.-L. Assessment of UVB-photoprotective and antioxidative activities of carrageenan in keratinocytes. *J. Appl. Phycol.* **2014**, *26*, 1813–1821. [CrossRef]
10. Nantel, F.; Denis, D.; Gordon, R.; Northey, A.; Cirino, M.; Metters, K.M.; Chan, C.C. Distribution and regulation of cyclooxygenase 2 in carrageenan induced inflammation. *Br. J. Pharmacol.* **1999**, *128*, 853–859. [CrossRef] [PubMed]
11. Tripp, C.S.; Blomme, E.A.; Chinn, K.S.; Hardy, M.M.; LaCelle, P.; Pentland, A.P. Epidermal COX-2 induction following ultraviolet irradiation: Suggested mechanism for the role of COX-2 inhibition in photoprotection. *J. Investig. Dermatol.* **2003**, *121*, 853–861. [CrossRef] [PubMed]

12. Pangestuti, R.; Kim, S.-K. Marine-derived bioactive materials for neuroprotection. *Food Sci. Biotechnol.* **2013**, *22*, 1–12. [CrossRef]
13. Moon, H.J.; Park, K.S.; Ku, M.J.; Lee, M.S.; Jeong, S.H.; Imbs, T.I.; Zvyagintseva, T.N.; Ermakova, S.P.; Lee, Y.H. Effect of Costaria costata fucoidan on expression of matrix metalloproteinase-1 promoter, mRNA, and protein. *J. Nat. Prod.* **2009**, *72*, 1731–1734. [CrossRef] [PubMed]
14. Kim, Y.-I.; Oh, W.-S.; Song, P.; Yun, S.; Kwon, Y.-S.; Lee, Y.; Ku, S.-K.; Song, C.-H.; Oh, T.-H. Anti-Photoaging Effects of Low Molecular-Weight Fucoidan on Ultraviolet B-Irradiated Mice. *Mar. Drugs* **2018**, *16*, 286. [CrossRef] [PubMed]
15. Hyun, Y.J.; Piao, M.J.; Ko, M.H.; Lee, N.H.; Kang, H.K.; Yoo, E.S.; Koh, Y.S.; Hyun, J.W. Photoprotective effect of Undaria crenata against ultraviolet B-induced damage to keratinocytes. *J. Biosci. Bioeng.* **2013**, *116*, 256–264. [CrossRef] [PubMed]
16. Maruyama, H.; Tamauchi, H.; Kawakami, F.; Yoshinaga, K.; Nakano, T. Suppressive effect of dietary fucoidan on proinflammatory immune response and MMP-1 expression in UVB-irradiated mouse skin. *Planta Med.* **2015**, *81*, 1370–1374. [PubMed]
17. Moon, H.J.; Lee, S.R.; Shim, S.N.; Jeong, S.H.; Stonik, V.A.; Rasskazov, V.A.; Zvyagintseva, T.; Lee, Y.H. Fucoidan inhibits UVB-induced MMP-1 expression in human skin fibroblasts. *Biol. Pharm. Bull.* **2008**, *31*, 284–289. [CrossRef] [PubMed]
18. Moon, H.J.; Lee, S.H.; Ku, M.J.; Yu, B.C.; Jeon, M.J.; Jeong, S.H.; Stonik, V.A.; Zvyagintseva, T.N.; Ermakova, S.P.; Lee, Y.H. Fucoidan inhibits UVB-induced MMP-1 promoter expression and down regulation of type I procollagen synthesis in human skin fibroblasts. *Eur. J. Dermatol.* **2009**, *19*, 129–134. [PubMed]
19. Ku, M.-J.; Lee, M.-S.; Moon, H.-J.; Lee, Y.-H. Protective Effects of Fucoidan against UVB-Induced Oxidative Stress in Human Skin Fibroblasts. *J. Life Sci.* **2010**, *20*, 27–32. [CrossRef]
20. Concepcion, M.R.; Avalos, J.; Bonet, M.L.; Boronat, A.; Gomez-Gomez, L.; Hornero-Mendez, D.; Limon, M.C.; Meléndez-Martínez, A.J.; Olmedilla-Alonso, B.; Palou, A. A global perspective on carotenoids: Metabolism, biotechnology, and benefits for nutrition and health. *Prog. Lipid Res.* **2018**, *70*, 62–93. [CrossRef] [PubMed]
21. Hashimoto, H.; Sugai, Y.; Uragami, C.; Gardiner, A.T.; Cogdell, R.J. Natural and artificial light-harvesting systems utilizing the functions of carotenoids. *J. Photochem. Photobiol. C* **2015**, *25*, 46–70. [CrossRef]
22. Shen, J.; Jiang, C.; Yan, Y.; Liu, B.; Zu, C. Effect of increased UV-B radiation on carotenoid accumulation and total antioxidant capacity in tobacco (*Nicotiana tabacum* L.) leaves. *Genet. Mol. Res.* **2017**, *16*, 1. [CrossRef] [PubMed]
23. Hupel, M.; Lecointre, C.; Meudec, A.; Poupart, N.; Gall, E.A. Comparison of photoprotective responses to UV radiation in the brown seaweed Pelvetia canaliculata and the marine angiosperm Salicornia ramosissima. *J. Exp. Mar. Biol. Ecol.* **2011**, *401*, 36–47. [CrossRef]
24. Heo, S.-J.; Jeon, Y.-J. Protective effect of fucoxanthin isolated from *Sargassum siliquastrum* on UV-B induced cell damage. *J. Photochem. Photobiol. B* **2009**, *95*, 101–107. [CrossRef] [PubMed]
25. Urikura, I.; Sugawara, T.; Hirata, T. Protective effect of fucoxanthin against UVB-induced skin photoaging in hairless mice. *Biosci. Biotechnol. Biochem.* **2011**, *75*, 757–760. [CrossRef] [PubMed]
26. Liu, Y.; Liu, M.; Zhang, X.; Chen, Q.; Chen, H.; Sun, L.; Liu, G. Protective effect of fucoxanthin isolated from Laminaria japonica against visible light-induced retinal damage both in vitro and in vivo. *J. Agric. Food Chem.* **2016**, *64*, 416–424. [CrossRef] [PubMed]
27. Chen, S.-J.; Lee, C.-J.; Lin, T.-B.; Liu, H.-J.; Huang, S.-Y.; Chen, J.-Z.; Tseng, K.-W. Inhibition of Ultraviolet B-Induced Expression of the Proinflammatory Cytokines TNF-α and VEGF in the Cornea by Fucoxanthin Treatment in a Rat Model. *Mar. Drugs* **2016**, *14*, 13. [CrossRef] [PubMed]
28. Matsui, M.; Tanaka, K.; Higashiguchi, N.; Okawa, H.; Yamada, Y.; Tanaka, K.; Taira, S.; Aoyama, T.; Takanishi, M.; Natsume, C. Protective and therapeutic effects of fucoxanthin against sunburn caused by UV irradiation. *J. Pharmacol. Sci.* **2016**, *132*, 55–64. [CrossRef] [PubMed]
29. Stahl, W.; Sies, H. β-Carotene and other carotenoids in protection from sunlight. *Am. J. Clin. Nutr.* **2012**, *96*, 1179S–1184S. [CrossRef] [PubMed]
30. Pangestuti, R.; Kim, S.-K. Biological activities and health benefit effects of natural pigments derived from marine algae. *J. Funct. Foods* **2011**, *3*, 255–266. [CrossRef]
31. Mok, I.-K.; Lee, J.K.; Kim, J.H.; Pan, C.-H.; Kim, S.M. Fucoxanthin bioavailability from fucoxanthin-fortified milk: In vivo and in vitro study. *Food Chem.* **2018**, *258*, 79–86. [CrossRef] [PubMed]

32. Carreto, J.I.; Carignan, M.O. Mycosporine-like amino acids: relevant secondary metabolites. Chemical and ecological aspects. *Mar. Drugs* **2011**, *9*, 387–446. [CrossRef] [PubMed]
33. Peinado, N.K.; Abdala Díaz, R.T.; Figueroa, F.L.; Helbling, E.W. Ammonium and UV radiation stimulate the accumulation of mycosporine like amino acids in Porphyra Columbina (Rhodophyta) from Patagonia, Argentina. *J. Phycol.* **2004**, *40*, 248–259. [CrossRef]
34. Oren, A.; Gunde-Cimerman, N. Mycosporines and mycosporine-like amino acids: UV protectants or multipurpose secondary metabolites? *FEMS Microbiol. Lett.* **2007**, *269*, 1–10. [CrossRef] [PubMed]
35. Barceló-Villalobos, M.; Figueroa, F.L.; Korbee, N.; Álvarez-Gómez, F.; Abreu, M.H. Production of mycosporine-like amino acids from Gracilaria vermiculophylla (Rhodophyta) cultured through one year in an Integrated Multi-Trophic Aquaculture (IMTA) system. *Mar. Biotechnol.* **2017**, *19*, 246–254. [CrossRef] [PubMed]
36. Gacesa, R.; Lawrence, K.P.; Georgakopoulos, N.D.; Yabe, K.; Dunlap, W.C.; Barlow, D.J.; Wells, G.; Young, A.R.; Long, P.F. The mycosporine-like amino acids porphyra-334 and shinorine are antioxidants and direct antagonists of Keap1-Nrf2 binding. *Biochimie* **2018**, *154*, 35–44. [CrossRef] [PubMed]
37. Hartmann, A.; Murauer, A.; Ganzera, M. Quantitative analysis of mycosporine-like amino acids in marine algae by capillary electrophoresis with diode-array detection. *J. Pharm. Biomed. Anal.* **2017**, *138*, 153–157. [CrossRef] [PubMed]
38. Navarro, N.P.; Figueroa, F.L.; Korbee, N. Mycosporine-like amino acids vs carrageenan yield in Mazzaella laminarioides (Gigartinales; Rhodophyta) under high and low UV solar irradiance. *Phycologia* **2017**, *56*, 570–578. [CrossRef]
39. Ryu, J.; Park, S.-J.; Kim, I.-H.; Choi, Y.H.; Nam, T.-J. Protective effect of porphyra-334 on UVA-induced photoaging in human skin fibroblasts. *Int. J. Mol. Med.* **2014**, *34*, 796–803. [CrossRef] [PubMed]
40. Yoshiki, M.; Tsuge, K.; Tsuruta, Y.; Yoshimura, T.; Koganemaru, K.; Sumi, T.; Matsui, T.; Matsumoto, K. Production of new antioxidant compound from mycosporine-like amino acid, porphyra-334 by heat treatment. *Food Chem.* **2009**, *113*, 1127–1132. [CrossRef]
41. Bhatia, S.; Sharma, K.; Namdeo, A.G.; Chaugule, B.; Kavale, M.; Nanda, S. Broad-spectrum sun-protective action of Porphyra-334 derived from Porphyra vietnamensis. *Pharmacogn. Res.* **2010**, *2*, 45. [CrossRef] [PubMed]
42. Daniel, S.; Cornelia, S.; Fred, Z. UV-A sunscreen from red algae for protection against premature skin aging. *Cosmet. Toilet. Manuf. Worldw.* **2004**, *129*, 139–143.
43. Ignat, I.; Volf, I.; Popa, V.I. A critical review of methods for characterisation of polyphenolic compounds in fruits and vegetables. *Food Chem.* **2011**, *126*, 1821–1835. [CrossRef] [PubMed]
44. Heo, S.-J.; Ko, S.-C.; Cha, S.-H.; Kang, D.-H.; Park, H.-S.; Choi, Y.-U.; Kim, D.; Jung, W.-K.; Jeon, Y.-J. Effect of phlorotannins isolated from Ecklonia cava on melanogenesis and their protective effect against photo-oxidative stress induced by UV-B radiation. *Toxicol. In Vitro* **2009**, *23*, 1123–1130. [CrossRef] [PubMed]
45. Ko, S.-C.; Cha, S.-H.; Heo, S.-J.; Lee, S.-H.; Kang, S.-M.; Jeon, Y.-J. Protective effect of Ecklonia cava on UVB-induced oxidative stress: In vitro and in vivo zebrafish model. *J. Appl. Phycol.* **2011**, *23*, 697–708. [CrossRef]
46. Kang, K.A.; Zhang, R.; Piao, M.J.; Ko, D.O.; Wang, Z.H.; Lee, K.; Kim, B.J.; Shin, T.; Park, J.W.; Lee, N.H. Inhibitory effects of triphlorethol-A on MMP-1 induced by oxidative stress in human keratinocytes via ERK and AP-1 inhibition. *J. Toxicol. Environ. Health Part A* **2008**, *71*, 992–999. [CrossRef] [PubMed]
47. Piao, M.J.; Zhang, R.; Lee, N.H.; Hyun, J.W. Protective effect of triphlorethol-A against ultraviolet B-mediated damage of human keratinocytes. *J. Photochem. Photobiol. B* **2012**, *106*, 74–80. [CrossRef] [PubMed]
48. Vo, T.S.; Kim, S.-K.; Ryu, B.; Ngo, D.H.; Yoon, N.-Y.; Bach, L.G.; Hang, N.T.N.; Ngo, D.N. The Suppressive Activity of Fucofuroeckol-A Derived from Brown Algal Ecklonia stolonifera Okamura on UVB-Induced Mast Cell Degranulation. *Mar. Drugs* **2018**, *16*, 1. [CrossRef] [PubMed]
49. Kim, K.C.; Piao, M.J.; Cho, S.J.; Lee, N.H.; Hyun, J.W. Phloroglucinol protects human keratinocytes from ultraviolet B radiation by attenuating oxidative stress. *Photodermatol. Photoimmunol. Photomed.* **2012**, *28*, 322–331. [CrossRef] [PubMed]
50. Piao, M.J.; Zhang, R.; Lee, N.H.; Hyun, J.W. Phloroglucinol attenuates ultraviolet B radiation-induced matrix metalloproteinase-1 production in human keratinocytes via inhibitory actions against mitogen-activated protein kinases and activator protein-1. *Photochem. Photobiol.* **2012**, *88*, 381–388. [CrossRef] [PubMed]

51. Piao, M.J.; Ahn, M.J.; Kang, K.A.; Kim, K.C.; Zheng, J.; Yao, C.W.; Cha, J.W.; Hyun, C.L.; Kang, H.K.; Lee, N.H. Phloroglucinol inhibits ultraviolet B radiation-induced oxidative stress in the mouse skin. *Int. J. Radiat. Biol.* **2014**, *90*, 928–935. [CrossRef] [PubMed]
52. Guinea, M.; Franco, V.; Araujo-Bazán, L.; Rodríguez-Martín, I.; González, S. In vivo UVB-photoprotective activity of extracts from commercial marine macroalgae. *Food Chem. Toxicol.* **2012**, *50*, 1109–1117. [CrossRef] [PubMed]
53. Kim, S.; You, D.H.; Han, T.; Choi, E.-M. Modulation of viability and apoptosis of UVB-exposed human keratinocyte HaCaT cells by aqueous methanol extract of laver (Porphyra yezoensis). *J. Photochem. Photobiol. B* **2014**, *141*, 301–307. [CrossRef] [PubMed]
54. Sánchez-Lamar, Á.; González-Pumariega, M.; Fuentes-León, F.; Vernhes Tamayo, M.; Schuch, A.P.; Menck, C.F. Evaluation of Genotoxic and DNA Photo-Protective Activity of Bryothamnion triquetrum and Halimeda incrassata Seaweeds Extracts. *Cosmetics* **2017**, *4*, 23. [CrossRef]
55. Mercurio, D.; Wagemaker, T.; Alves, V.; Benevenuto, C.; Gaspar, L.; Campos, P.M. In vivo photoprotective effects of cosmetic formulations containing UV filters, vitamins, Ginkgo biloba and red algae extracts. *J. Photochem. Photobiol. B* **2015**, *153*, 121–126. [CrossRef] [PubMed]
56. Boulho, R.; Le Roux, J.; Le Quémener, C.; Audo, G.; Bourgougnon, N.; Bedoux, G. Fractionation of UV-B absorbing molecules and of free radical scavenging compounds from Solieria chordalis by using centrifugal partition chromatography. *Phytochem. Lett.* **2017**, *20*, 410–414. [CrossRef]
57. Kim, H.M.; Lee, D.E.; Park, S.D.; Kim, Y.T.; Kim, Y.J.; Jeong, J.W.; Lee, J.-H.; Jang, S.S.; Chung, D.K.; Sim, J.-H. Preventive effect of fermented Gelidium amansii and Cirsium japonicum extract mixture against UVB-induced skin photoaging in hairless mice. *Food Sci. Biotechnol.* **2014**, *23*, 623–631. [CrossRef]
58. Hyun, Y.J.; Piao, M.J.; Kim, K.C.; Zheng, J.; Yao, C.W.; Cha, J.W.; Kang, H.K.; Yoo, E.S.; Koh, Y.S.; Lee, N.H. Photoprotective effect of a Polyopes affinis (Harvey) Kawaguchi and Wang (Halymeniaceae)-derived ethanol extract on human keratinocytes. *Trop. J. Pharm. Res.* **2014**, *13*, 863–871. [CrossRef]
59. Bedoux, G.; Hardouin, K.; Marty, C.; Taupin, L.; Vandanjon, L.; Bourgougnon, N. Chemical characterization and photoprotective activity measurement of extracts from the red macroalga Solieria chordalis. *Bot. Mar.* **2014**, *57*, 291–301. [CrossRef]
60. Piao, M.J.; Kang, H.K.; Yoo, E.S.; Koh, Y.S.; Kim, D.S.; Lee, N.H.; Hyun, J.W. Photo-protective effect of Polysiphonia morrowii Harvey against ultraviolet B radiation-induced keratinocyte damage. *J. Korean Soc. Appl. Biol. Chem.* **2012**, *55*, 149–158. [CrossRef]
61. Piao, M.J.; Hyun, Y.J.; Oh, T.-H.; Kang, H.K.; Yoo, E.S.; Koh, Y.S.; Lee, N.H.; Suh, I.S.; Hyun, J.W. Chondracanthus tenellus (Harvey) hommersand extract protects the human keratinocyte cell line by blocking free radicals and UVB radiation-induced cell damage. *In Vitro Cell. Dev. Biol.-Anim.* **2012**, *48*, 666–674. [CrossRef] [PubMed]
62. Piao, M.J.; Hyun, Y.J.; Cho, S.J.; Kang, H.K.; Yoo, E.S.; Koh, Y.S.; Lee, N.H.; Ko, M.H.; Hyun, J.W. An ethanol extract derived from Bonnemaisonia hamifera scavenges ultraviolet B (UVB) radiation-induced reactive oxygen species and attenuates UVB-induced cell damage in human keratinocytes. *Mar. Drugs* **2012**, *10*, 2826–2845. [CrossRef] [PubMed]
63. Kim, A.D.; Piao, M.J.; Hyun, Y.J.; Kang, H.K.; Suh, I.S.; Lee, N.H.; Hyun, J.W. Photo-protective properties of Lomentaria hakodatensis yendo against ultraviolet B radiation-induced keratinocyte damage. *Biotechnol. Bioprocess Eng.* **2012**, *17*, 1223–1231. [CrossRef]
64. Song, J.H.; Piao, M.J.; Han, X.; Kang, K.A.; Kang, H.K.; Yoon, W.J.; Ko, M.H.; Lee, N.H.; Lee, M.Y.; Chae, S. Anti-wrinkle effects of Sargassum muticum ethyl acetate fraction on ultraviolet B-irradiated hairless mouse skin and mechanistic evaluation in the human HaCaT keratinocyte cell line. *Mol. Med. Rep.* **2016**, *14*, 2937–2944. [CrossRef] [PubMed]
65. Piao, M.J.; Yoon, W.J.; Kang, H.K.; Yoo, E.S.; Koh, Y.S.; Kim, D.S.; Lee, N.H.; Hyun, J.W. Protective Effect of the Ethyl Acetate Fraction of Sargassum muticum Against Ultraviolet B–Irradiated Damage in Human Keratinocytes. *Int. J. Mol. Sci.* **2011**, *12*, 8146–8160. [CrossRef] [PubMed]
66. Cseri, L.; Razali, M.; Pogany, P.; Szekely, G. Organic Solvents in Sustainable Synthesis and Engineering. *Green Chem.* **2017**, 513–553.
67. Heo, S.-J.; Park, E.-J.; Lee, K.-W.; Jeon, Y.-J. Antioxidant activities of enzymatic extracts from brown seaweeds. *Bioresour. Technol.* **2005**, *96*, 1613–1623. [CrossRef] [PubMed]

68. Kim, S.; Wijesekara, I. Development and biological activities of marine-derived bioactive peptides: A review. *J. Funct. Foods* **2010**, *2*, 1–9. [CrossRef]
69. Athukorala, Y.; Kim, K.-N.; Jeon, Y.-J. Antiproliferative and antioxidant properties of an enzymatic hydrolysate from brown alga, Ecklonia cava. *Food Chem. Toxicol.* **2006**, *44*, 1065–1074. [CrossRef] [PubMed]
70. Hifney, A.F.; Fawzy, M.A.; Abdel-Gawad, K.M.; Gomaa, M. Upgrading the antioxidant properties of fucoidan and alginate from Cystoseira trinodis by fungal fermentation or enzymatic pretreatment of the seaweed biomass. *Food Chem.* **2018**, *269*, 387–395. [CrossRef] [PubMed]
71. Camel, V. Microwave-assisted solvent extraction of environmental samples. *TrAC Trends Anal. Chem.* **2000**, *19*, 229–248. [CrossRef]
72. Hahn, T.; Lang, S.; Ulber, R.; Muffler, K. Novel procedures for the extraction of fucoidan from brown algae. *Process Biochem.* **2012**, *47*, 1691–1698. [CrossRef]
73. Yuan, Y.; Macquarrie, D. Microwave assisted extraction of sulfated polysaccharides (fucoidan) from Ascophyllum nodosum and its antioxidant activity. *Carbohydr. Polym.* **2015**, *129*, 101–107. [CrossRef] [PubMed]
74. Flórez-Fernández, N.; López-García, M.; González-Muñoz, M.J.; Vilariño, J.M.L.; Domínguez, H. Ultrasound-assisted extraction of fucoidan from Sargassum muticum. *J. Appl. Phycol.* **2017**, *29*, 1553–1561. [CrossRef]
75. Haq, M.; Chun, B.-S. Characterization of phospholipids extracted from Atlantic salmon by-product using supercritical CO 2 with ethanol as co-solvent. *J. Clean. Prod.* **2018**, *178*, 186–195. [CrossRef]
76. Haq, M.; Ahmed, R.; Cho, Y.-J.; Chun, B.-S. Quality Properties and Bio-potentiality of Edible Oils from Atlantic Salmon By-products Extracted by Supercritical Carbon Dioxide and Conventional Methods. *Waste Biomass Valorization* **2017**, *8*, 1953–1967. [CrossRef]
77. Sivagnanam, S.P.; Yin, S.; Choi, J.H.; Park, Y.B.; Woo, H.C.; Chun, B.S. Biological properties of fucoxanthin in oil recovered from two brown seaweeds using supercritical CO_2 extraction. *Mar. Drugs* **2015**, *13*, 3422–3442. [CrossRef] [PubMed]
78. Roh, M.K.; Uddin, M.S.; Chun, B.S. Extraction of fucoxanthin and polyphenol from Undaria pinnatifida using supercritical carbon dioxide with co-solvent. *Biotechnol. Bioprocess Eng.* **2008**, *13*, 724–729. [CrossRef]
79. Conde, E.; Moure, A.; Domínguez, H. Supercritical CO_2 extraction of fatty acids, phenolics and fucoxanthin from freeze-dried Sargassum muticum. *J. Appl. Phycol.* **2015**, *27*, 957–964. [CrossRef]
80. Saravana, P.S.; Getachew, A.T.; Cho, Y.-J.; Choi, J.H.; Park, Y.B.; Woo, H.C.; Chun, B.S. Influence of co-solvents on fucoxanthin and phlorotannin recovery from brown seaweed using supercritical CO_2. *J. Supercrit. Fluids* **2017**, *120*, 295–303. [CrossRef]
81. Meillisa, A.; Siahaan, E.A.; Park, J.-N.; Woo, H.-C.; Chun, B.-S. Effect of subcritical water hydrolysate in the brown seaweed Saccharina japonica as a potential antibacterial agent on food-borne pathogens. *J. Appl. Phycol.* **2013**, *25*, 763–769. [CrossRef]
82. Gereniu, C.R.N.; Saravana, P.S.; Chun, B.-S. Recovery of carrageenan from Solomon Islands red seaweed using ionic liquid-assisted subcritical water extraction. *Sep. Purif. Technol.* **2018**, *196*, 309–317. [CrossRef]
83. Saravana, P.S.; Tilahun, A.; Gerenew, C.; Tri, V.D.; Kim, N.H.; Kim, G.-D.; Woo, H.-C.; Chun, B.-S. Subcritical water extraction of fucoidan from Saccharina japonica: optimization, characterization and biological studies. *J Appl. Phycol.* **2018**, *30*, 579–590. [CrossRef]

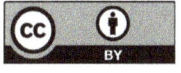

© 2018 by the authors. Licensee MDPI, Basel, Switzerland. This article is an open access article distributed under the terms and conditions of the Creative Commons Attribution (CC BY) license (http://creativecommons.org/licenses/by/4.0/).

MDPI
St. Alban-Anlage 66
4052 Basel
Switzerland
Tel. +41 61 683 77 34
Fax +41 61 302 89 18
www.mdpi.com

Marine Drugs Editorial Office
E-mail: marinedrugs@mdpi.com
www.mdpi.com/journal/marinedrugs

www.ingramcontent.com/pod-product-compliance
Lightning Source LLC
LaVergne TN
LVHW071949080526
838202LV00064B/6711